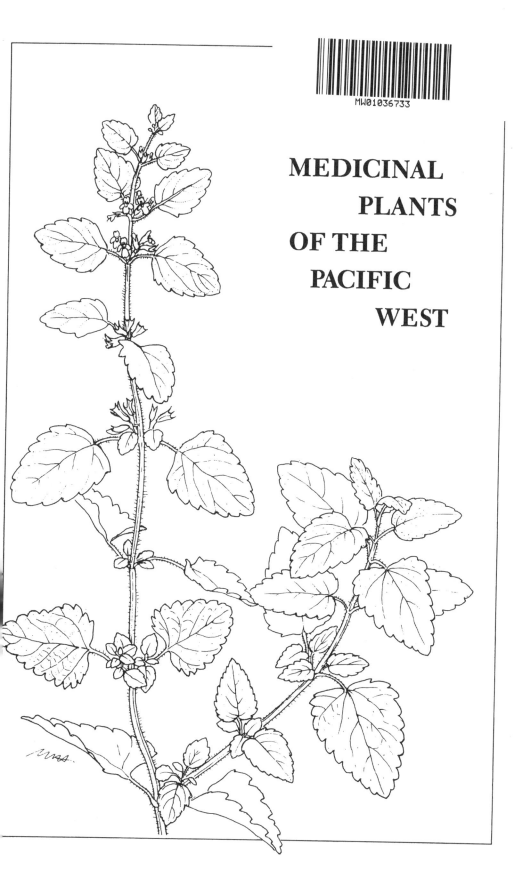

MEDICINAL
PLANTS
OF THE
PACIFIC
WEST

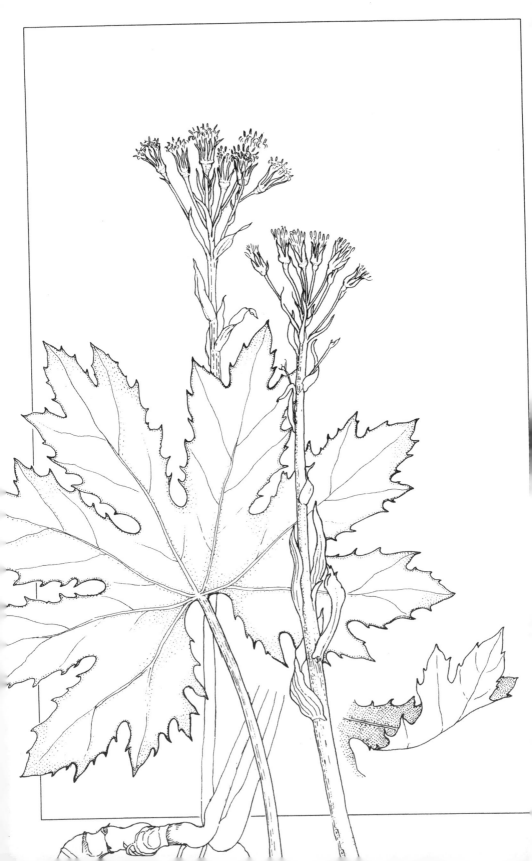

MEDICINAL PLANTS
OF THE
PACIFIC
WEST

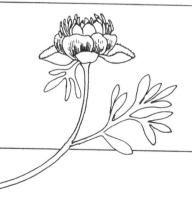

Michael Moore
Illustrated by MIMI KAMP

MUSEUM OF NEW MEXICO PRESS
SANTA FE

Museum of New Mexico Press edition
10 9 8 7 6 5 4 3 2

Book design by Jos. Trautwein
Text drawings and photographs copyright ©1993 by Mimi Kamp
Maps by Michael Moore

Manufactured in the United States of America

Library of Congress Cataloging-in-Publication Data

Moore, Michael
    Medicinal plants of the Pacific West / Michael Moore—1st ed.
        p. cm.
    Includes bibliographical references and indexes.
    ISBN 978-0-89013-539-6
    I. Medicinal plants—West (U.S.)   1. Title
RS164.M616   1993
615' .321'079—dc20   93-280
                                                        CIP

Museum of New Mexico Press
P.O. Box 2087
Santa Fe, New Mexico 87504
www.mnmpress.org

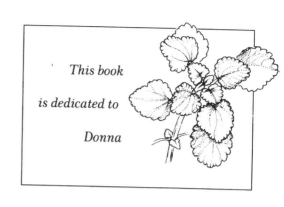

This book

is dedicated to

Donna

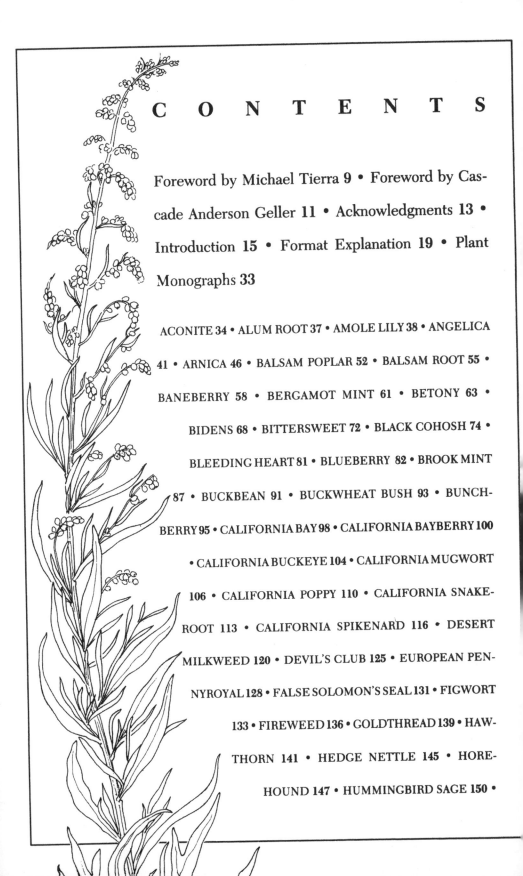

C O N T E N T S

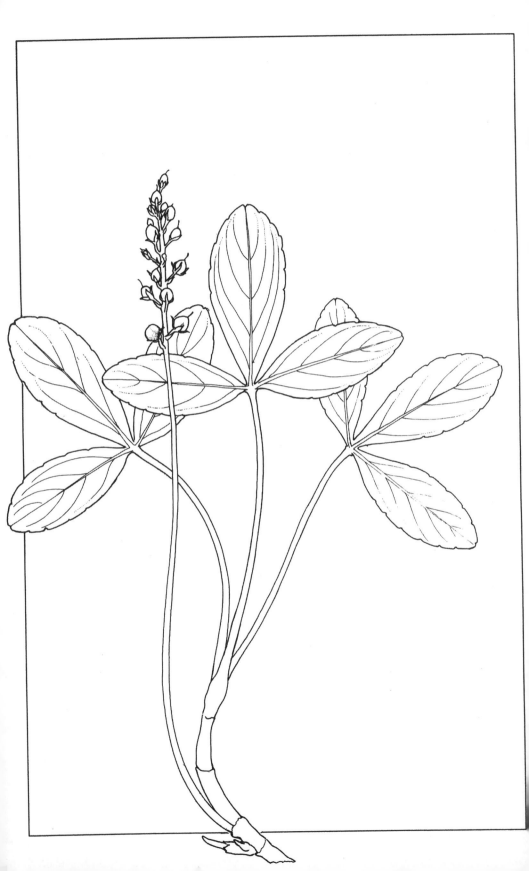

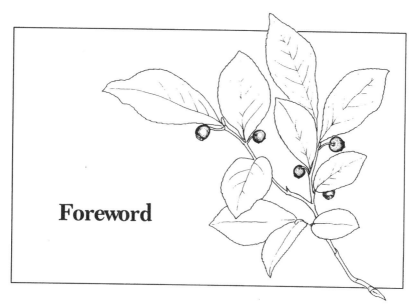

Foreword

It must have been in 1968 that my natural curiosity, or rather curiosity for the mysteries of nature, drew me into an herbal apothecary shop at a mountain craft fair in Topanga Canyon in the Malibu hills outside of Los Angeles. With bundles of dried herbs hanging everywhere, and strange potions and salves with their handwritten labels, the shop made me feel like I had happened onto a time warp, and was now in the cabin of an Ozark mountain trader or backwoods shaman rather than at a fair in Topanga Canyon.

I vaguely remember not staying long, since at that time I didn't even know what an herb was, let alone that they had any practical purposes. My dawning infatuation with herbs was not to occur until at least a couple of years later, when I moved to a wilderness community in the mountains of northern California. Before leaving the shop, I did notice a big burly bear of a man sitting behind the counter, maybe a little concerned that perhaps I or one of my transitional, beatnik-becoming-hippie companions might be tempted to appropriate an herbal potion or concoction without payment.

It was more than twenty years later at an herbalists' gathering at Breitenbush, Oregon, that Michael Moore reminded me of my first unwitting steps into the world of herbs—or more specifically into his herb world at the time. It has been an ongoing jest between us, signifying that his interest in herbs predated mine, or for that matter just about any other mid-twentieth-century herbal renaissance herbalist I know of. In the same spirit of lighthearted banter, I have tried to assure him that neither I nor my companions illegitimately appropriated any of his potions back in 1968.

There has to be practical value to this historical dribble, so for the sake of excuse let's say it serves to establish Michael Moore's longtime dedication and involvement with herbs, and by default, his well-earned qualifications for writing this important work, the latest in a series intended to express his personal experience in gathering, preparing, and prescribing the medicinal plants of the entire North American continent.

In 1968, I only knew of Michael as an outstanding trumpet player and frequent solo and ensemble performer in the classical avant-garde music scene that was happening in the shadow of the late twentieth-century composer Arnold Schönberg, on the UCLA campus. Being a pianist and composer myself, I was also involved in the fringe of what was then called the New Music Workshop of UCLA.

True to the tenets of the mid-twentieth-century avant-garde art scene from which both he and I emanate, Michael has made his life a personal art form that can challenge many conventional concepts of being. In this he also conforms to the prevailing individualistic and cantankerous nonmodel of most self-made, mid-twentieth-century pioneers of the herbal renaissance: those of us who, over the years, have had to resort to creatively surreptitious ways to practice the art of herbal medicine in a politically unfavorable climate. In Michael's case one senses, however, that his contradictory and often paradoxical nature masks a gentleman with great personal sensitivity and intelligence.

Even so, if you have the distinction of encountering Michael Moore, say as a student in one of his many seminars or herbal field trips that he offers each year throughout the country, at first glance you are more likely to think that you are in the presence of a mountain biker than a renaissance man, errant genius-herbalist, author, and composer who has had several symphonies commissioned and performed by the Orchestra of Santa Fe.

One of the many things that soon betrays his inner gentleness and refinement is that one seldom encounters a harsh critical word from him in either his teaching or writing. He is more than likely to give others the benefit of his doubts even when he refers to such dubious diagnostic measures as muscle testing, biokinesiology, and iris diagnosis as "reasonable tests in some circumstances, but notoriously erroneous in overdiagnosing real squiggly-squirmy parasites."

The point is, of course, that Michael knows enough self-taught anatomy, physiology, physiopathology, botany, and biochemistry to have medical doctors knocking at his door to learn how herbs work on the human body. Beyond this, his knowledge of these erudite subjects is so consummate that it allows him to poetically juggle complex physiological concepts in often amusing and quizzical ways. This you will readily perceive in his writing.

Therefore, this particular opus, *Medicinal Plants of the Pacific West*, is not just another dry text of scientific ethnobotanical erudition. Like his previous works, it is seasoned with Michael's unique droll humor and witticisms. This gives it the advantage of any good book—that is, of being able to hold our interest even when it must appropriately navigate through paragraphs of potentially deadly standard botanical classifications. In addition to the welcome humor, we can appreciate the authority of Michael's twenty-five-plus years of personal herbal experience as he informs and guides us throughout all the steps of locating, harvesting, and preparing each herb for use.

Michael's book invites you to accompany him through the coastal foothills, mountains, and canyons of the Pacific West, and to discover the many medicinal botanicals that abound in this area, one of the world's richest terrains.

Michael Tierra, O.M.D.
Santa Cruz, California

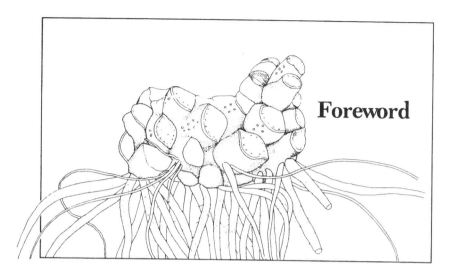

Foreword

Somebody had to do it. My version is still stashed in a box in the closet, perhaps someday to have a life of its own. Now, at last, I have one very excellent book to refer to on the herbs of the Pacific states.

When I first migrated to the West, on the heels of Richard Nixon's galloping success at reelection, feeling ashamed of being an American and looking to lick my wounds in the wilds of the towering volcanos, I sought an herbal guide to take on the trail with me. Alas, there was none. I even had some trouble finding a really good western wildflower guide. So I left the country for a year or so and came back with the intention of writing a trail guide for herbalists. Well, I kept adding to it, and then felt I should wait until I was more mature, or something, and the next thing I knew, fifteen years had gone by. Now I am more mature but have even less time to write.

Fortunately, Michael Moore has taken the time to complete a very good book. Every one of his books is excellent because Michael is a rarity who really knows his subject and can convey serious information in a lighthearted style. He knows what herbalists want and need to know about plants because he is one of the best herbalists in this country. He walks on and off the paths of his life really paying attention to plants and not just the lovely or showy species, but the seemingly insignificant but potent little allies that the whole world is full of.

Michael seems to tell us all he knows about these herbs: how to identify them, when and how to harvest and prepare them, what known constituents they contain—and I love his habitat descriptions because they are so accurate. But even if you never intend to wildcraft or prepare a single herb from scratch, and all you ever want to do is know how to use herbs for medicine, then you are still holding one of the best books you could ever buy on this subject. Michael is well versed in using herbs for medicine, and it is a blessing for all of us that he is writing down his understanding of this. So much information about how to use plants for healing has been lost due to arrogance and ignorance on the part of marauding newcomers that any shred of knowledge that can be saved from someone actually working with herbs is extremely important.

There is a whole lot that could be said about herbs, and there are a whole lot of books that are saying this and that about herbs. My library shelves are overflowing with herb books. It seems that in recent years, more and more of my herbal reading is coming from Europe, Germany in particular. There seems to be more respect given to herbal medicine there, but there is also a sterility to the writing that leaves an empty feeling. Michael's books, on the other hand, are full of life—lusty and bold you might even say, without being pretentious. I'm sold on them. *Medicinal Plants of the Mountain West* became one of my favorite books as soon as I was lucky enough to get a copy. Recently, on a trip to the Sonoran Desert, I was really able to break in my copy of *Medicinal Plants of the Desert and Canyon West*, and as I suspected, it was very useful. Then there is *Los Remedios: Traditional Herbal Remedies of the Southwest,* which I refer to often and which has helped me, on a couple of occasions, to aid M.D.s with Spanish-speaking patients who were taking an herbal remedy that the doc was suspicious of. *Medicinal Plants of the Pacific West* has been long-awaited, and my copy will soon look very used. In fact, I find the best bet with these kinds of good field guides is to have two copies—one for the office and one for the field.

Thank you, Michael Moore, for the good books and the chance to tout your good work. I only hope that the wild spaces we've walked and studied and harvested in—and all of their resident green beauties and furry, scaled, and winged beasties—will thrive in the coming years as the American West becomes ever more settled. May we, as a people, have the courage, ability, and wisdom to save the little wildness this country has left.

Cascade Anderson Geller
Portland, Oregon

ACKNOWLEDGMENTS   I would like to thank the folks who have been with me in the Pacific West over the years: Michael and John from Topanga, Velia and the elusive Ray, Shalom, Nina, Michele, Chavela, Anne, Big Stuart, Emerald Valley Rosemary, Oregon Ed, Tierney, Sue and Carol (formerly Cue and Sarol), Doc Terry, CDC George, Halsey, Mimi, and Donna. From Red Crane Books, thanks to Carol, retired Drummer Dennis, and Ann for editing the book, and (is this our *fourth* book? really?) Jim Mafchir. Some technical thanks to Adam Seller, Steve Dentali, Robyn Klein, Steven Foster, Ed Smith, Cascade Anderson Geller, David Winston, and James Green. Each of them added to my knowledge or aimed me down a road for this particular book. I would like to thank Michael, Cascade, and Susun for reviewing the manuscript. Many other friends have added to my cauldron and nature, but these are those that helped in this particular book about the Pacific Coast. And I want to thank Mimi for finding the plants and putting them on paper—the muse of Bisbee Junction strikes again.

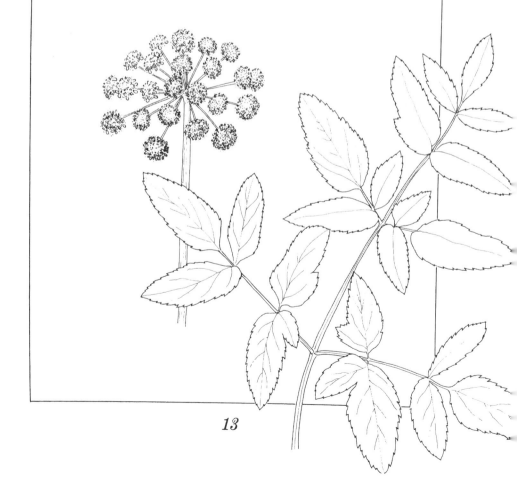

13

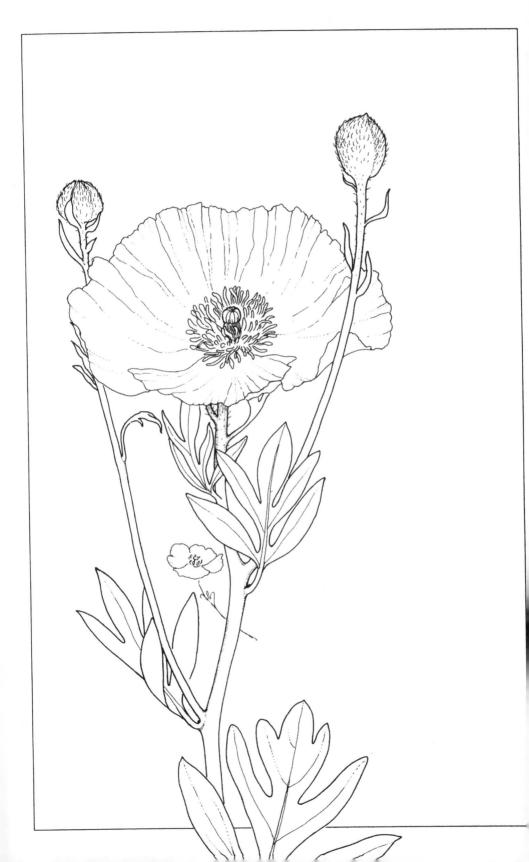

INTRODUCTION

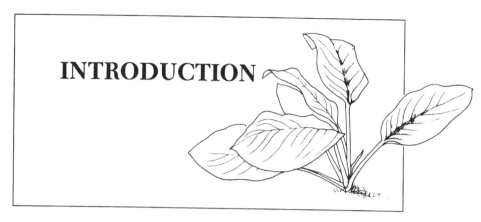

This book is meant to be used by intelligent, sensible people who want to learn about and use the medicinal plants of the Pacific region, who want to get out and *do* something—get out of the hive cities, the concrete, the subtle degradation of product and service marketing.

Many of us feel that an increasingly costly medical system has conversely become inept at disease prevention or health continuity in its pursuit of diagnostic sophistication and hard science. We have found that it is better to prevent disease ourselves, through diet and lifestyle, and use less invasive alternative therapies *first*, resorting to Standard Practice Medicine when we *really* get sick. We also wish to be able to treat ourselves for minor disorders or constitutional weaknesses, and use homeopathy, supplements, glandular extracts—and especially herbs.

Every health food store and co-op has a vast array of patent formulas, teas, capsules, loose herbs, and other genial geegaws, with books telling you how to use them. There will be ten different Echinacea preparations from different manufacturers, all claiming supremacy. There will be Chinese patent medicines, Ayurvedic preparations, flower essences, and aromatherapy products; there will be homeopathic remedies, some in high potency, some mixed with actual herb extracts, and some hybrids that may have Chinese, Ayurvedic, homeopathic, and Western botanicals all tossed together—maybe even with some freeze-dried thyroid gland and a chelated amino acid as well. There are food supplements and vitamins that have plant medicines thrown in, herbal preparations with vitamins added. You can get some new herbs as ground capsules, tinctures, "chelated" extracts (whatever those are), with or without alcohol or glycerin (if so, what keeps them from spoiling?); as isolates, standardized extracts, freeze-dried, even potentized. What *is* all this stuff?

I am an old-fashioned herbalist. I want to know where the plant can be found; how it can be gathered and when; how common or rare it is; in what kind of circumstance the plant will make the best therapeutic; how it is to be processed, dried, or preserved; and how long it will stay good. Once I know these things, I will know the plant well enough to be able to purchase it in commerce or reject it in commerce. Then, I will need to know its physiologic and pharmacologic effects; how it affects healthy people; how it may help sick people; what its possible side effects are, contraindications; the proper and improper doses; and so forth. For the plants within this book (as in my previous books), I have given the best information I can regarding all these latter factors.

Some of you will have your own experiences with some of these plants as medicines or tonics. Be that as it may, if you are going to use botanicals, *you first have to know the plants*. Herbal medicines are biologic agents. If you allow that they have a proper place in self-treatment or alternative practice, then you should have a damn good idea of what they are before using them. Although some of the plant medicines that are marketed are prepared by knowledgeable herbalists, there is still a whole lot of absolute junk out there. Most manufacturers use plant materials from commerce, and these may be alright sometimes, but are frequently horrible.

Herb brokers in North Carolina will pay $4.00 a pound for whole-dried "Kansas Snakeroot," and $1.25 a pound for "Missouri Snakeroot." The first is *any* species of Echinacea, usually dug along roadsides, the second is *Parthenium integrifolium*, or Prairie Dock, a vaguely related plant with large, grey-pithed tubers that have been used in the trade for one hundred years to adulterate the first plant. This substitution is so widespread that extensive German studies on Echinacea had to be completely redone several years ago because the plant material used as *Echinacea angustifolia*, obtained through normal crude drug sources, was 80% Prairie Dock. Skullcap, Goldenseal, Siberian Ginseng, and Panax Ginseng are other plants that are frequently not what they seem.

There are a growing body of manufacturers who rely on organic growers and knowledgeable wildcrafters for their plant sources, and these folks take pride in their quality. But most of the herb products in the health food industry are made from what retailers have purchased wholesale by the pound, after the wholesalers have purchased in 100- or 1,000-pound lots from the brokers or importers, who have paid measly prices to poor folks in Appalachia, or slave prices to third world, *really* poor folks, for oftentimes iffy-quality herbs. Someone who takes care that their food is organic (or at least clean) tries to drink clean water, wants to avoid air and landfill pollution, wants their kids to get a reasonable education, and tries to live a generally clean life should realize that their herbs, taken for self-treatment, offered to patients, or viewed as self-empowering agents of personal change, can be *junk*. That's why I write these books and teach my classes. If you only end up with ten or fifteen plants that you know well and trust, then you are indeed blessed. That is all a *curandera* uses most of the time, that is most of what a good Chinese herbalist needs, that is most of what an old Eclectic M.D. used, and that is the number of plants I imagine traditional healers have mostly relied on for fifty thousand years. Even the professional homeopath, the aristocrat of remedy proliferation, will dispense no more than one or two dozen different remedies 99% of the time. You don't *need* a whole bunch of different plant medicines if you are going to use them in the arena of tonics or subpathologies, where herbs are appropriate. You just need to know the ones you gather, and know them intimately. This isn't a playing card collection I am talking about, where the *most* is the *best*. Herbs can be compared to over-the-counter pharmaceuticals—how many different aspirin preparations are needed in one medicine cabinet, or how many different brands of hydrogen peroxide would you keep on hand? Similarly, how many different expectorants, bitter tonics, urinary tract astringents, or stomach-soothing herbs does a family *really* need? Nor is having a bunch of expensive herb stuff from the health food store a substitute for knowledge. Our consumer society tries to convince us that quantity is a substitute for quality. Nonsense. Learn a few good plants, collect them yourself, get to know them yourself, in the true sense of the amateur. Know, too, that what herbs do best can generally be found in plants that grow in your state or province. Of course, there are many exceptions. Nothing smells as fine as good Lavender, nothing quite matches Dong Quai, Vitex, or Cotton Root for functional reproductive imbalances, and nothing else can quite substitute for some good Echinacea.

In this book, I have tried to give the complete characteristics of each plant, as if it were the only plant there is. That way, although something may be the ideal remedy for a problem, you may still use the plant described to help. For example, Yerba Santa is a great plant for drying out drooling sinuses, and Bidens is great for lower urinary tract irritation, but if you only have gathered one of them, it is a reasonable substitute for the other. This way, your ten or fifteen plants will cover the problems that are the central strengths of plant medicines.

This is a list of things to keep in mind when using this book:

1. *Be sure of the plant you are picking.*

2. *If the herb makes you sick, take less or throw it away.*

3. *If it doesn't work, use more or forget it entirely.*

4. *Trust your judgment, not mine. You're there, I'm not.*

5. *That which stimulates can irritate; that which can help, can hurt.*

6. *Just because it's "natural" doesn't necessarily make it better.*

7. *If you don't get better, or get worse quickly, call your doctor.*

8. *Pick what you need and protect the rest.*

Some of the plants in this book are "little drugs," and have clear and understandable functions—to inhibit certain organisms, decrease inflammation under certain circumstances, suppress specific types of smooth muscle spasms, and so forth. Those of you with a medical background will understand their implications and perhaps find them less toxic adjuncts where stronger medications might otherwise have to be used. Those of you with backgrounds in Traditional Chinese Medicine or Ayurvedic Medicine may find that the tonic and strengthening effects of other plants in this book fit your philosophy of diagnosis, and can use them in place of some of your imported and expensive remedies. And I hope what I am sharing gives all of you the right tools to use your plant medicines with self-empowering confidence.

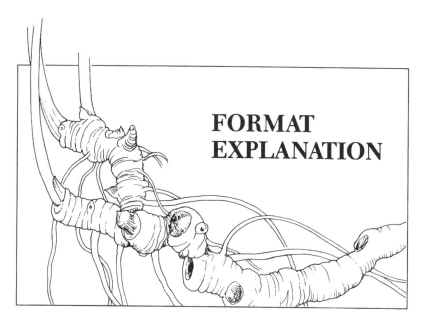

FORMAT EXPLANATION

COMMON NAME I have listed the primary plants under the most common name used in the Pacific region, when they are addressed as medicinal plants. Aconite and Hypericum may be referred to as Monkshood and St. John's Wort in field guides, but the first names are more common when they are discussed as herbs. The common name Alkali Heath is widely used, but *Yerba Reuma* is the name used when it is dealt with as a traditional Mexican *remedio*. Many monographs deal with several distinct plants in the same genus: Betony is the common name I use, but different species, with the same basic uses, may be known as Indian Warrior, Lousewort, or Elephant's Head, yet are all lumped together as Betony. Conversely, Mints, the *Mentha* genus, are listed separately as Lemon Mint, Spearmint, Peppermint, Brook Mint, and European Pennyroyal because they are each used differently. Personally, I would just as soon put both Manzanita and Uva Ursi in the same monograph, but few people think of them as being virtually identical, so they are listed separately. An option, of course, is to list everything by the Latin names, but this is a book for general, not technical use; so common names it shall be.

LATIN NAME Although the original intent of Latin naming was to create a universal, inviolate nomenclature, this is often open to riotous discussion amongst botanists. With the information explosion of the last decade or two, and extensive integration of plant science information from Eastern Europe and Asia tossed into the pot, taxonomy and nomenclature are going through some changes. I have tried to do a balancing act between the most widely used scientific names in the current Pacific floras, those in the most popular field guides, and what is presently accepted but not yet reflected in revisions of major floras. Besides, for me the Mints will always be Labiatae (not *Lamiaceae*), and Oplopanax is more fun to say than Echinopanax.

OTHER NAMES These are other names in general usage or found in widely used books, including English, Spanish, and Native American names. Also listed are alternate Latin names found in current texts or older herb or pharmaceutical books still in use.

MAPS Each herb has a thumbnail distribution map, reflecting its range within the Pacific West. If the habitat is described as being in lower foothills, between 2,000 and 4,000 feet, then those areas within the shaded part of the map that lie between those extremes are where the plant will be found. The approximate range shown is based on herbarium specimen localities, other people's distribution maps, and my own observation (where they differ). Where several species are described in the text, the map reflects the distribution of *all* of them; if I have mentioned in passing an atypical species that is not a usable herb or a rare species that I feel shouldn't be gathered, their distribution is not included, if they lie outside the general boundaries of the primary plants.

APPEARANCE I have attempted to describe the salient features of the plant or plants in question, particularly as they appear in the field. I have used few botanical descriptions and less taxonomy, so any of you trained in botany should attempt to not grind your teeth. I am dealing with the physical, morphologic patterns—the smell of the leaf, the panache, and the shape of root and stem growth. I have focused on the physical characteristics that dominate when the plant is collectable or when it is in its optimal circumstances. I have further emphasized the aspects that will make it easier to tell it apart from other similar plants, and the special circumstances peculiar to each plant, whatever they are.

Naturally, the ideal approach is to go out with a field botanist or herbalist familiar with plants. Most areas have native plant societies, wildflower groups, or botanical gardens that give afternoon walks, and there are herb stores and herbalists scattered here and there in our area that give medicinal plant walks from time to time; so just ask around.

HABITAT This will always be approximate, since plants, like people, want to live wherever they can. Plant communities have always been changing, anyway. Some plants can only grow in certain types of soil, within old-growth diversity, or within specific limits of rainfall, coastal fog, and the like. Cities, land development, and grazing alter this drastically, with the result that some plants are now found only in widespread pockets between towns, and others, formerly both lowland and forest plants, are now only found in the uplands; and still others thrive *because* of people (think "weeds").

Again, I have tried to emphasize the peculiarity of each individual plant's distribution, as it exists at this writing. For example, a plant such as White Sage is only found in a few counties in southern California and Baja California, but it is very common within that range, and the harvesting of the leaves has little effect on it anyway. Black Cohosh, on the other hand, is found in an immense part of the Northwest, but often in small stands, widely separated; and you will have to do some backcountry hiking to find much of it. If the leaf weren't almost as useful as the root, I wouldn't have included it at all. At least one plant, Yerba Mansa, is only mentioned in the supplemental section because, although very abundant and *very* useful, in our area it is mostly found in the wretched, polluted lowlands of the California agribusiness valleys.

Plants with barbed seeds can be expected almost anywhere; some plants, like Hypericum, follow us, and have an expanding range, and some, like California Poppy, can burst out of cultivation to establish new communities. Habitation, therefore, has to be approximate. Some plants can be completely frustrating to locate, and you might consider checking herbarium specimens, both for general appearance and for recent localities. Universities, junior colleges, botanical gardens, state and county extension services, and even the U.S. Forest Service often maintain such a collection. You may not wish to announce your intentions when you inquire. I am not insinuating that you should be sneaky about it; perhaps *circumspect* is a better word. Development, highways, logging, grazing—all these activities bite deeply into our plant communities, but the careful harvesting of plants for medicinal use leaves no footprints if done properly; still I would recommend circumspection. (Alright, be sneaky.)

In general, plant localities for southern California, Silicone Valley, Sacramento Valley, and the Seattle-Vancouver corridor should be viewed with great skepticism, unless developments nearby are less than ten years old. These areas have been extensively altered because of human development, and whole communities of plant and animal life have disappeared. On the other hand, suburban weeds like Bidens and Oxeye Daisy are more common than ever.

CONSTITUENTS These are substances, either single compounds or complexes, that seem to be responsible for the plants' activities. I have made little effort to define the nature of many of the compounds, but have for the most part merely listed them. In any case, many of the effects and uses of herbs may not derive from the so-called bioactive constituents, and may not be reducable to substances but rather to all parts acting as a gestalt. For example, when using Digitalis as a crude drug, it is vitally important to know both the constituents and their proportions in a given shipment. The drug activity is the direct result of these factors. A very different heart medicine, Hawthorn, has effects that cannot be monitored very well by individual compounds, and predictable medicine derives from a predictable quality of the herb.

Of course, a bunch of the plants in this book contain specific substances that clearly are responsible for specific actions; the more alkaloids in California Poppy, the stronger the effects from the same dose; Oregon Grape and Goldthread have high levels of the yellow alkaloid berberine, and the differences between them as therapeutics is the result of different secondary alkaloids. So, once again, I am treating each plant in the same manner, but the relative importance of each plant part is as diverse as are the plants themselves. The known constituents may be what do things, or they may have little or no part in the therapeutic use. If this information helps a few of you readers and users with technical backgrounds, fine; if the names impress some of you and make your left brain respect the plant more, fine; if they hold no meaning or interest for you, so be it; I feel all three ways on different days of the week.

COLLECTING Make a point of picking only plants growing in prime locations. Individual plants with many insect holes and obvious poor health are probably located at the extremes of their preferred growing conditions and may also have distinctly atypical biochemistries. Several noted exceptions, such as California Bayberry and Red Root, may be more potent when growing in stressed circumstances, but they *are* exceptions. Always check around after you have located a needed plant. There may be a whole field of it over the next rise or around the bend in the road. On the other hand, it may be the only one in the whole valley—and should be left alone. Furthermore, a plant common in one state may be a rare, protected plant in the next state, so check first if in doubt.

Certain conservation practices are always necessary. If a plant grows in large stands, never pick more than a third of the plants. If it is a large, solitary bush or tree, never pick more than a fourth of the foliage or twigs and do so preferably from the borders of the plant, leaving the older, central growth to regenerate outwards. If you are digging roots, dig no more than half of the immediately visible plants and the largest of the group, leaving the younger ones to grow and reseed. Fill up your holes if they are deep, and fill up your holes even if they aren't.

I have taken great pains in this particular book, far more than in others, to delineate the *specific* problems and moralities of collecting herbs in the Pacific West. There are *lots* of folks living here, the pressure on the land is great, and more of you will use this book than my others. I have excluded many plants because I could see no way to rationalize a collecting procedure that would *not* harm the species. I included two marginal plants, Black Cohosh and Trillium, only because the foliage alone could be used, and not the traditional roots. Further, preparing a fresh plant tincture will often provide much greater therapeutic value from less plant material. Besides, this book is not aimed at professional wildcrafting for commerce, but for our discrete harvesting. If our species of Black Cohosh, rather than the far more abundant eastern species, were to enter the vast crude drug trade, the dried roots of *every* existing plant would not be sufficient for the amount of one year's commerce. Since an herb collector in North Carolina is paid something like seventy cents a dried pound for the abundant *Cimicifuga racemosa,* collecting *C. elata,* an infinitely more elusive plant, might yield 1 or 2 pounds in a full dawn-to-dusk day. All these factors protect the plants.

In order to further protect the plants, when collecting, throw a chunk or two of budding rhizome back in the hole, spread the seeds around the area or other similar areas if they are mature, and bring back a bulb or two for your garden if they are dormant. Wherever you gather, presume that you will come back the next year to the same place and find the plants still healthy. Don't make the common mistake of looking many days for a plant, finding it finally, and taking a whole load of it back with you—it's like you are punishing it for your frustration. And most of it will go to waste.

Remember, know a few plants well, know what you will need, and don't try for the record number of shopping bags full of later unused (or in a year, maybe unknown) dried herbs you bring back from a picking trip. I have held that record for twenty years—I warn and scold from experience.

DRYING METHODS

Method A This is the preferred method for drying aboveground foliage that forms distinct stems. The stems are cut below the lowest green leaves or bark, bundled facing the same direction, then bound 1 or 2 inches from the cut ends with #31, #32, or #33 rubber bands (⅛ inch wide). Twine or wrapped wire may be used for a few low-moisture plants such as Mormon Tea or Yerba Reuma, but most herbs will shrink and fall out. If the plants are unusually dirty or sticky, such as Yerba Santa, they may be washed under cool water, squeezed gently, rinsed, shaken free of excess water, fanned out, and hung to dry. Washed bundles, and especially succulent herbs that are bundled, must be smaller in circumference to prevent spoilage. In reality, very few herbs need to be washed if they are gathered clean, and away from the roads. Annual herbs grow quickly and absorb little environmental pollutants. Perennial herbs growing up from extensive roots, such as Nettle or Yarrow, may live for many years, storing environmental toxins and metals in increasing quantities each year, and sending them up to the foliage during the green months. Check your area for agribusiness, mining, and other sources of toxic substances; if they are upstream or upwind, go elsewhere.

Herbs must *never* be dried in sunlight; instead, they should be hung from hooks or nails in shaded areas with adequate ventilation until both the tops and the bottoms are brittle-dry. Many bulky, drier plants can simply be dried loosely in paper bags, and I mention this in the text where appropriate. If you live in the San Francisco area or along Puget Sound, the moisture rolls in at night, and the plants in the garage that are dry in mid-afternoon will get rehydrated at night. Most dried plants contain water-activated enzymes, and allowing this cycle of dry and moist to continue will reduce your herbs to little more than compost. Dry them inside, use a dehydrator (*not* the oven or microwave), or rely on preparations made in the field. The end point of drying botanicals has always been to finish with herbs that resemble the living plant in color and texture. The Lemon Mint that you picked was virulent dark shiny green with purple stems, but the stuff you bring in next month from the garage has turned olive-drab grey-black. Not good.

After drying, herbs may be stored in a variety of ways, but the bundles are usually broken down, stripped of leaves and/or flowers, and discarded or cut up. For most herbs in bloom, the flowering half of the bundle is chopped into regular short segments with pruning shears or kitchen shears. The remaining lower half of the stems is stripped of leaves, the leaves kept, and the stems discarded. This is general; the many specific peculiarities of each plant are mentioned in the text.

Canning jars and cleaned reused jars are the optimum storage containers. Coffee cans, plastic bags, even paper bags may also be appropriate, and with some delicate plants, freezing the dried herb is best. I have covered a number of special circumstances with regard to many of the plants, but if in doubt, use the jars. Storage should be in a cool, dark area. And, most importantly, *label everything*. It is best to include when and where you picked the plant as well, even listing preparation and dosage directions. Memory is fleeting. I also hold the record for mystery plants and mystery tinctures accumulated in a single year, so I speak from *vast* experience.

Method B This is a simple method for drying small roots, seeds, fruit, resins, and leaf bunches. Use the lower half of cardboard cartons that beer and soda cans are shipped in. They are nearly always sliced along the sides and the cans stacked inside in half-box flats, discarded after the canned drinks are sold. They are clean, your local convenience store may have a four-foot-high stack waiting (just for you) inside the front door, and they can be reused many times. Place the herbs loosely along the bottom of the flat, fill another, stack it at a right angle to the first, and so forth. You can bring a lot of flats back with you this way, the back seat filled wtih six layers, four across, the windows open, and the air drying them as I speak . . . just watch out for sudden stops, and make sure the top layer doesn't start to blow out the window.

When they are dry, store as above or as specifically described for that herb. Always remember that it takes a lot longer to process the herbs you gather than it does to gather them in the first place. If you slaughter a chicken, you don't put the carcass aside to dress later in the week—you do it now! If you dig roots or pick herbs that need to be washed or sliced or bundled, do it now! If you are going to tincture them fresh, do it now! If you want to dry the herb, process it as *soon* as it is dry.

STABILITY This defines how long you can expect a gathered plant to stay reasonably strong or what characteristics it must retain to still have potency. The rule of thumb is that green herbs are good for a year, and roots and barks for two years; but the exceptions are many, and they are listed in the text where applicable. Salves and oils, if they contain an antioxidant, are good for several years, and, with few exceptions, tinctures last for years.

PREPARATIONS

Teas: Cold Infusion Suspend 1 part (by weight) of the herb in cloth or paper towel in 32 parts of water at room temperature for at least six hours, preferably overnight, squeezing out the excess tea from the herb packet when finished. It is best to moisten the dry herb first before suspending it; gravity does the rest. The substances that dissolve in the water are heavier than water, sink to the bottom of the jar, and set up a slow displacement current. The water containing more solubles is heavier than the water containing less solubles, so there is always a rise towards the top of weaker tea, always a draw downwards from the suspended herb. It is a very efficient method and, as it uses no heat, the least altering to plant constituents of any tea process.

Teas: Standard Infusion Boil 32 parts of water, remove it from the heat, and steep 1 part by weight of the herb in the water for one-half to one hour, depending on the density of the botanical. Pour through a strainer, and add additional water (poured through the herb) until the original 32 parts is reached.

Teas: Strong Decoction Bring to a boil 1 part (by weight) of the herb in 32 parts of cold water. Continue boiling for ten minutes, remove from the heat, and cool until it is body temperature. Strain, and add enough water, if needed, to make 32 parts of tea.

Teas: Weak Decoction Follow the directions above, but use ½ part, by weight, of herb.

> NOTE: In making the first three teas, you will have a solution that represents the approximate strength of each fluid ounce having the water-soluble parts of 1 gram of herb. The cold infusion preparation is somewhat more efficient at extracting dense storage compounds, since the extended submersion in water allows both enzyme activity and the reabsorption of water by hydrolysis and digestion, making some poorly soluble constituents dissolvable. When preparing teas, make no more than a day's worth at one time. After a couple of days, the dissolved substances in the tea may begin to recombine, precipitate, or salt out; and if stored even longer, spoilage can occur. Plants that need to be made into tea anew each time are noted in the monograph, as are any other special tea preparations.

Eyewash: Wherever the making of eyewashes is mentioned, keep two important factors in mind. First, make the tea with isotonic water (neutrally saline) by using clean or distilled water (1 quart) combined with a slightly rounded *measuring* teaspoon of table salt (½ teaspoon per pint, ¼ teaspoon per cup). Second, make a fresh batch of tea each time you use the eyewash, or, at the very least, discard the unused eye solution after four hours. If you have irritated and inflamed eyes, the last thing you need is to wash them with dirty tea.

Sitz Bath: Make the tea as per the directions, pour it into a tub that you can sit in; *then* add the rest of the water to get a comfortable temperature. Adding hot, steaming tea to a gallon or so of warm water makes it too hot; if you need a sitz bath, the last thing you need is to poach your privates. If the directions call for adding tincture, then fill the tub with warm water and add the tincture last. If no specific directions are given, make a pint of standard infusion tea. If you have no round tub and use the bathtub, double the amount of tea or tincture used, since you will need much more water to bring the level to your hips. Friendly advice: if you haven't done one of these before, put the tub inside your bathtub. You have *no* idea how little room there is for water in a round tub after even the scrawniest person fills it with their rump, and you will probably overfill it the first time. Have an overripe tomato or vinegar-filled water pistol with you if you live in a relaxed household; if you sternly retaliate against the first person to come in and make some wise-assed comment about your inglorious situation, you will nip the problem in the bud.

Salves: Method A This is an efficient method of making salves out of plants that are not very oil soluble, by using alcohol as an intermediate solvent. Grind up 1 part (by weight) of herb, place it in a container with a top, moisten it thoroughly with ½ to ¾ part (by volume) of pure ethanol or 90% rubbing alcohol, and let it set covered for at least two hours. Place it in a blender, cover it with 7 parts (by volume) of vegetable oil (preferably olive), and blend the hell out of it. Blend it until the side of the top is warm, turn it off, and pour it through a cloth inside a strainer placed over a bowl. Squeeze out all the oil and toss the remnants. As an example, grind 3 ounces of Oregon Grape leaves, moisten the mixture with 1½ ounces of Everclear (95% ethanol), let it set for two hours, scrape it into a blender, add 21 ounces of olive oil, and blend it for five minutes while you lay a piece of cheesecloth over the strainer on a mixing bowl; when you find that the glass container is warm, turn the blender off, pour the mean green slurry into the cloth, let it drain while stirring with a rubber spatula, grab the sides of the cloth, and squeeze out the rest of the oil. At this point you will have 17 or 18 ounces of dark green oil, impregnated with Oregon Grape alkaloids—and green hands, green spatula, green bowl, green strainer, green blender top, and a cloth-covered oily mass to discard.

Although you can keep the oil in that form, to make a salve, dissolve 1 ounce of beeswax for every 5 ounces of finished oil in a double boiler or in a pan over a *very* low heat. With the example above, you would add 3½ ounces of beeswax with the 17 to 18 ounces of Oregon Grape oil, heat them together until the beeswax has melted, and pour the mix in the baby food or jelly jars that you should have nearby. (Didn't I mention that? Sorry.) You use the Oregon Grape herb instead of the root for oil extraction, because the leaf contains simpler compounds in less dense cells. You can get the active alkaloids out of the leaf, but little or none from the root; that's just the way it is.

Salves: Method B This is for those herbs that are readily soluble in oil. Grind 1 part of the herb, blend it with 7 parts of vegetable oil until warm, pour into a jar, and set aside for a week. Pour it back into the blender, blend until warm, strain, and proceed as above for adding beeswax.

> NOTE ON SALVE-MAKING: If you make a salve with beeswax, it oxidizes or turns rancid very slowly and will be good for a couple of years. If you keep it as an oil, you will need to use olive or sesame oil, neither of which gets rancid. Several of the herbs, such as Balsam Poplar buds, are themselves antioxidant and need no special attention. If you want to use an inexpensive oil, such as corn or sunflower, add ½ ounce of ground and dried Chaparral leaves (*Larrea tridentata*) to each quart and let it set for a month, or add 1 ounce of gum benzoin per quart, shake it up, and let it set. These prepared oils can be used for any salve-making; just label them well to avoid other uses—Chaparral-flavored vinaigrette is loathsome.
>
> If you plan on making many salves, find a beekeeper in your area. Pharmacies will charge a buck an ounce, a beekeeper no more than four dollars a pound—usually less. Conversely, a pharmacy may be able to sell you a whole bunch of small, brown plastic jars, complete with Nixon-proof caps, since they dispense pills in them. If you wish glass salve containers, check with your local bottle or packaging wholesaler. Also, cultivate the friendship of new parents; they often have lots of baby food jars just going to waste.

Poultice: This is a hot, moist mass, consisting of a base (Marshmallow root, powdered Mallow leaves, Comfrey root, clay, Flax, Kudzu, and so forth) and one or more active substances (such as a tea, herb powder, or tincture), that is placed on any part of the body, usually held between two pieces of gauze or cheesecloth, and changed or covered with a hot, wet towel when cool. This aids pain, congestive inflammation, tissue damage, and skin distension. It also aids in absorption of the herb constituents into the skin, and absorption of edema and waste products through the skin and into the poultice. Poultices always help but are seldom employed in medicine anymore; so it's up to us.

FRESH PLANT TINCTURE Take 1 part, by weight, of the fresh plant, just gathered and rinsed, chop it into small pieces, place it in a clean glass jar with a good lid, cover the chopped herb with 2 parts of 95% ethanol (pure grain alcohol like Everclear), screw the lid on after making sure the herbs are compressed enough in the jar that the alcohol comes up to the top of the herb, and set it aside for seven to ten days. If you use a standard quart canning jar, you can stuff 10 or even 11 ounces of herb in the jar, and the addition of 20 or 22 ounces of alcohol will cover it to the top. There may not be quite enough room for the last couple of ounces of liquid, but after settling for a day, the level of alcohol in the jar will have lowered and you can now add the balance. You will usually find that 12 ounces of fresh root can be covered with 24 ounces of alcohol to fill a quart jar completely. When you try to compress 10 ounces of really bulky foliage, like

California Bay or Maidenhair Fern, resist the temptation to use a trash compactor; you can do it . . . you *can* do it.

The alcohol dehydrates the cells of fresh plants; all living constituents contain water, and the alcohol draws the substances into the surrounding liquid until, by the time you drain off the fininshed tincture, it has a deep, radiant color, and the herb remainder is yellowish, dusty white, and exhausted of its constituents, color, and essence. Succulent roots, such as Balsam Root and Lomatium, will be exhausted but may retain too much residual tincture. If you have access to a hydraulic juice press, slurry up the fully steeped tincture and root pieces, pressing all the tincture out. Some people blend the fresh herb with the alcohol at the start, and then let it set for a week or two; but this ruptures the cell walls, prevents the process of dehydration, releases a number of inactive starches and structural compounds into the tincture, and increases the formation of insoluble compounds formed between active (dehydrated) and inactive (ruptured) substances. Nothing is fixed with plants, and this is probably alright with some herbs, but I don't know any specifics; so I chop and steep, not blend and steep.

Pure grain alcohol is available from liquor stores all over the western U.S., except California (and it is not sold in British Columbia as well). This tincturing method needs 190 proof (95%) alcohol to work properly; 80 or 100 proof (40% or 50%) is quite inferior in its ability to extract, so Californians will have to go to bordering states to get it, and Canadians will have to sneak it across the border in empty water jugs (although I would never suggest anyone break the law—honest, really). I have used 157 proof Myers Rum *in extremitus*, and it works fine, but I always had the urge to pour the finished tincture over little round raisin cakes or mix it with Coca-Cola; and frankly, the scent of fresh California Bay tincture riding tentatively over that of double-distilled rum was evilly perverse.

Folks in southern California can always go into Mexico and pick up a liter of Victoria brand *puro de cana* (pure grain alcohol) for three or four bucks; you can bring a liter a month, legally and tax-free, back into the U.S. It may be possible to bring more at one time, paying the duty at the border, but *please* check first. Also, bring a big, 800-page Stephen King tome to read while you wait in line to be glint-eyed by U.S. customs officials. Better yet, park on the Yankee side, walk over the border to the second (not the first) liquor store on the Mexican side, buy the bottle, and walk back through to the U.S. This whole border process is guaranteed to make even a church organist or Mormon elder fumble guiltily, wondering if it is illegal to have once seen part of *Easy Rider* on cable television (without inhaling).

DRY PLANT TINCTURE This is the classic one of grinding the herb, weighing the coarse powder, adding the solvent, putting the mixed gloop into a canning jar, and shaking it twice a day for two weeks, letting it set a day, pouring the standing tincture, and squeezing the cloth-wrapped marc as dry as your wrists can make it. This is a fine and time-honored method, producing a full strength tincture (usually); it has always been a proper alternative method to percolation (see below).

To outline by example, here goes. Grind and sift 4 ounces of *Arnica cordifolia* leaves and flowers. According to this book, you need to make a 1:5 tincture with

50% alcohol (with the balance always presumed to be water); when you make a steeped dry tincture (this way), you add the menstruum (half alcohol and half water in this case), 5 parts (20 fluid ounces) with the Arnica, 1 part (4 ounces) —and that is what you steep and shake in a jar for two weeks. You may only be able to remove 12 or 13 ounces (with strong hands), but that extractable tincture has a strength of 1:5. Unfortunately, all the moisture still in the marc that you discard is *also* 1:5 tincture. If you can borrow a hydraulic juice press or an old lard press, you may be able to end up with 16 or 17 ounces of tincture. Remember, you put *in* the 5 parts of menstruum (solvent)—20 ounces in this case; what you get *out* depends solely on the efficiency of your squeezing methods.

An acetum, or vinegar tincture, uses standardized apple cider vinegar as the solvent, instead of an alcohol-water menstruum.

Percolating a dry plant tincture, on the other hand, takes twenty-four hours; you *finish* with the full 20 ounces of 1:5 tincture, and the extraction is actually more effective. Percolation is the official process and is a neat, low-tech, no-heat method, but requires a special percolator glass cone and a bit of hands-on practice that is difficult to describe (like line dancing) but easy to *do*. The whole procedure is explained, rationalized, and illustrated impeccably in any edition of Remington's *Pharmaceutical Sciences*. Every pharmacy has a copy behind the counter (in many states it is required), so you might ask to Xerox those pages or borrow an outdated edition. Otherwise most libraries will have one. If you can't locate an old glass percolator cone, have the lower inch cut from the bottom of some empty 24-ounce Perrier bottles at a glass shop, and have the edges ground. Set the cone or bottle upside down in the top of a quart wide-mouth Mason jar, with the cap available to screw onto the bottom (former top) if you need to control the rate of drip; according to Remington, this gives you a crude but effective percolator cone. Follow the Remington directions, using a common herb for starters, and do a couple batches until you get it right. It won't help to ask a pharmacist to show you how; any pharmacist under sixty years of age is unlikely to have ever percolated a botanical tincture since his or her third year lab test, if then. We are on our own, in case you haven't noticed.

MEDICINAL USES Several considerations must be kept in mind when using herbs to remedy a physical imbalance or disease. Acute illnesses, those with quick onset, strong symptoms, and a self-limiting nature, should be treated simply, using one or two herbs. The purpose of botanicals here is to give comfort, speed defense reactions, and limit and define the course to prevent complications or prolongation. Common sense is paramount, since the remedies may not be sufficient or may cause an overreaction. The use of salicylate herbs (Balsam Poplar, even Licorice Fern) may turn a fever into chills. Conversely, stimulating the fever, as with Wild Ginger or Yarrow, can be an excess on occasion. Any reaction which itself denigrates or impedes the body's strength must be avoided, since one of the main validities of good herbal therapy is its ability to aid and augment defense responses without hindering them with toxicity.

Since the pharmacology of most herbs is so diffused, they are rarely able to supplant, sidestep, or suppress body defenses or reactions in the manner of many drugs. Although these same drugs will have distinct secondary toxicities, often very dangerous ones, they can be so focused and emphatic in their benefits that they can supply imperative benefit for those unable to regain internal equilibrium

—save lives if you will. Properly used, their value outweighs their danger. Physicians are often opposed to things like herbs; they have spent their professional lives dealing with the knowledge that the most commonplace prescription has many side effects *at the proper dosage*, and they bear the ultimate responsibility to weigh value against danger. It is only natural for them to presume that herbs have similar dangers *at the proper dosage* and should not be so widely used by nonprofessionals. If the dangers that accompany therapeutic doses were the same for herbs as drugs, this whole book would be flagrantly immoral.

The proper use of herbs in most cases is for the subclinical stage of a disease, for a person in normal health, and they are not going to be of value if the imbalance progresses to a full overt disease response. Conversely, most existing drugs, with toxicity at therapeutic levels, work poorly for subclinical problems that have not "ripened" yet; the side effects are greater than the benefits. If you figure on getting better, use herbs to help; if you think you are *really* getting sick, it doesn't help to take a lot more of the same herbs until *they* make you sick as well. The therapeutic window for herbs will always be below their adverse effects. Excessive quantities of an herb sufficient to cause a toxic reaction simply compromise basic health without supplying the synthetic defenses offered by proper drug therapies.

Put it this way: most herbs are used to strengthen the innate defenses, and attempt to stimulate natural healing; if they make you sick, this weakens you, and it is harder to get well on your own. If you get really sick, and can no longer be expected to recover unaided, or without organ damage, drugs can intervene and turn the decline around. They may sicken you, but you are not relying on your defenses at that point; your sickness is draining you, and the drug shield is far more positive than its side effects are negative. When you turn the corner, *then* you will heal by yourself.

Medicine is still the way to go for many conditions; it has always been most adept at the upper end of pathologies, but in recent years it has come to ignore the lower end, even to the point of seeming to deny that the subclinical (not yet treatable) state exists. "If you're not sick, you're healthy." This is not really the belief of Medicine, mind you, but that's the way it works in real life. De facto, not de jure, is the medical reality. Use herbs for the lower end, and see the doc for the upper end of human discomfort.

For chronic illness, more complex combinations are usually more effective than single remedies, with small regular doses preferable to erratic larger doses. The dose should be small enough that it produces no overt symptoms. You first need to use one or more herbs that can be expected to help the main symptoms. If you *only* use them, the imbalance may lessen for a while, but attacking the problem directly will eventually wear out their value. Chronic disease is often helped initially during the "honeymoon" period, but, whether using herbs, drugs, acupuncture, or diet, a single-minded approach wears out, the imbalance returns, and you need to move on to something else. For example, chronic sinusitis with periods of acute pain followed by periods of little or no pain will never be "cured" by any agent that simply suppresses the sinus inflammation. Chronic disease usually arises out of both inherited and constitutional imbalances coupled with lifestyle. Once you have acquired chronic sinusitis, then any body or emotional stress that comes along will be likely to cause the condition to worsen.

You don't need some sinus irritation to directly start the pain; it flares up from such unrelated problems as bad food, family fights, constipation, a death in the family, or an IRS audit. Just like old Doc Selye wrote down fifty years ago, once you have a chronic disease, *any* stress is currency. That's why, if you are going to use an herb or two specifically aimed at the problem, you have to use other herbs to lessen metabolic stress as well. They don't affect the sinuses, but they should decrease the stress of the person who *has* the sinusitis. If you lessen the symptoms *and* lessen the stress, the therapy "has legs." Besides, if you stir up the metabolism for any length of time, it is important that you stimulate the body's ability to break down and excrete the waste products you stir up. If you have chronic sinusitis, such a formula, using plants from this book (and others) might go as follows:

1. SPECIFIC *Bidens, Composition Powder (under California Bayberry), Oxeye Daisy, or Yerba Santa*

2. LAXATIVE *Oregon Grape, Sweet Root, or Cascara Sagrada*

3. LIVER STIMULANT *Bittersweet, Buckbean, California Mugwort, California Snakeroot, Oregon Grape, or Dandelion Root*

4. DIURETIC *Buckwheat Bush, Nettle, or Oxeye Daisy*

5. LYMPHATIC *California Bayberry, Figwort, or Red Root*

6. NERVINE *Betony, Hypericum, Lemon Balm, Stream Orchid, or Valerian*

And, if you have cold hands and feet, a tendency for low blood pressure, and hate the cold and damp, you should add:

7. CIRCULATORY STIMULANT *Bittersweet, California Bayberry, Devil's Club, or Wild Ginger*

In conclusion, number 1 should be an herb or herbs dealing with the active symptoms of the chronic problem and should be the largest component. The rest, numbers 2 to 6, and if necessary, number 7, are "satellite" or tonic herbs to facilitate and diffuse. None of the support herbs should be present in palpable quantities; that is, the laxative should not have a pronounced laxative effect, the nervine should not be in enough quantity to cause drowsiness, and so forth. The rest of the formula is only to aid making changes that can occur as a result of the specifics. Unlike acute disease, the course of chronic illness is slow and submerged, and, even if the sinusitis stops after a few weeks of such a formula, you *still* have the weakness, and you may need to return to the herbs next year. The secondary herbs can be of your choice, but a good tonic possesses little overt drug potential; so it would *not* be wise to use Aconite for the nervine, as an example.

Always use an herb that has a mild effect whenever possible, and one whose various properties seem to suit your constitution in general. If you are under medical care for your problem and are taking regular medication, don't presume to use herbs on a regular basis; you may interfere with liver metabolism of the drugs or add more stress to your kidneys or skin. Try to follow one approach at a time. Extended use of any biologically active substances is not appropriate during pregnancy, and that includes a bunch of herbs, no matter how subtle they seem to be. Even such widely used prebirth strengtheners as Raspberry leaves and Squaw Vine are probably best used in the last trimester only. Of course, if I were a woman with some kids, I might feel differently; I cannot speak from experience.

Most chronic problems not of direct genetic cause will generally derive from imbalances in lifestyle, an improper diet, emotional or spiritual instability, and stress. The end result (chronic disease) can be considered partially genetic and partially lifestyle- and stress-related—the result of negative habits of body function or response. The best time to instigate therapy on any or all of these levels, including herbal, is during periods of change. For some people, the spring or fall season is most auspicious; for others, it might be when moving to another place, leaving a relationship, having a child, changing jobs, religion, or diet. In any case, wait until you have completely recovered from an acute episode to start the herbs.

A combination of drug and herb therapy can be useful, useless, or disastrous, and it is far too unpredictable to deal with here in great detail, except where specific contraindications are mentioned. An herb such as Nettle, with little systemic effect other than as a source of nutrients and moderate astringency, may be useful as a food supplement. Otherwise it is safest to leave each to its separate realm.

Some specific problems should be mentioned. Like aspirin, the salicylate herbs should never be combined with anticoagulants. These include Balsam Poplar, Licorice Fern, and even Red Root, as well as Alder, Birch, Aspen, Pipsissewa, and Pyrola in the supplemental section. Herbs with pronounced sedative effects, like their drug counterparts, should not be consumed with alcohol. More complex and unpredictable drug approaches such as anticholinergics, adrenergic blockers, anticonvulsants, and postoperative medications should be taken only under the closest supervision and not combined with herbs. Even as gentle an astringent as Buckwheat Bush can alter the rate of intestinal absorption or bind and block the drug. Laxatives and liver herbs may alter the rate of absorption or excretion of prescription drugs and affect their predictability. Much study has gone into determining the fate and absorption rates of drug therapy, and doses are set based on normal metabolizations. Herbal laxatives and liver stimulants can only interfere.

The time of day and mode of use affects the strength of reaction to many herbs. Sedatives and laxatives work best when their use coincides with normal patterns of sleep and defecation. A bitter tonic or stomachic works best when taken shortly before meals or before a predictable discomfort. Potential stomach irritants may need to be taken on a full stomach; herbs meant to work quickly, on an empty stomach. An herb used for recurring symptoms that give advance warning (such as migraine headaches or PMS) or which are part of a predictable stress (such as insomnia or hangovers) works better when taken *before* the discomfort has settled in. It is easier and takes less therapy to prevent a known problem than to try to stamp it out after it starts.

In dealing with young children a great deal of caution must be used, since defense responses can become excessive or prove inadequate very quickly. In young children and infants, the speed of infection may not be quantitatively different than in adults, but an organ or system can be compromised much sooner because of the considerably smaller volume of resistant tissue. The toxins produced by the same volume of bacterial infection in an adult and a child represent very different proportions of body volume. One should be especially cautious in totally relying on home remedies for small children when the sickness is febrile, eruptive, or involves diarrhea or the eyes, ears, or mouth. Any lung infection should be approached conservatively. The most fanatically devout follower of natural healing methods should still take an infant or young child to a physician when there is any doubt at all; the course of some diseases can be quick, volatile, and unpredictable. Small life-forms, be they plants or people, react quickly and without sophistication. The high fever, nausea, and vomiting may be the same for mild sniffles or viral meningitis. The acquired immunity of a two year old is not extensive, and most infectious responses are against new microbes. You can't tell how serious the organism is, only how strongly the child responds; so play it safe. Children respond very well to the simplest, most benign herbal remedies, but the majority of the plants in this book should not be used for little children; the diaphoretics and the stomachache medicines—the Yarrow, Mints, Lemon Balm—are the things for kids, as are the herbs indicated for topical use.

Similarly, certain modifications should be used in treating the aged. They are usually more sensitive to herbs and drugs, and smaller quantities should be used, from one-half to two-thirds as much. Special care should be taken when an herb has a nauseating or cathartic effect. Herbs that I refer to as alteratives and those described as parasympathetic or cholinergic stimulants should be used with care. The equilibrium of health is often more delicate in the aged, with small irritation causing great discomfort. Most of the illness of age is the direct result of chronic disease, so most preparations should be given using the chronic-disease format listed above.

Rare diseases *are* rare, and most discomforts and illnesses can be helped with herbs; even serious problems usually *had* a window of herbal use early on. Still, the ideal circumstance is to know (or be) a physician who will allow for the validity of herbal medicine, yet act as a screen for more serious problems. Lacking that, get to know your body and use common sense.

Even though drug therapy and surgery may not always be the best approach, and even though medicine treats less serious illnesses poorly, the *best* diagnostician for the nuts-and-bolts problems we have with our bodies is the physician. And the best advice about prescription drugs comes from the drug specialist, a pharmacist.

ACONITE
Aconitum columbianum
page 34

ARNICA
Arnica latifolia
page 46

AMOLE LILY
Chlorogalum pomeridianum
page 38

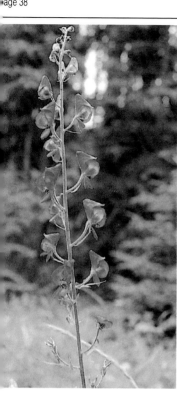

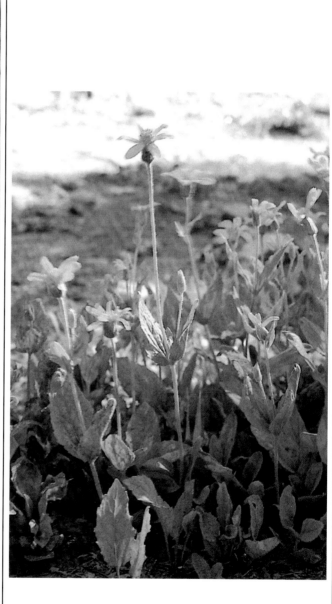

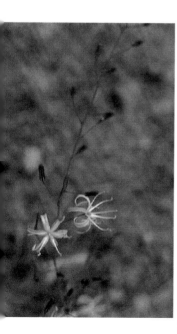

BALSAM ROOT
Balsamorhiza sagittata
page 55

BANEBERRY
Actea rubra
(in fruit)
page 58

BANEBERRY
Actea rubra
(in flower)
page 58

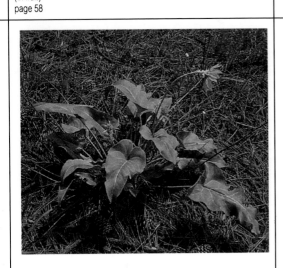

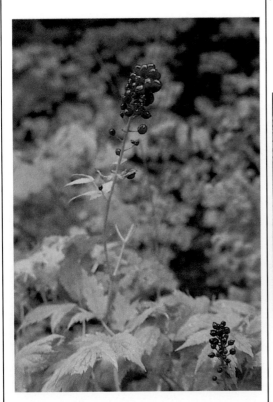

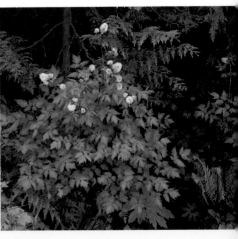

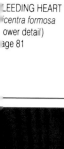

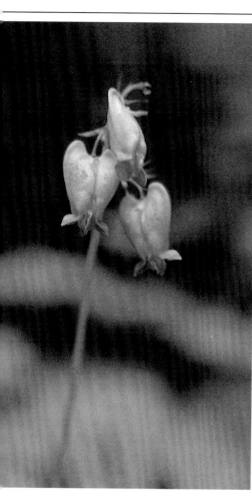

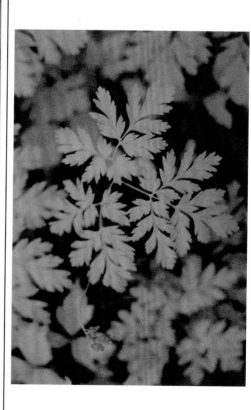

BLACK COHOSH
Cimicifuga elata
page 74

CALIFORNIA BUCKEYE
Aesculus californica
page 104

BUNCHBERRY
Cornus canadensis
page 95

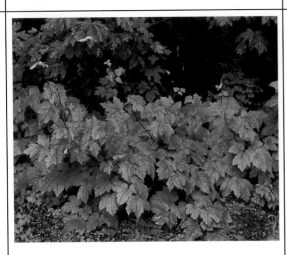

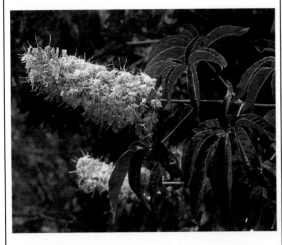

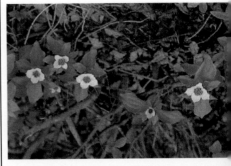

CALIFORNIA SPIKENARD
Aralia californica
page 116

DEVIL'S CLUB
Oplopanax horridum
page 125

FALSE SOLOMON'S SEAL
Smilacina stellata
page 131

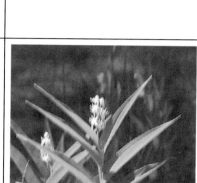

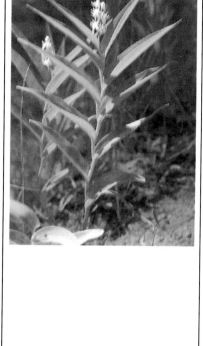

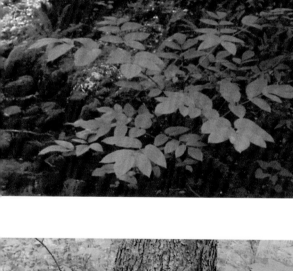

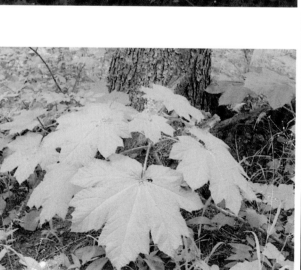

FIREWEED
Epilobium angustifolium
page 136

HUMMINGBIRD SAGE
Salvia spathacea
page 150

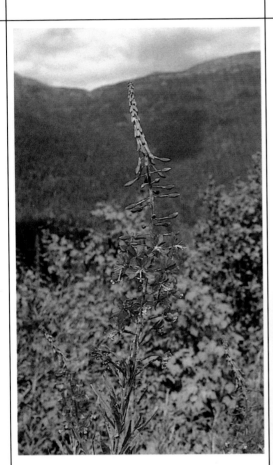

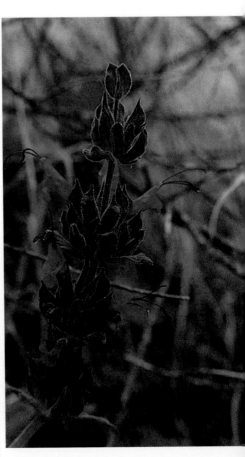

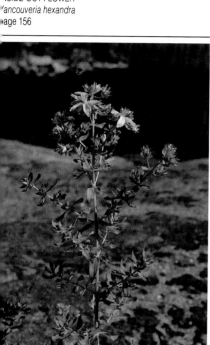

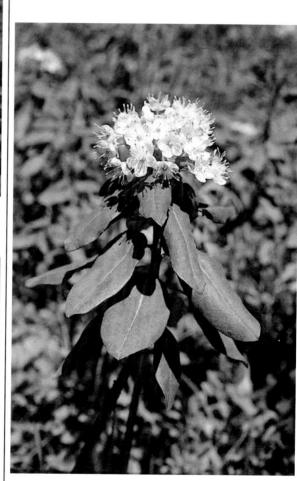

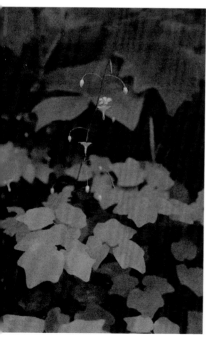

LICORICE FERN
Polypodium glycyrrhiza
page 163

LOMATIUM
Lomatium dissectum
page 167

MAIDENHAIR FERN
Adiantum pedatum
page 174

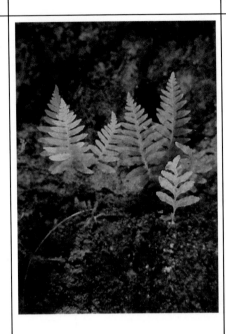

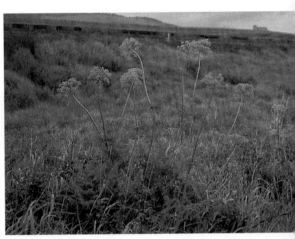

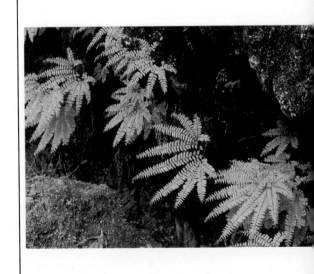

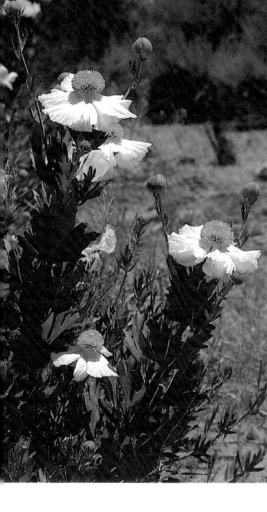

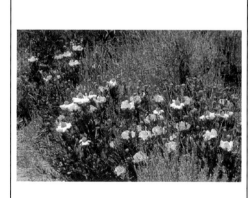

NETTLE
Urtica dioica
page 185

PEARLY EVERLASTING
Anaphalis margaritacea
page 197

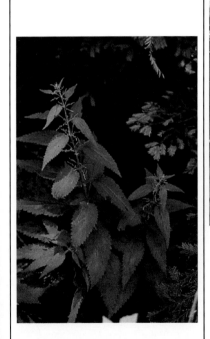

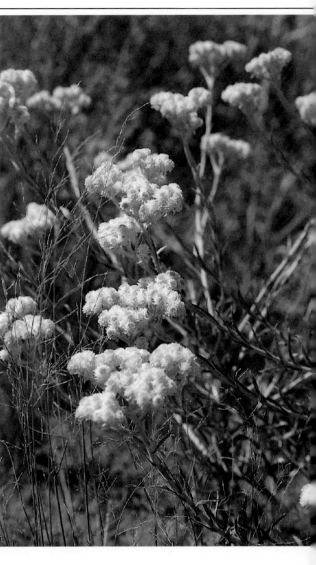

PRICKLY POPPY
Argemone corymbosa
page 206

PRICKLY POPPY
Argemone corymbosa
(flower detail)
page 206

RED CEDAR
Thuja plicata
page 209

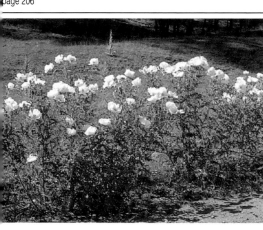

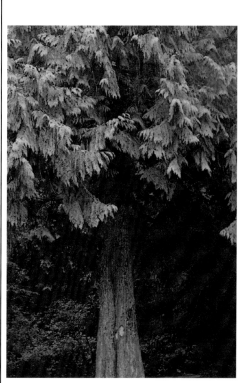

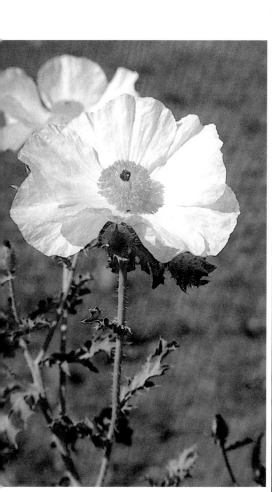

REDWOOD
Sequoia sempervirens
page 219

SALAL
Gaultheria shallon
page 221

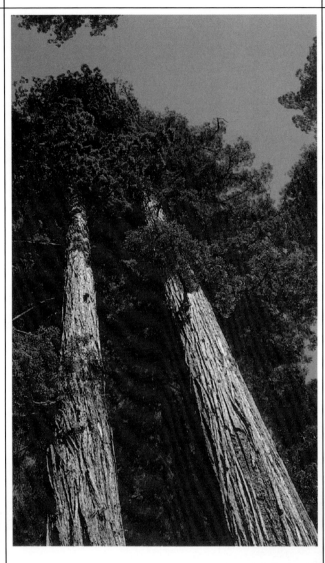

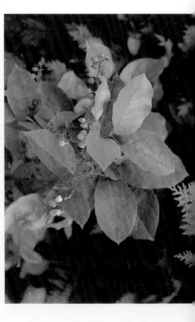

SARSAPARILLA
Smilax californica
(open growth)
page 224

SARSAPARILLA
Smilax californica
(viny growth)
page 224

TRILLIUM
Trillium ovatum
page 239

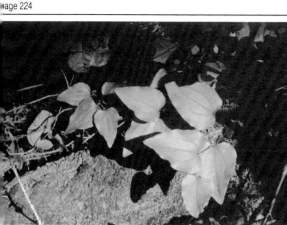

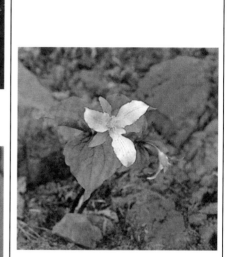

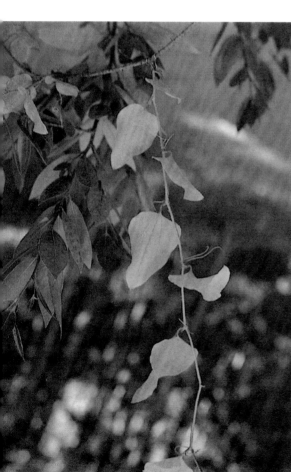

WESTERN COLTSFOOT
Petasites palmatus
page 253

WESTERN SKUNK CABBAGE
Lysichiton americanum
page 263

VANILLA LEAF
Achlys triphylla
page 250

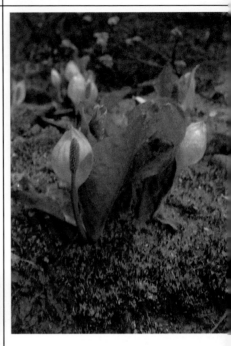

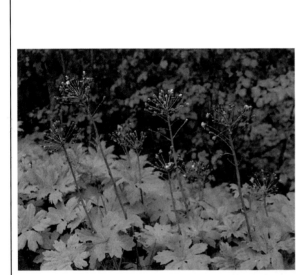

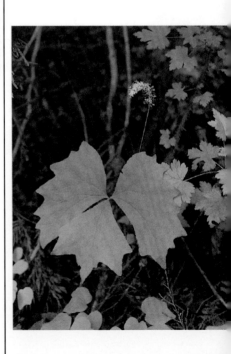

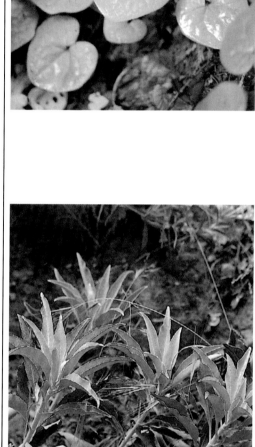

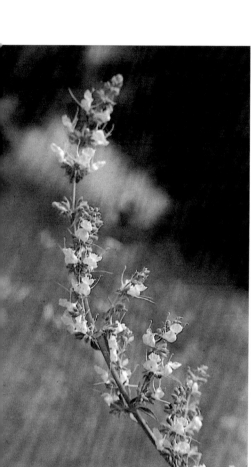

YERBA BUENA
Satureja Douglasii
page 278

YERBA BUENA
Satureja Douglasii
(detail)
page 278

YERBA DEL LOBO
Helenium hoopesii
page 281

YERBA SANTA
Eriodictyon californicum
page 285

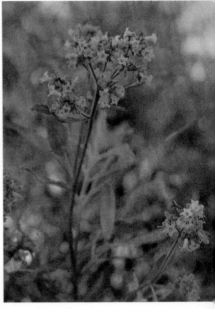

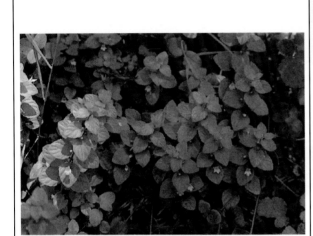

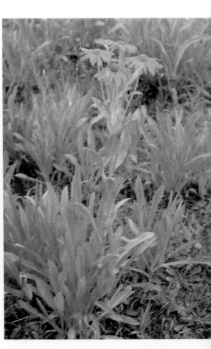

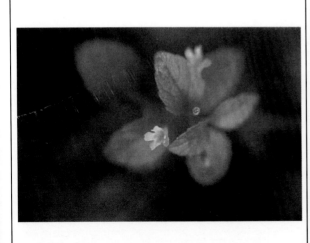

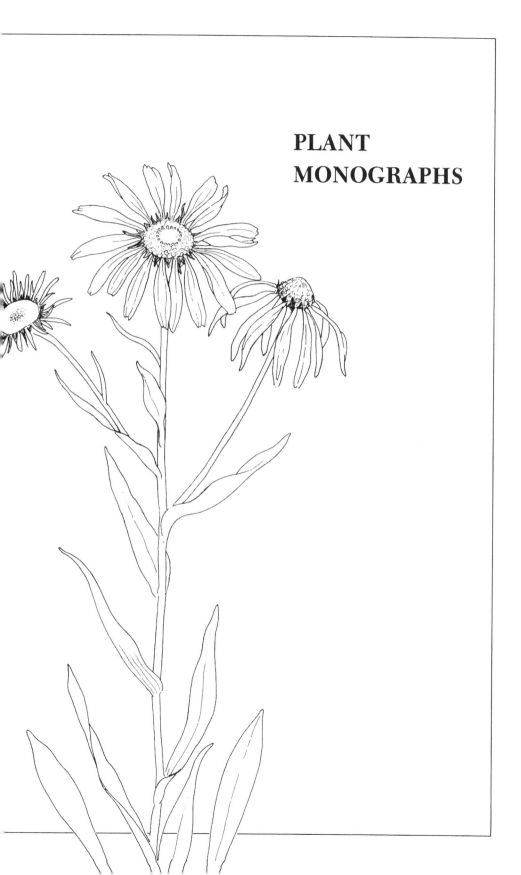

**PLANT
MONOGRAPHS**

Aconite   *(Poisonous)*

Aconitum columbianum   (Ranunculaceae)
OTHER NAMES   Monkshood, Wolfsbane; *A. fischeri*, etc.

APPEARANCE When in flower from July to September, this is one of the most elegant plants of the mountains. Its height is from 2 to 8 feet, and it usually grows in dispersed stands. The striking flowers are dark blue to midnight blue, from ½ to 1 inch tall. They form loose racemes off of many terminal branches and resemble a Larkspur without the spur, the upper flower petal distinctly arched or hooded. Smaller plants may only have a single terminal flower group. The leaves are sharply divided into three or five segments resembling a Wild Geranium leaf, with the basal leaves sometimes 4 inches across, and the alternate stem leaves decreasing in size and complexity towards the top.

This is a complex and variable plant, intermixing in Alaska and Siberia with at least one Asian species. It is periodically divided into other species and varieties and then revised back into the single one. Some races have yellow-purple flowers, some isolated colonies form little aerial bulbs along the stem leaves or lower flowers, and some colonies grow almost as vines; but by and large the form mentioned is nearly universal.

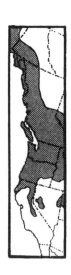

HABITAT Aconite likes fresh water, and grows in shady drainage and by creeks in moist coniferous forests, often next to Willows or the shaded lower edges of wet meadows. It grows in the north coastal range from Humboldt and Trinity counties in California; north to Alaska; from Tulare County northwards in the Sierra Nevada; up the Cascades; and from central Oregon northwards in all the ranges. It grows across and down into the Rocky Mountains, and is common in higher elevations of Arizona and New Mexico as well. Further, it is found at high elevations in eastern and western Nevada, and in the central ranges from the Toiyabes to the Ruby Mountains.

CONSTITUENTS Aconitine, aconine, iso-, pseudo-, benzoylaconitine, and a bunch of lesser and variable aconite-type steroidal alkaloids, including aconitic, succinic, malonic acids, and so forth. Nearly all of the activity derives from the first two alkaloids, although chemists have gleefully isolated dozens and dozens of minor variations on a theme (aconitine) produced by the many variations in the Aconites.

COLLECTING Let's face it: Aconite is a poisonous plant. The aboveground plant is weaker, and the roots are *really* nasty; so in my low-tech, submedical plant usage I only employ the fresh herb in flower, or the carefully dried flowering tops, leaves and all. If you are using the dry herb, Method A, process into coarse sections and store in a tight jar, protected from light.

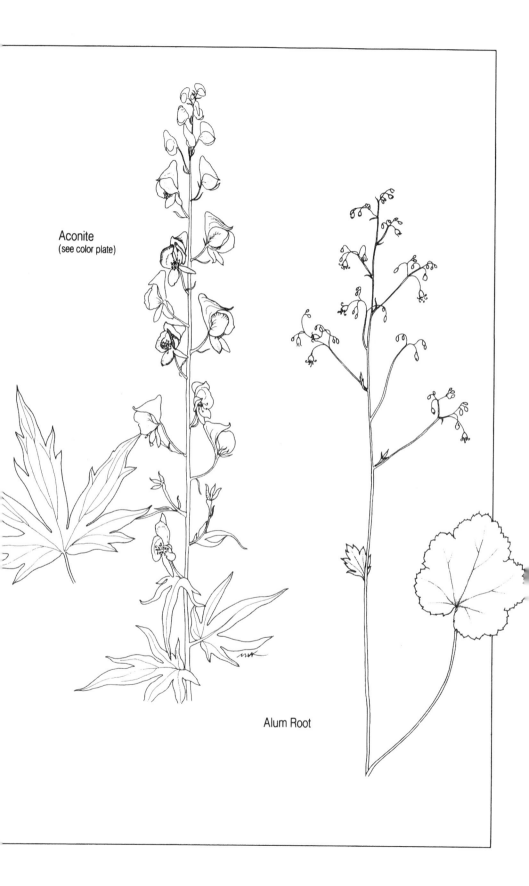

Aconite
(see color plate)

Alum Root

STABILITY The various tinctures and liniments, three or four years, the dried plant only about a year.

PREPARATION Fresh Herb Tincture, 1:5 (grain alcohol or 90% isopropyl alcohol); Dry Herb Tincture, 1:10, 70% alcohol. Aconite Liniment is prepared by percolating or macerating the dried herb, at a ratio of 1:2, in 90% isopropyl alcohol, and dissolving 5% camphor crystals, weight to volume. If you make 10 ounces of the 1:2 tincture, dissolve ½ ounce of camphor in it.

MEDICINAL USES The safest and most practical use of Aconite is for *pain.* Topically, the various forms may be applied to any surface where the skin is unbroken, as with Arnica usage. For nerve-derived pain with some local or nerve inflammation and a sense of heat, as in the case of neuralgia, sciatica, and bruises, Aconite liniment or tinctures may be applied with a cloth moistened by it and held against the part for a few minutes. Herpes zoster pain (shingles) responds well to Aconite topically, even when there is a moderate amount of vesicular eruption. Apply the tincture, let it dry, and then cover the area of inflammation with a mild salve or dusting powder. The pain is further decreased with some Motherwort (*Leonurus cardiaca*) tea or tincture.

The fresh herb tincture can be used internally, but be careful not to take excessive quantities: take only 3 to 6 drops at a time! It should be used by the strong and vigorous with acute inflammation, not by the tired, depressed, or those with chronic disease. The small doses help to modify fever that includes pain, irritation, and inflamed mucosa and eyes, and is accompanied by a rapid, wiry pulse. The few drops may be repeated every three hours as long as you feel hot and excited; when you feel better, stop its use. I have taken 10 to 12 drops when needed without ill effect; but I am here, and weigh 250 pounds, and you are there— so *please* act with caution. The first symptom of taking a little too much is a sense of slight tingling in the mouth and fingers. Older docs and pharmacists who remember Aconite as a medication may cringe at any recommendation for internal use. My defense is that this is the *herb,* not the far stronger *root,* and the amount recommended is easily a tenth of the dosage formerly used as a cardiac sedative. This follows the low doses of the Eclectics and approaches Homeopathy.

CONTRAINDICATIONS Aconite is not recommended externally or internally during pregnancy, and don't use it internally if you are tired, rundown, or cold. Also, as always in treating fevers yourself, once the fever passes, be sure of what made you sick. If the fever continues or keeps returning in the evening, see the doc of your choice. Aconite helps to moderate the excessive *symptoms* that some strong folks get, not the actual *cause* of the fever. The cause may need medical attention.

Alum Root

Heuchera glabra, H. micrantha, etc. (Saxifragaceae)

OTHER NAMES Mountain Saxifrage

APPEARANCE The various species of Alum Root are all similar in appearance and in use; the two species above are the most common in the Pacific Coast area. The leaves are all basal, palmately cleft, look like a garden or wild Geranium leaf, and emerge from the end of long petioles. They form little bunches before and after blooming, the leaves arching over, with older ones becoming discolored towards red or purple. The roots are long and fibrous-tuberous, with dark, chaffy bark and flesh that is pinkish. The flowers are borne on long and slender extended stems, a few along the upper edges in some conditions, branching off into smaller side panicles in other conditions. They are small, puffy cups, with five petals and stamens, usually light pink. Since you want to gather the roots in late summer and fall, the most you will see of the flowers is an occasional tan stem hanging down from the basal leaves. Mountain Saxifrage is a lovely plant for any rock garden, if you want to transplant some roots in fall.

HABITAT *Heuchera micrantha* grows on coastal hillsides and rocky cliffs from north of Santa Barbara in California to Oregon; and then, along with other species, up to nearly timberline from the Sierra Nevada northwards to British Columbia; and east to the west side of the Lochsa-Selway drainage in Idaho. *Heuchera parvifolia* is found in the mountains from Idaho, Alberta, and Utah, east and south into the Rockies. *Heuchera glabra* is a plant of moist stream banks and moist mountainsides, from the Mount Hood area of the Oregon Cascades, northwards through the coastal and central mountains of Washington, north through British Columbia to the whole Alaska coastal area and the Aleutians. If you find Valerian growing on moist rocky hillsides, you will find Alum Root. Look for rock slides and glacial deposits.

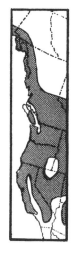

CONSTITUENTS Tannin, phlebotannins, and other polyhydric phenols, with galloyl glucosides.

COLLECTING Gather the leaves and roots in August and September, the roots as late as November. Scrape off the dark chaff on the roots, and after they have partially wilted, slice the roots into thin cross-sections and finish drying, Method B. Bundle the leaves to dry, Method A.

STABILITY The dried leaves are good for at least a year. The dried root, either sliced or powdered, lasts at least two years or more.

PREPARATION Fresh Root Tincture, 1:2; add 5% glycerin to the finished tincture. Dry Root Tincture, 1:5, 50% alcohol, 40% water, 10% glycerin;

use 30 to 60 drops up to four times a day, internally; otherwise use the tinctures externally at full strength or dilute with equal parts of water. The Cold Infusion, 1 to 2 fluid ounces up to four times a day, internally; for a douche or enema, 4 fluid ounces, with a cup of warm water. For a first aid tincture, add an equal part of a strong antimicrobial plant tincture that is not alkaloidal, such as Lomatium, Usnea, Yerba Mansa, White Sage, or California Snakeroot. The high levels of astringent phenols in Alum Root will bind and precipitate out alkaloids in such plants as Oregon Grape root. The powdered root can similarly be mixed in equal parts with an antimicrobial herb that is stable as a powder, such as Oregon Grape root, Yerba Mansa, or Lomatium.

MEDICINAL USES Alum Root is a good, solid astringent. It contains a variety of tannin complexes and maintains a widely dispersed effect that makes it more usable than nearly all of our astringents. Internally, the tincture, tea, or compounded tincture is an excellent mouthwash for sore gums and sore throat, and the tea or tincture is very good for stomachache or ulcer pain. It is a very useful astringent for diarrhea, especially when combined with an antispasmodic like Silk Tassel, Peony root, or Angelica, and an intestinal antimicrobial like Usnea, Oregon Grape root, or Balsam Root. The weak tea is an excellent douche or enema for short-term mucus membrane inflammation, such as candidiasis or bacterial vaginosis.

The powdered plant is a very soothing dust for chafing and blistering, and, along with Bistort Root, is our best hemostatic, stopping bleeding quickly and helping to prevent infection. I like it best when combined with an antimicrobial herb, but even by itself it is disinfecting. The powder is a good way to stop shaving nicks, particularly if you use only the root; the powdered leaf works fine, but will look weird stuck to your chin, whereas the light tan root doesn't show much.

OTHER USES The dried leaf or root slices can be added to pickled fruits and vegetables to keep them crisp and colorful.

Amole Lily

Chlorogalum pomeridianum, etc.   (Liliaceae)
OTHER NAMES Soap Plant, California Soap Plant; *Amole*

APPEARANCE From spring to late fall, Amole Lily wears a wreath of 1- and 2-foot-long basal leaves that are grasslike, wavy-margined, and have a ridged central vein. In spring the plant puts up a tall, leafless flower stalk, tough and distinctly more robust than the leaves. The plant bears

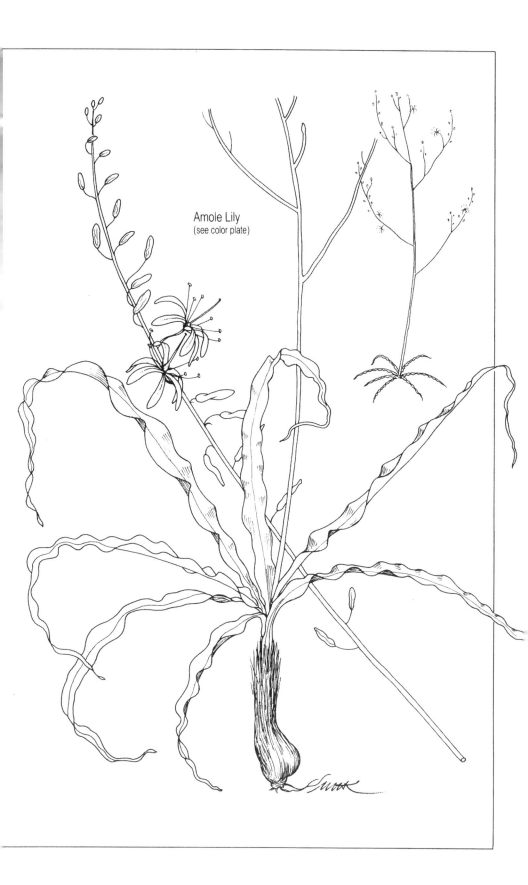

Amole Lily
(see color plate)

an open panicle of a few (or in moist years, many) small, white, six-petaled lily flowers, slightly fragrant, which open in the evenings. The bulb is shaped like a long onion and is covered densely with a thick coat of protective brown fibers, the surviving strings from previous years' bulb layers. By summer or fall these fibers may be visible, poking out of the ground below the basal leaves, especially the down-slope edges in the common hillside habitats.

These lilies are usually found in colonies. The leaves are easily overlooked in the spring, since they are often covered with the typical hillside grasses of southern California. By summer, however, the grasses are brown, and the green leaves and desiccated flower stalks are more clearly visible. The moist centers of the bulbs have a slightly onionlike smell. There are several other species of *Chlorogalum*, but *pomeridianum* is by far the most common, representing the vast majority of biomass of the seven species of the genus. It is also the soapiest.

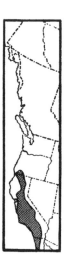

HABITAT Amole Lily is found on dry open hills and in foothills and nearby flatlands, usually in the same general localities as Buckwheat Bush, Manzanita, and the several wild Sages of California. If you find a few plants down in the valley, walk up the foothills to find the main stand; if you find some on a ridge, follow the hill down to the main colony. Amole Lily grows up and down the western edge of the Sierra Nevada, along the coastal ranges from Sonoma County south to Baja California; inland to the western edge of the Imperial Valley, as far east as Tehachapi Pass; and in the hilly country between the central valleys and the coast. It is found sporadically in Oregon as far north as Coos County along the drier hillsides slightly in from the coast.

CONSTITUENTS Saponins, principally chlorogenin and amolonin.

COLLECTING Gather the bulbs from late summer to fall. Except in the driest years (when you shouldn't be gathering anyway because the plants are having a hard enough time trying to survive without water, and don't need more trouble from uncompassionate harvesters), look for the largest plants, and just dig those, leaving all the younger ones to carry on. The larger bulbs produce taller and thicker stalks, which may still be standing. Otherwise, the bigger, older plants have longer, more numerous basal leaves, and start to turn yellow-beige, while the younger plants are still somewhat green. I have harvested stands in the Santa Monica Mountains for years in this fashion, without depleting the colony.

The fall bulbs transplant easily into your garden. If you dig up some little bitty bulbs by accident, don't feel guilty; just transplant them. The fresh bulbs are far better than those you have dried and can be stored for months in a refrigerator. You can store them even longer if you layer them sideways, pack them with slightly moist sand or inert mulch, and then cover and put them in a dark place.

STABILITY Two months in a refrigerator, six months or more when packed. Once you have stripped and sliced a bulb, and stored the remainder in the refrigerator, it will not last more than a week. If you go away and forget about it, it will eventually rot and produce an amazingly foul smell. This is not good, believe me.

PREPARATION Strip the bulb of hair, grate or slice thinly several table-spoons of the inner bulb into a piece of cheesecloth, fold it over, and rub it in a cup of warm water until it foams well. The herb in the cloth can be rubbed directly into the hair, the soapy water added gradually. Let the soap stay in the hair for five or ten minutes and rinse.

MEDICINAL USES In addition to being an excellent hair treatment in its own right, the regular use of the Amole Lily shampoo is as an effective treatment for seborrhea, dandruff, and scalp tineas such as cradle crap and barber's itch. For added antifungal effects, add a tablespoon of the fresh leaf tincture of Thuja or Cypress to the water, or use a cup of strong tea of Oregon Grape root or leaf to help make the soap. Always make a fresh batch of Amole Lily shampoo each time, as it wears out. The treatment is also fairly effective for mange and other skin infections of dogs and cats, although many cats find the scent objectionable.

OTHER USES The outside hairs of the bulbs are durable but soft, and, if lightly oiled, can be made into excellent brushes and small brooms.

Angelica

Angelica arguta, A. pinnata, etc.   (Umbelliferae)
OTHER NAMES   Lyall's Angelica, Kneeling Angelica, Small-Leaf Angelica; *Osha del Campo*

APPEARANCE There are literally dozens of different Angelica species in the Pacific West, but most are difficult to find or identify and are not all that common outside of widely dispersed stands in obscure or threatened localities. Of the typical medicinal Angelicas, these two species are the most common, widespread, and predictable. *Angelica hendersonii,* a rough and chunky little member that grows along coastal bluffs from Monterey, California, to southern Washington, is also common, but peculiar and atypical in its constituents and less reliable than the other two. *Angelica arguta* is a large plant, with bipinnate or tripinnate aromatic leaves that have a blue-green or grey-green color and a slightly rough texture. The flowers are usually white, but I have seen them with a rose tinge; the seeds are round and winged with the common three ridges on the lateral surfaces. The seeds taste a little like celery and a little like cardamom. The root is large, often divided into big branches, light grey-brown skinned, and cream-colored soapy-aromatic inside. Under most circumstances, the larger plants grow out in raggedy mats (especially in the open), with tall but languid flowering stalks, sometimes 6 to 7 feet tall, but usually 3 or 4 feet in height, and not too much taller than the foliage, except in younger plants.

Angelica pinnata is a smaller plant that spreads less than *A. arguta*. It is more likely to be a 3-foot flowering stem with several basal leaves, less likely to spread out from the root to form a cluster of basal leaves and several flowering stems. The leaves are mostly pinnate, with only the lowest leaflets likely to divide again. The flowers are white to light pink and form nearly round, flattened seeds, also with the three little lateral groves, and with a leaf, seed, and root scent similar to the previous species. The roots tend to be smaller and more carrotlike, and are less likely to form root masses; but they are just as strong a medicine.

Another species, *Angelica genuflexa*, forms large mats, with odd dull green leaves that arch back from the lowest pair of leaflets to the tip; hence the common name Kneeling Angelica. The roots are very strong, but the seeds tend to be rather bitter.

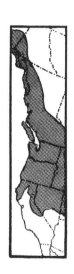

HABITAT *Angelica arguta* grows on slopes, in foothills, in well-drained meadows, and along rocky river and stream banks, usually in dispersed stands. It can be found in the north coastal range and Klamath Mountains of California (unpredictable); southwest and central Oregon (common); east of the Cascades from Washington through eastern Oregon, northern Nevada, Idaho, and western Montana; down into Utah and western Wyoming; and north into southeastern British Columbia and southwest Alberta.

Angelica pinnata grows in moist, shady, and biodiverse places, from Idaho and western Montana down into northern Nevada and Utah, as well as all along the moist edges of the Great Basin.

Angelica genuflexa is rare in northwest California; occasional in the coastal ranges of Oregon and Washington; found more abundantly in northern Washington, British Columbia east to the Selkirks and into Alberta; and north through the Panhandle, across Alaska, and into Siberia, where it interbreeds with (or becomes) *Angelica polymorpha*, the main Angelica that is cured into Dong Quai, a very important Chinese herbal medicine.

I used to pick *Angelica tomentosa* and *Angelica lineariloba* in the southern Sierra Nevada, and the first one in the coastal range from Santa Barbara northwards. In the last fifteen years there seem to be fewer and fewer clean localities for them, and the drought of the last half of the 1980s seems to have cut them back extensively; so I have stopped picking them completely, and would discourage any of you from the same.

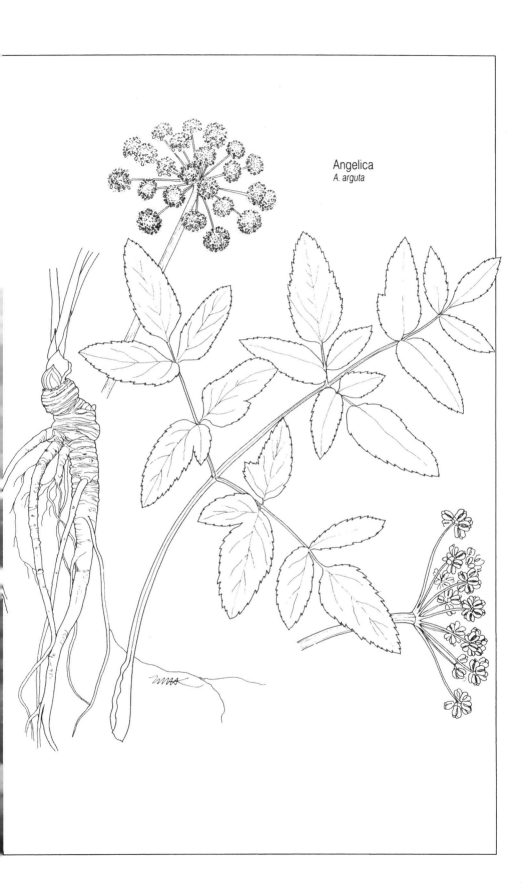

Angelica
A. arguta

CONSTITUENTS Although not directly extracted from these three plants, expect about 1% volatile oil with phellandrene, pinene, linalool and borneol (with variants), angelic acid, angelicol, ancelicin, osthol, osthenol, umbelliferone, and a flavone, archangelenone. Other constituents will vary, but these are the primary ones, nearly universal in the temperate Angelicas.

COLLECTING Collect the seeds before they fall and preferably when a little green; dry Method B. The roots are best from the time that the seeds are nearly mature to the time that the leaves still retain some green but are nearly dead (usually October). If you are drying the root, slice it lengthwise like you would to make carrot sticks, chopping them up for tea only when you are going to *make* the tea. In my experience, chopping up the root into pieces results in rapid deterioration of the volatile constituents. Dry Method B.

STABILITY Seeds, to eighteen months, lengthwise root slices to two years.

PREPARATION *Seeds:* Dry Tincture, 1:5, 65% alcohol; for tea, a scant teaspoon steeped until warm, or a few added to other teas, such as Peppermint or Catnip, as a stomach antispasmodic. *Root:* Fresh Tincture, 1:2, 15 to 30 drops; Dry Tincture, 1:5, 65% alcohol, 30 to 60 drops (ad lib). The Tea: a rounded teaspoon, as an infusion, steeped until lukewarm.

MEDICINAL USES The seeds, in any form, are primarily useful for acid indigestion with stomach pain or for the sensation of a full, uncomfortable belly. The seeds are also exceptionally effective for nausea and vomiting, not so much to suppress necessary nausea, as from bad food, but to stop the dry heaves or extended nausea that can continue long after there is any food to eject. If a fever accompanies the nausea, the seeds can also be used to stimulate sweating. The root can be used similarly, although the seeds are distinctly more superficial in their constituents and have a stronger effect on the stomach and esophagus. The root's main value is its strong, but not depressive, antispasmodic effects. I have seen it help asthma that is dry, spastic, and instigated by anger, fear, and frustration. It isn't strong, so you need to take a number of doses over several hours, but it has the advantage of producing no sedation or (as in inhalers) no stimulation. A good Lobelia tincture should be tried first, but if it doesn't help within one or two minutes, go to the Angelica.

For intestinal cramps, with gas and gurgly borborygmus (the sensation of gerbils in wet suits surfing goofy-foot down your transverse colon), for menstrual cramps that seem partially intestinal, and for the two-day killer flatus you get from eating undercooked lentil loaf at the yoga conference, use Angelica root. Try it for PMS that has a predominantly colon effect, with constipation, poor fat digestion, hemorrhoids, and abdominal bloat. Although not particularly a stimulant to the uterus, avoid fresh root tincture and seeds during pregnancy.

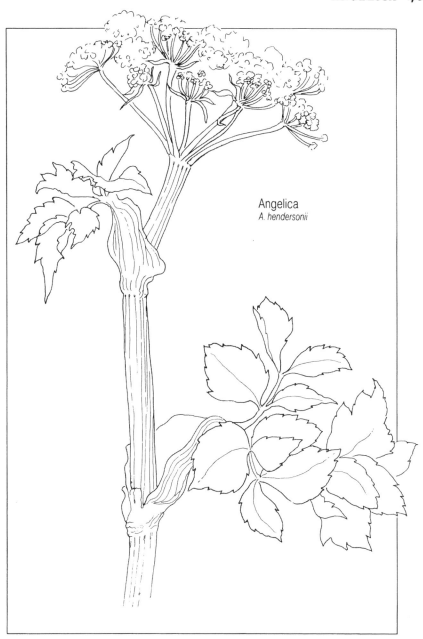

Angelica
A. hendersonii

OTHER USES Candied Angelica root, made from genteel garden Angelica grown in England or Connecticut is a tasty perversity. Trying to make candied roots from our tough and grim wild Angelicas is . . . terrible. The dried leaves can be a nice addition to rice and barley soups.

Arnica

Arnica cordifolia, A. latifolia, etc.   (Compositae)
OTHER NAMES   Heartleaf Arnica, Broadleaf Arnica, Mountain Arnica, Leopard's Bane

APPEARANCE Our various Arnicas are many and confusing. Some may be hybrids; some are found in small stands here and there over six states and others just reach into our area from the northeastern part of the continent. The flowers of some are supposed to nod but don't always, or have rayless flowers mixed with rayed ones on the same plant. The two species listed above probably make up two-thirds of the total biomass of the Pacific Arnicas and are the ones I always go looking for. *Arnica cordifolia* (Heartleaf Arnica) is a plant of predominantly basal-leaf growth. The heart-shaped leaves form large patches in shady locations, expanding by lateral root growth. Colonies send up a few flowering stems along sunny edges of the colony and bloom in golden abundance in moist, warm years. As with most Arnicas, the stem leaves are narrower than the basal leaves, and they are opposite. The flowers are bright, buttery yellow. The ray flowers number up to a dozen and have an extended, pointy flair that makes them readily identifiable. The basal and stem leaves are light, downy green, undulating, and have small serrations along the margins that may not be obvious until you flatten a leaf out to examine it. By midsummer some of the basal leaves start to turn yellow and light brown, making identification especially easy from a distance. Most of the Heartleaf Arnica blooms between late June and mid-July, with the neat yellow blooms turning into fluffy flyaway flowers (say that three times quickly, if you can). Broadleaf Arnica (*Arnica latifolia*) resembles *Arnica cordifolia* in most respects, but the foliage is less downy, the leaf serrations are more distinct, and instead of a round, undulating panache, the shapes are more pointed, the veins more pronounced, and the opposite stem leaves nearly as large as the basal leaves. Broadleaf Arnica is also less likely to form extensive lateral basal-growth. *Arnica latifolia* is likely to have one or more sets of paired flowers branching from the upper leaf axils, particularly towards late summer. *Arnica cordifolia* rarely has more than the single terminal flower.

Many other Arnicas occur; some forms, such as *A. mollis, A. longifolia*, and *A. diversifolia*, are taller (up to 2 feet in height, twice as tall as the first two species), with many pairs of pointed leaves along the flowering stem, and form dense stands of crowded plants. *Arnica parryi* is a spare, delicate plant with large triangular basal leaves; thin, lanceolate opposite stem leaves; and small, oval, yellow flowers that lack ray petals, and which usually nod downwards from long, paired petioles. Still, the first

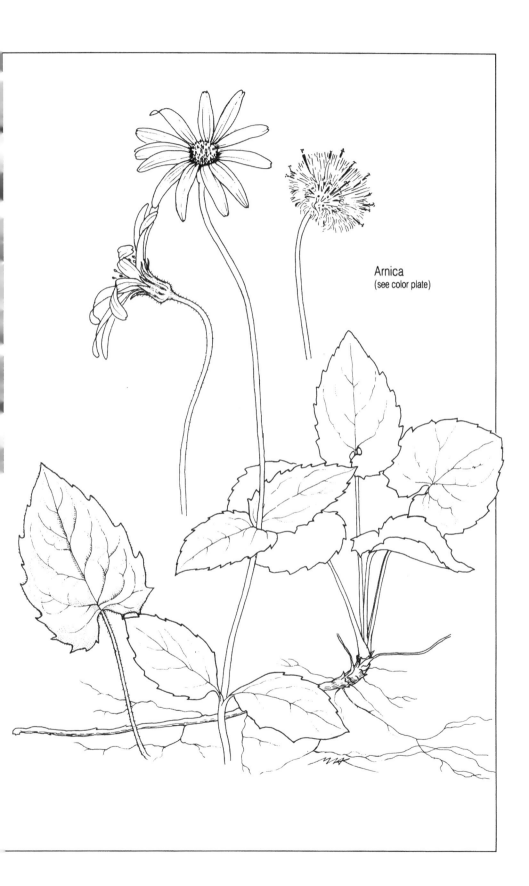

Arnica
(see color plate)

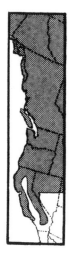

two species are far the most common. Remember: Arnicas grow in the mountains, usually have large basal leaves, stem leaves that are always paired, and have bright, gold-yellow sunflowers (except for *A. parryi*).

HABITAT Heartleaf Arnica grows in the high mountains of southern California and is joined by Broadleaf Arnica in the north coast range and the northern stretch of the Sierra Nevada. In California the Arnicas are found above 5,000 feet in moist, old-growth forest, and at 9,000 feet, a whole gaggle of other Arnicas appear. In Oregon, Washington, British Columbia, Alaska, Nevada, Idaho, and Montana, the two main species are abundant, especially in higher main forests and subalpine forests, whatever the altitude. The other main DYC (damn yellow composite) in the same localities are the related Senecios, which have alternate leaves and, frequently, scalloped margins on the lower or basal leaves. If you get up in the high mountains in early or midsummer, find small yellow sunflowers with opposite leaves, growing in colonies, that are downy, sticky, or somewhat aromatic when crushed, you got yourself some Arnica.

CONSTITUENTS Volatile oils (aerial parts) and resins (root) containing fatty acids and aromatics, including thymol, thymohydroquinone, arnicin, arnidendiol, arnidiol, arnisterin, and a whole bunch of carotenoids and flavonoids. Traces of a couple of alkaloids have been found in the genus, but the Arnicas are fortunately lacking the toxic alkaloids found in their close cousins the Senecios.

COLLECTING The flowers, the part traditionally used for medicine, should be gathered in early bloom, usually from mid-June to early July. They fluff up when dry, producing nose-irritating fiber. I find it easiest to collect the whole flowering stems, lay them loosely in paper bags, flowers first, and leave them there until they are dry. All parts of the plant are active. Both the flowers and the root are official drug plants in British pharmacy. After late July (or even late August in the highest altitudes), when the flowers have bloomed, seeded, and fluttered away, gather the still green basal leaves and the lateral rhizome/roots. The fresh preparations can be made from either the flowers, the flowering stalks, or a leaf-root combination. Commercial Arnica consists of the dried flowers of (usually) *Arnica montana,* the European species. The bright yellow flowers manage to reach us looking like fluffy brown stuffing removed from an ancient sofa left in the backyard for twelve years. I have no idea how such a lovely plant obtains such a state. I have been unable, in two decades, to reduce the Arnica I have gathered to the morbid lifelessness of the Arnica I have purchased in normal commerce. I have a friend in Montana who has cultivated the European species and dries the flower in the usual fashion, producing fluffy, yellow-white medicine just like our native stuff. Maybe they use special life-sucking machines especially developed for the herb trade and politicians. Unlike the latter, I am sure the international herb trade means well.

STABILITY The dried flowers are good for two years if stored in a cool, dry place totally out of the light. The dried whole plant and root may stay potent even longer: if kept intact until use, a large amount of Arnica gathered in a banner year could be dried and kept stable for years if sealed in an airtight container and stored in a freezer, although it is such a useful plant you will probably use it before that.

PREPARATION Whole fresh plant, fresh flowers, or fresh root are all made as Fresh Tincture, 1:2; Dry Herb Tincture, 1:5, 50% alcohol; or Dry Root Tincture, 1:5, 60% alcohol. If you have a few root segments along with the whole dried plant, 50% alcohol is quite adequate. If the tincture is made predominately from the more resinous root, use the higher alcohol percentage mentioned. The Oil or Salve is made Method A, using only the aerial parts and/or flowers. Oil extraction of Arnica presents the same problem as with many other plants. Even with the use of a small amount of alcohol as an intermediate solvent, root constituents are made up of such complex storage compounds that they are not very soluble; the foliage and floral constituents are simpler and more soluble. This dichotomy exists with other herbs, such as Echinacea, Goldenseal, Oregon Grape, and Yerba Mansa; all make a really spiffy oil and salve when you use the herb, but their roots are virtually insoluble.

MEDICINAL USES The primary uses for Arnica have remained unchanged for centuries. The tincture, oil, salve, tea, or bruised fresh plant is used externally for bruises, hyperextensions, arthritis, bursitis, and myalgia. Arnica works by stimulating and dilating blood vessels, particularly the specialized capillaries that control whether blood is piped into the small peripheral capillary beds or is shunted over to small veins, bypassing more widespread blood dispersal. Good, diffused blood transport and circulation into injured, bruised, or inflamed tissues helps speed up resolution and removal of waste products. Arnica does not have the anesthesia of menthol or Wintergreen or the counterirritation property of other aromatic balms, and should not be expected to have their immediate effects. Instead, in a few hours or overnight, it aids in removing the congestion that results from a bruise, sprain, or hyperextension. In osteoarthritis, the stimulation supplied by Arnica is a small but significant aid in increasing the absorption and drainage of the hyaline cartilage, lessening some of the early and chronic congestion of the joints that leads, gradually, to the overgrowth of bony cartilage characteristic of osteoarthritis. In rheumatoid arthritis, a highly variable condition with many elements of immunologic disfunction, including overt autoimmunity, it is wise to try using Arnica on the swollen joints for two or three days. If it helps the inflammation and shortens the length of morning stiffness in the primary joint, you will usually find that it can be used regularly without any problem. If it starts to overheat the joint or redden the skin below the surface, *stop*.

Arnica stimulates activity of macrophages, the big white blood cells that perform much of the cleaning and digestion in injured tissues. Macrophages act as bridges between the blind, instinctive, seek-and-destroy resistance of the innate immunity and the antibody, learned-and-remembered, defenses of the acquired immunities. With most rheumatoid arthritis, it helps to increase scavenging and cleansing of the enlarged joint with Arnica, but sometimes the macrophage stimulation can distinctly aggravate the local inflammation and dilation of blood vessels.

Arnica has always had a reputation for being "scary," since every once in a while it induces a strong adverse skin reaction, with subcutaneous inflammation and pain. In reality, this is almost always when it is used for a person with rheumatoid arthritis who already has exaggerated macrophage activity. How do you know? Trial and error. If you have RA, you may wish to try Arnica even if you risk a strong, but usually short-term, skin reaction. To lessen the potential, mix 1 part of the tincture with 2 parts of commercial Witch Hazel extract. For the rest of its external uses, Arnica is nearly always safe and devoid of skin reactions, although it should be avoided when the skin is scratched, abraded, or broken; broken skin can increase the likelihood of Arnica-induced inflammation. Although other herbalists (past and present) have recounted problems, the *only* instance where I saw Arnica cause a skin reaction was on a man with rheumatoid arthritis that was very reactive to his consumption of tomatoes, potatoes, and chiles—members of the Nightshade family. All in all, the classic use of Arnica is for joint, muscle, and cartilage pain that is aggravated by movement and helped by rest. Usually when something just sits there and throbs, you need to apply cold to the area, or an aromatic balm—or take an aspirin. After a day or two, however, it may stop throbbing and only hurt when you use it. That is an Arnica moment.

Arnica, with or without some Witch Hazel, is an invaluable aid for chronic, obstinate sore throat, especially the kind that lingers as a raspy-gurgly half-cough like an old hair ball after you got over the chest cold and went back to work. Put 1 teaspoon of the tincture and ½ teaspoon of salt in 8 ounces of water, gargle a small amount, swish it around, and spit it out. Do this every hour for the rest of the day. With the antimicrobial effects, macrophage stimulation, and vascular stimulation, Arnica should clear up those boggy throat membranes in no time at all. For chronic tonsilitis, add 2 teaspoons of Red Root tincture to the Arnica, salt, and water.

Arnica can be used internally with great benefit, as long as you are physically strong, have no blood vessel, liver, or kidney disease, and you use it sparingly. If you dumped your mountain bike backwards down a slope and didn't hurt anything too much (except your ego), but you are sore all over and you know that tomorrow you will wish you were dead, take 10 or 15 drops of Arnica tincture in a little water. Repeat it again in the evening, and the day-after-you-dump aches and pains will be markedly less. Charlie Jordan, the well-known New Mexican herbalist, started using the tincture in this manner with his rugby team. He would pull apart the scrum, find some teammate twisted up into a Beetle Bailey pretzel (complete with cartoon birdies tweeting overhead), give him a squirt of Arnica, and watch him snap back into a physically alert state. Using a little Arnica internally after you have been thrashed, bumped, or banged up will aid in dispersing the disorganized fluids out of the injured muscle or joint and lessen the volume of trapped and eventually congested blood and fluids that will stare back at you in the mirror the next day. I am not talking about broken bones or bubbling chest wounds, but rather the type of injury that results when the shelf falls on you as you are moving or the baseball bat hits you in the knee at a softball game.

CONTRAINDICATIONS Do not continue topical use if the preparation causes a rash. Do not use topically at the same time you are using aromatic balms or DMSO, or if the skin is seriously abraded. Do not use internally if you are pregnant, have chronic intestinal inflammation, or have any overt disease involving blood vessels, blood clotting, heart function, the liver, or the kidneys. If the problem is of the kind that Arnica is helpful for, but you have these conditions, try using homeopathic Arnica preparations. Although homeopathy is usually thought of as being used for conditions that can be mimicked by large amounts of the same substance that is attenuated for the remedy, some herbs act the same above as below. Hypericum (St. John's Wort), Arnica, and some Anemones can be used in small tincture doses for the same symptoms they are used for in homeopathy. This may not seem an important observation to you, but take my word for it: it will get the fur flying in debates between herbalists and homeopaths. This is my book, you own it, and I can say what I want to. The author's tyranny will deny equal time to homeopathy.

OTHER USES In Janice Schofield's delightful book *Discovering Wild Plants*, she has a recipe for a very effective foot powder that uses Arnica:

> *1 cup white or blue clay*
>
> *½ cup dried whole Arnica*
>
> *½ cup dry Devil's Club root bark*
>
> *½ cup dry Plantain herb*

Grind the herbs into a fine powder and mix thoroughly with the clay.

Balsam Poplar

Populus balsamifera, P. trichocarpa (Salicaceae)

OTHER NAMES Black Cottonwood, Balm of Gilead, Western Balsam Poplar; *Tacamahac; Populus balsamifera,* var. *balsamifera, Populus balsamifera,* var. *trichocarpa*

APPEARANCE Practically speaking, these two Poplars/Cottonwoods are varieties of the same species. They interbreed extensively, basically forming a single amorphous species, with the northern stands having a smaller, squatter shape and two-part capsules, the southern stands having a taller, slimmer appearance, with fuzzy, three-part capsules, and the trees in British Columbia, Washington, and Alberta being genetic shake-and-bake, with fuzzy two-part capsules and various admixtures thereof. Full-grown trees are from 30 to 100 feet in height, deciduous, with deep grey and yellow-grey, furrowed bark, and with broad, open-crowned foliage. It is the largest broad-leafed tree in the Pacific West. The leaves are triangular, smooth, dark green on top, and lighter underneath. They are broad, but without the exaggerated heart-shape of Fremont Cottonwood's serrated leaves (southern California through New Mexico) or the fluttery, heart-shaped leaves and smooth, light bark of the high mountain Aspen. The fall leaves are darker, more golden green than Fremont Cottonwood (straw yellow) or Aspen (dazzling yellow). The winter/spring leaf buds are resinous, aromatic, and reddish brown wads of oily goo, and when dried have the unfortunate appearance of dead cockroaches, dipped in beeswax and lightly browned.

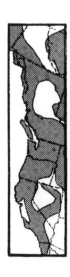

HABITAT The archetype *P. balsamifera* is found from virtually all of Alaska, south to central British Columbia, and all the way east to the Atlantic Coast of Canada, dipping south into the Great Lakes area and the Northeast U.S.; and down the Continental Divide as far as north-central Colorado. It is a tree of alluvial valleys, from nearly the coast to almost timberline. The other type, *P. trichocarpa,* grows from coastal southern Alaska to northern Baja California; east to southwestern Alberta and western Montana; over into Idaho, Utah, and Nevada; on both sides of the Cascades; south into all the major mountain ranges of northern California; and into the drainages of the higher ranges of southern California. Look for it by rivers, in moist valleys, at the edges of natural lakes, or in canyon bottoms; it is common and widespread throughout the wet areas of the Pacific West.

CONSTITUENTS A soft balsamic resin, a yellow volatile oil, principally humulene; gallic acid, malic acid, salicin, populin, mannitol, chrysin, fixed oil, tectochrysin, arachidonic acid, trichocarpin, and bisabolol.

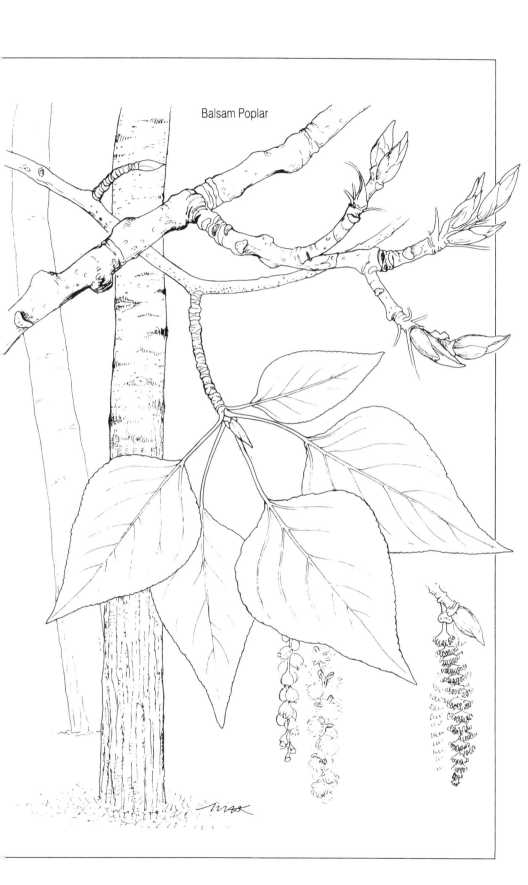

Balsam Poplar

COLLECTING Gather the leaf buds in winter or early spring, while they are still sealed and pointed. The whole budding twigs contain the resins, not just the buds; and if you are going to make the external preparations, gather the branch tips heavy with buds, and use all of it. For internal use and cough mixtures, the buds only are best. Schofield makes the sensible observation that gathering the buds at freezing temperatures keeps the resins hard and the buds easier to handle. If this isn't possible, take the gooey mass back home, freeze it, and separate the pieces while brittle for drying. For use in fresh plant preparations, process the buds and twigs within a couple of days. Otherwise, the buds need to be dried, since they will mold. Even with all their oleoresins, the buds still contain a fair amount of water, and, laying in flats, may take a week or two to completely dry and be ready to store.

STABILITY Properly dried buds will stay potent for at least a couple of years.

PREPARATION Fresh Plant Tincture, 1:2, 30 to 60 drops, Dry Plant Tincture, 1:5, 70% alcohol, 15 to 30 drops, both up to four times a day. The oil may be extracted in several ways. For fresh buds, slowly boil 1 part by weight of crushed plant in 4 parts by volume of water, simmering for about an hour. Add 1 part by volume of vegetable oil, let the mixture stand until cool, stirring several times, and decant off the oil from the water and exhausted buds. The vegetable and bud resin are lighter than the water, dissolve together, and float on top. Pure resin is too potent for topical use, and the steeped oil can be used as it is. The dry buds can be blended with 10 parts olive oil, poured into a jar for a couple of days, reblended, and strained. For burns, animal fat is preferable to vegetable oil, and you have a choice of lard or butter. If using butter, clarify it first by melting it and pouring the butterfat off the top; use unsalted, sweet butter, as salted butter is often partially rancid. Use 1 part by volume of crushed fresh or dry buds, and cook over a very low heat in 2 parts of lard or butterfat for at least three or four hours. I find it best to let the mixture harden overnight, reheat it the next day, and then pour the salve into jars, straining through a cloth draped over a sieve or colander. The buds themselves are antioxidant, so no Larrea, gum benzoin, or vitamin E oil is necessary, as the herb itself will prevent rancidity.

MEDICINAL USES The salicylates, relatives of aspirin found in Balsam Poplar, act topically as anti-inflammatory agents; and the aromatic resins act as vasodilators, antimicrobials, and stimulants to skin proliferation. This gives the oil or salve a huge range of uses. First, the oil, salve, or tincture can be applied to sprains, hyperextensions, and arthritic joints. It is helpful for pain from inflammation or congestion (hot or cold), and, although Arnica or Yerba del Lobo may be better for pain that occurs only on movement, Henbane may be more useful for dull, constant aching, and Hypericum may be better for neuralgia, Balsam Poplar is a simple, reliable, and predictable pain and swelling treatment if you don't feel in the mood for such fine points of specificity. Besides, it can be combined with any one of those herbs by using the steeped oil to make a second-step oil (or salve) using the alcohol-steep of Method A, with the other herb (or herbs) being dissolved in the Poplar bud oil. With Hypericum, make the combination of equal parts of the steeped oil of *both* plants.

This latter combination is an excellent hemorrhoid treatment, and the lard or butter salve can be used by itself as well. The salve has been used for burns by Native Americans and Europeans for millenia. It lessens pain, keeps the surface antiseptic, and also stimulates skin regeneration.

Finally, the tincture is a very effective therapy for chest colds, increasing protective mucus secretions in the beginning, when the tissues are hot, dry, and painful. Later, it increases the softening expectorant secretions when the mucus is hard and impacted on the bronchial walls, and coughing is painful. Further, the aromatics are secreted as volatile gases in expiration. This helps to inhibit microorganisms and lessen the likelihood of secondary, often more serious, infections.

Balsam Root

Balsamorhiza sagittata   (Compositae)
OTHER NAMES   Arrowleafed Balsam Root

APPEARANCE This is a handsome plant, usually growing in stands, with long-petioled basal leaves shaped like arrowheads and silvery green in color. The flowers are yellow sunflowers, usually extending past the leaves on long basal stems. Larger plants may have dozens of bright yellow flowers in the spring, and meadows and hillsides with Balsam Root in bloom are astonishingly lovely. In summer and fall the large, silvery green leaves are the identifying mark. This plant resembles, and may grow with, Mules-Ears (*Wyethia* species), but the latter is lance-shaped and smooth-leaved, with some species having stems bearing leaves, others having foliage with a yellow tinge; none has the large, deep, grey-yellow resinous roots of the Balsam Root. There are several other species of *Balsamorhiza* in the Pacific West, but *B. sagittata* is by far the most common, widespread, and useful.

HABITAT This plant grows in the mountains and foothills around the Great Basin; on both sides of the Sierra Nevada, Panamints, and Nevada

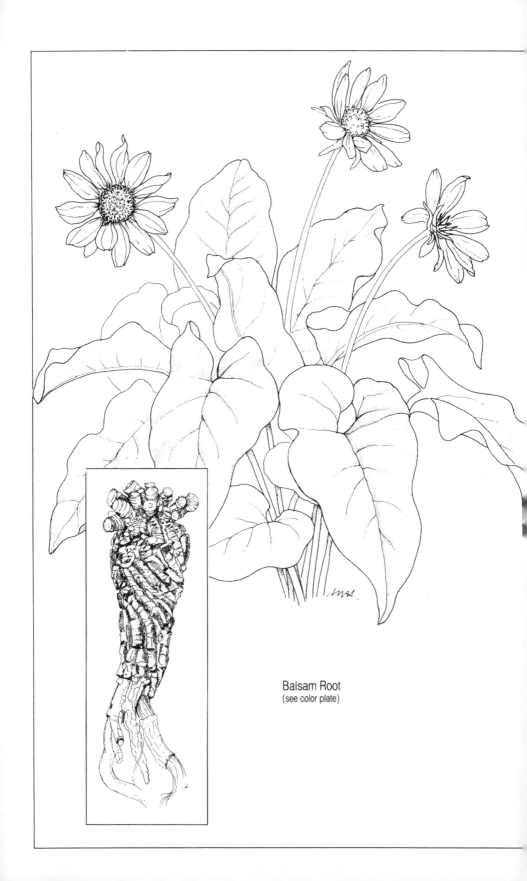

Balsam Root
(see color plate)

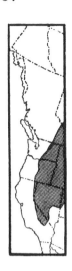

ranges; northwards in Oregon and Washington; east of the Cascades, into eastern British Columbia, Idaho, and Utah; and down the Rockies from Alberta south. It grows in open clearings, on dry hillsides, in dry meadows and passes, sometimes in partial shade, often in the open. It is frequently found on open hillsides above creeks; if so, it is an easily seen indicator plant when you are looking for *Lomatium dissectum* as well; they are complementary plants in their respiratory and anti-infective uses, so it can be very convenient when you find them growing together.

CONSTITUENTS Although not much studied, the leaf stem and root sap contain flavonoids, including 6-hydroxy-kaempferol, 7-methyl-ether, terebinthine principles in the root, resins, inulin, heterotetraglycans, and conjugated caffeic acids similar to the Echinacea group.

COLLECTING Gather the leaves in late spring to midsummer, bundle by the long petioles, and dry Method A. The roots can be gathered anytime, but spring roots are juicier, oilier, and better for use as an expectorant; late summer and fall roots are better for use as an antimicrobial and immunostimulant. If you plan to use the fall roots for a fresh root tincture, clean them of chuff, brush the dirt off with a wire brush, chip off the dark brown, corky bark, soak the whole roots in water for three or four hours, drain, and *then* slice them up for the tincture.

STABILITY The powdered leaves are good for at least a year, the dried root for at least two years, fall roots for longer.

PREPARATION The powdered leaves as a poultice, with hot water and hot towels on top, the powdered leaves as a salve, Method A. Fresh Root Tincture, 1:2, Dry Root Tincture, 1:5, 65% alcohol, 20 to 50 drops in hot water, both up to four times a day. Although not as efficient, a Standard Decoction, 2 to 3 ounces several times a day, can be used. A very good cough syrup can be made with the fresh roots, especially when dug in the spring. Add 1 part of the finely chopped fresh root by volume to 4 parts by volume of honey. Heat to a slight boil, maintaining the low heat for an hour or two. Allow to cool overnight, warm over some heat until liquified the next morning, and pour through a strainer. You can vary the cough syrup by replacing part of the Balsam Root with some fresh Lomatium, Angelica, or Osha, as long as the volume ratio is 1:4. Pour the warm syrup into a jar and store at room temperature. Take a teaspoon as needed.

MEDICINAL USES Balsam Root is a simple disinfectant-expectorant, and can be used both at the beginning of a sore throat and to stimulate the loosening of mucus when getting over bronchitis or any pulmonary disorder.

The powdered leaf, as a poultice or salve, will stimulate healing and regranulation of mild burns and chronic skin sores and ulcerations. The whole plant is an effective first aid for skin infections, and the root is a practical antifungal for skin tineas, from cradle crap to athlete's foot. The root is also a mild immunostimulant, stimulating white blood cell activity, and you can combine it with our other immunostimulants (Astragalus, California Snakeroot, Thuja, Devil's Club, and Yerba Mansa) along with a dash of Lomatium as an antiviral, taking a couple of squirts of the mixture two or three times a day as an immunotonic.

OTHER USES The dried seeds, roasted lightly in the oven, can be ground, hull and all, and added to muffins, breads, and granola.

Baneberry

Actea rubra   (Ranunculaceae)

OTHER NAMES   *A. arguta, A. spicata,* var. *rubra, A. rubra,* var. *arguta,* etc. It is also spelled *Actaea.*

APPEARANCE Baneberry is a big, happy forest plant, with large dark green leaves, divided several times into twos or threes, with the leaflets sharply toothed and strongly veined. The several leaves are on long, wiry stems, and if you lift them up, you'll notice that they branch out from stems arising from the root, and are not basal leaves arising from the root itself. Baneberry's close relative Black Cohosh has larger leaves that are somewhat basal, with larger leaflets that are sandpapery to the touch. The leaves of Baneberry average from 12 to 18 inches long, half the length of the far less common Black Cohosh. The flowers are white, forming broad, short, and stumpy puffs maturing into a fat cluster of bright red, succulent berries that soon fall, often leaving one or two stuck to the otherwise empty pincushion flower stalk. Mature plants, from the root to the top of the stalk, are usually 2 feet tall and about the same diameter. In dry years they will not set flowers, and stands in deep shade seem to never bother at all.

Although most of our Baneberries are red, white varieties also occur; otherwise the plants are the same. Folks from back East may be confused, since *Actea pachypoda,* or White Baneberry, is a different species than *Actea rubra,* or Red Baneberry (the same species as ours). They look so similar, how can you tell, in Upper Peninsula Michigan, if the plant with white berries is White Baneberry or white-berried Red Baneberry? It is a puzzlement. Back home again, the root of our plant is a small, warty, scaly, and dense rhizome with wiry rootlets, dark reddish brown on the outside, cream-colored inside, with a pith that darkens after it is exposed to the air. Baneberry plants are usually found in dispersed stands, sometimes in dense patches.

HABITAT Baneberry can be found in moist, biodiverse woodlands, from

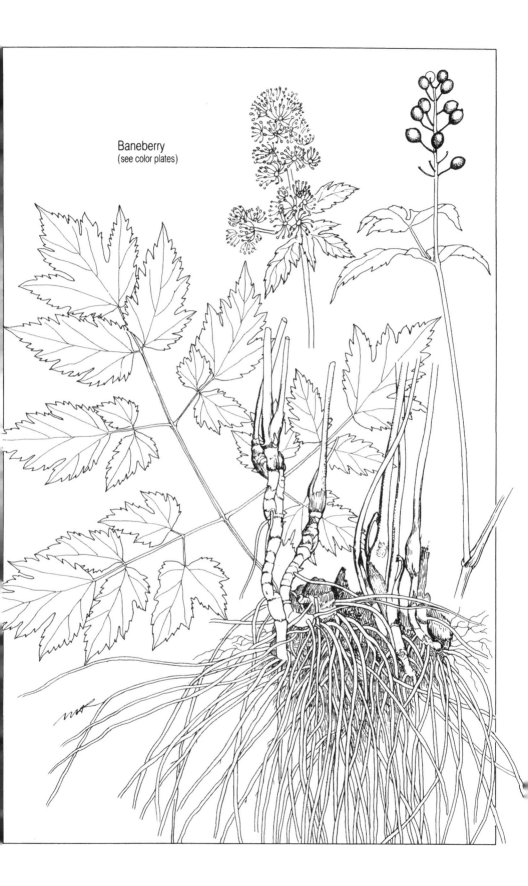

Baneberry
(see color plates)

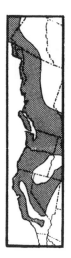

the San Bernardino Mountains of southern California, north to Alaska, and east to the Atlantic Coast. It likes shade, moist and rich dirt, and can grow down to the water in shaded streams and back up against dark hillsides in other areas. The further north you go, the more it may grow in the open, until in British Columbia and Alaska it may be found in nearly full sunlight. Otherwise, further south, it may take several minutes to adjust your pupils to the deep shade that hides the dozen plants you are surrounded by. Although Baneberry does not need old-growth forest as much as such plants as Trillium, Licorice Fern, or Black Cohosh, it is still most abundant in clean places.

CONSTITUENTS The dried root contains nearly identical components to Black Cohosh, namely 20% resins, made up of cimicifugin, cimigenol, and actea-type glycosides. However, it does not seem to contain the estrogen-mimicking compound found in Black Cohosh.

COLLECTING Gather the root after the berries are matured, or, in unflowered stands, in August or September. The root dries into dense, tough masses, so slice or snip the fresh root into small sections, and dry Method B.

STABILITY The dried root should be stable for several years.

PREPARATION The dry root for internal use as a Dry Tincture, 1:5, 70% to 80% alcohol. The dose should be 10 to 20 drops, up to three times a day. For external use as liniment, macerate 2 ounces of the ground root with 1 ounce of powdered Tobacco and a scant tablespoon of African Cayenne in a pint of 70% rubbing alcohol for a couple of weeks and strain. You might wish to add a dram or teaspoon of Wintergreen Oil or Sweet Birch Oil to the finished liniment.

MEDICINAL USES Internally, the root has the same uses as listed under Black Cohosh, with the exception of estrogenic. That means it functions the same way as an anti-inflammatory, peripheral vasodilator, antispasmodic, and sedative. Although I had long considered Baneberry to be somewhat toxic, I have changed my mind in recent years. The constituents in the root are nearly the same as in Black Cohosh, although the resins seem a little stronger on a weight basis; hence the lower recommended dose. The *berries* are apparently quite toxic and have given this plant a bad reputation. The liniment is very useful for swollen, painful sprains and contusions. The root is locally analgesic, the Tobacco is anti-inflammatory, the Cayenne provides counterirritant heat, and the oil (if used) contains methyl salicylate, a useful analgesic and counterirritant. If you use the oil, you need to moderate how often you use the liniment, as the Wintergreen or Sweet Birch oils can be absorbed into the skin and cause a little dizziness or constipation.

CONTRAINDICATIONS Not for use during pregnancy, as well as the other conditions that are listed under Black Cohosh.

Bergamot Mint

Mentha citrata   (Labiatae)

OTHER NAMES   Lemon Mint, Orange Mint

APPEARANCE Bergamot Mint grows in stands, connected by roots, and will cover a stream bank or sandbar with dozens or hundreds of 2- to 5-foot-tall stems. The whole plant is dark, shiny green; with roundish opposite leaves; square, stout, and sometimes semi-inflated stems; and bright pink or lavender terminal flowers. The flower heads are usually puffy and in one mass, but they can form terminal rings and even intersperse with leaflets down the stem. In ideal growing circumstances, plants may form large mats, with submerged stems becoming roots and with stoloniferous swellings bearing rootlets. This is a horticultural hybrid, sterile (I think) and reproducing through flooding. The leaf scent is pungent—lemony and exquisite. It closely resembles its relative Peppermint in all aspects, except for its scent, larger size, and more southern distribution.

HABITAT Bergamot Mint is found erratically in the Santa Monica Mountains, in moist areas around Antelope Valley, and here and there in coastal creeks from Los Angeles County north to Washington. It grows in the Willamette Valley and lower creeks west of the Cascades in Oregon; it can be encountered in the most unlikely places. I have no idea how it has established itself in some of the localities I have found it, growing in places such as Oregon or northern California coastal creeks that seem to drain no habitation, trickling down from little isolated mountains near nothing else. I have encountered stands in the northwest drainage of the Sierra Nevada of California and further south near Lake Isabella. Unpredictable. You just have to get in the habit of checking bends in creeks, dribbles, and trickles—suspicious stands of dark, close-growing plants in and next to water. It might be Bergamot Mint, or Peppermint, or Spearmint—or it might be some gross weed like Epazote. If you don't look, you won't find. So be it.

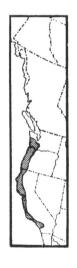

CONSTITUENTS Citral, l-limonene, d-limonene, menthol, menthone, and a whole bunch of other related aromatics that will vary with the growing circumstances.

COLLECTING Gather whole stems in mid- or late summer, dry Method A, and strip off from largest stems against the grain.

STABILITY The herb is good as long as it smells good. If stored as whole leaves, it may last two years.

PREPARATION As a simple tea, ad libitum. You can make a great flavoring extract by tincturing the fresh leaves, 1:2, or a liqueur by adding some maple syrup to the tincture until it tastes as you wish.

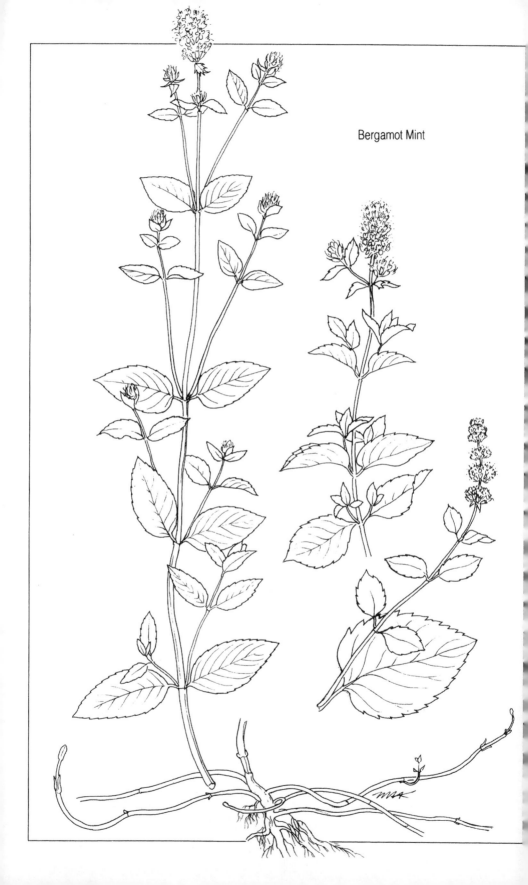

Bergamot Mint

MEDICINAL USES Some people will find that Bergamot Mint settles indigestion even better than Peppermint; if not, add some *to* Peppermint to improve the taste of that simplistic stalwart. It improves the taste of Lemon Balm, which always seems to smell better than it tastes, and it is equally complementary to the marginally unpleasant taste of Sage and Pitcher Sage. The stems are aromatic and can be added to tea blends; thrown on fires for incense; added to a sauna; or added to Thai or Chinese cooking when Lemon Grass is called for, and removed before serving. Or try a Bergamot Mint Julep, and add it to Mediterranean cooking that calls simply for Mint. Similarly, add some leaves to a batch of lemonade or limeade; try mixing the tincture with Peppermint Oil for mint jelly; add it or the liqueur to the punch bowl; or throw a dash into fruit salads. The leaves can be added to oolong or Darjeeling tea to give them that Earl Grey flavor, which is derived from the oil of Bergamot, a citrus fruit that this mint is named after. Further suggestions: lemon chiffon pie, cheesecake, Key lime pie, grasshoppers, and so forth. Lovely stuff.

Betony

Pedicularis spp. (Scrophulariaceae)

OTHER NAMES Indian Warrior (*P. densiflora*), Elephant's Head (*P. groenlandica*), Little Elephant's Head (*P. attollens*); Lousewort (general name)

APPEARANCE The Pacific West is the heartland of the *Pedicularis* genus, particularly in the north; there are fourteen species in Alaska alone. By and large, the most common can be lumped into four groups.

Group One. Elephant's Head and Little Elephant's Head are upright plants of the high meadows; they are unbranching and have little flowers that look like an elephant's head. Elephant's Head (*Pedicularis groenlandica*) has few basal leaves, the stem leaves are short and fernlike, and the flowers are a striking magenta or purple-pink, with the "trunk" extended down and out in front of the three-lobed "ears." The plants are a foot tall on the average and generally have single stalks. The foliage is smooth (glabrous). Little Elephant's Head (*Pedicularis attollens*) is generally smaller, with fernier leaves, and is usually downy on the upper leaves and the inflorescence. The flowers are white or light pink, and the "trunk" extends no further than the lower lobes of the corolla. The plant tends to form multiple stems more than the previous species.

Group Two. These are short plants, with a large rosette of fernlike leaves and short, central spikes of rather large flowers. Indian Warrior (*P.*

densiflora) has leaves up to 6 inches long, and short, chunky flower spikes up to a foot in height, densely covered in bright red, inch-long flowers. After wet California springs, Indian Warrior supplies the scarlet color found on hillsides covered with wildflowers; the blue color is Lupine, orange is California Poppy, and the yellow is several other plants. *P. semibarbata* has basal leaves also up to 6 inches in length, and shorter spikes of gold-yellow flowers, often barely rising above the leaves. *P. centranthera* also has fernlike basal leaves, with short spikes of purple or purple-tipped white flowers, up to an inch in length. The whole plant tends to have a purplish tinge, particularly in the spring.

Group Three is the same but taller. *P. bracteosa* usually has several or many simple stems from the same root (sometimes tuberous), with many fernlike leaves, both basal and (in some varieties) a stem rosette. The flowers are usually yellow-pink, but may be from white to purple. *P. parryi*, a similar basal-leaved plant from the Rocky Mountains (where it is usually yellow) is found in Idaho and western Montana as a purplish yellow flowered plant. Both of these plants have shorter basal leaves, more extended flowering stalks, and run up to 3 feet in height.

Group Four is simply *P. racemosa,* an open, many stemmed plant of 2 feet in height, with lanceolate leaves. The fernlike nature of other Betony leaves is only evident by tiny crenulations, or teeth, on the leaves. The flowers are from white to yellow, the stems and the leaves are often purplish, and the flowers may even have purplish veins. The flowers have a sharp sickle-shaped, downwards beak nearly touching the lower, spread lobe of the corolla, and their overall appearance is lopsided-goofy. In general, much of the variation in flower color of the last three groups, and even their morphology differences within a species, can be explained by their semiparasitic nature. Not only can their constituents be varied by the nature of their host plant, but so can their growth and appearance.

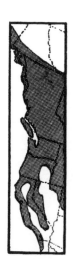

HABITAT *Group One* is found in high mountain meadows that have considerable winter snow cover. *P. groenlandica* is found from California to Alaska and eastwards; *P. attollens* grows even higher in the mountains (up to 12,000 feet) in California and the southern Cascades of Oregon. Generally, both grow in meadows covered in Sedum, Bistort, and Marsh Marigold.

Group Two, P. densiflora, a spring bloomer, grows along the coastal ranges and foothills from Baja California to southern Oregon. *P. semibarbata* is found in the Yellow Pine (Ponderosa) belt of the Sierra Nevada and Cascades of California, and in extreme southern Oregon, as well as the higher southern California ranges and western Nevada. *P. centranthera* is occasional in eastern Oregon and Washington, Nevada, Utah, and down the Rockies. It is a plant that can be found in the dry lower mountains of Pine and Oak.

Group Three, P. parryi, is a plant of the moist higher forest, from Idaho

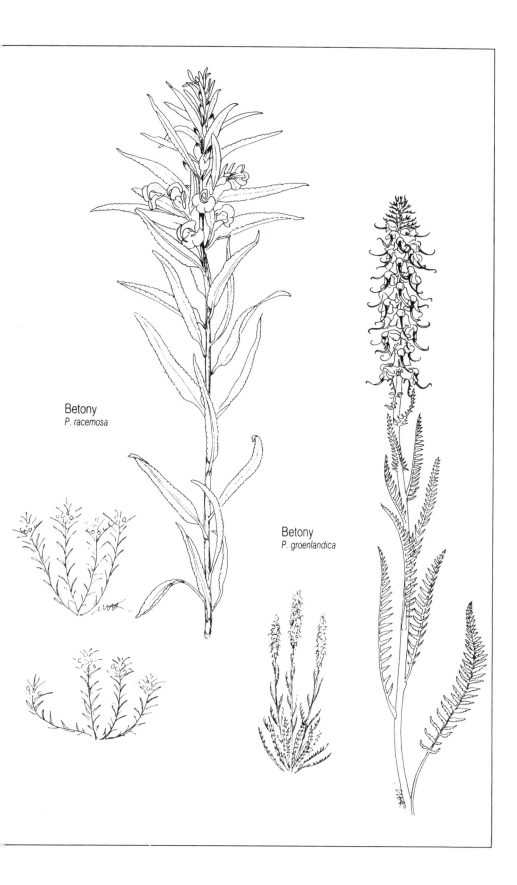

Betony
P. racemosa

Betony
P. groenlandica

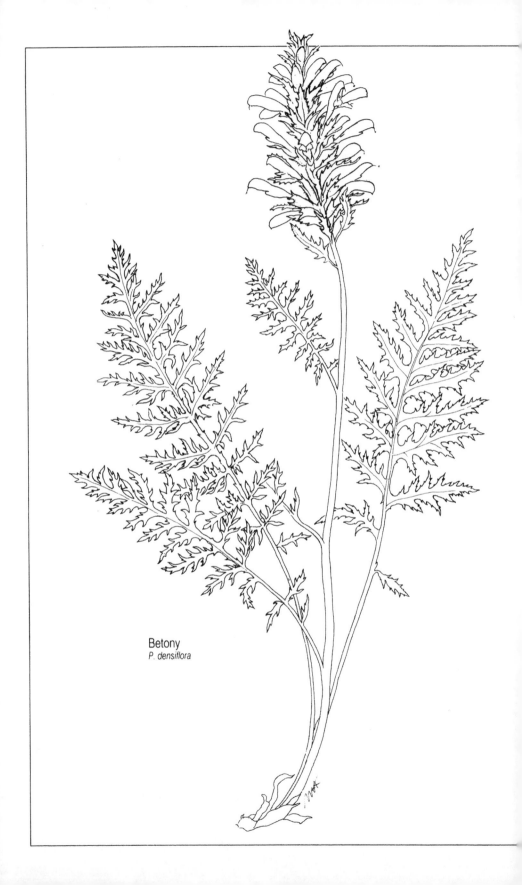

Betony
P. densiflora

and Montana south through the southern Rockies and the high inner ranges of Nevada and Utah. *P. bracteosa*, in its various forms, grows in the moist middle mountains from the southern edge of the Cascades in California (where it is sometimes referred to as *P. flavida*), all the way to British Columbia, all across the Pacific Cordilleran ranges, and down to the Colorado high country.

Group Four, P. racemosa, grows from the northern coastal range and Sierra Nevada Range in California, northwards to British Columbia—and generally with the same range as *P. bracteosa*, but extending further south into Arizona and New Mexico. It likes Douglas Fir, Red Fir, and Spruce forests, at whatever elevation they occur. The flowers tend to run towards pink in the area west of the Cascades, towards cream, and even yellow, in the Great Basin ranges and the Rocky Mountains.

CONSTITUENTS This is a big problem, for it seems difficult to figure out exactly what the Betonys contain and what is derived from the larger plants on which they are sometimes parasitic. As an example, *Pedicularis bracteosa* and *P. groenlandica* may tap into *Senecio triangularis*, a big, happy Ragwort found in similar moist mountain areas; if so, they will contain toxic *Senecio* alkaloids and should not be used. *P. bracteosa, P. parryi*, and others may tap into Pines and Spruces, with pinidinol present; if so, the herb will act atypically by warming the skin and stimulating urine. *P. racemosa* is nearly always parasitic upon Spruce; but in dense colonies, some will be dark purple in foliage (very parasitic and high in pinidinol) and others will be bright green, with very little purple, and relatively autonomous in their constituents.

Whenever picking a Betony, check to see if it is autonomous or parasitic, and if it is parasitic, make sure it is tapping into something benign like an Oak. This gives you Betony constituents (whatever *they* are) and not some other plant's secondary compounds that may be toxic. Using a *Pedicularis* growing on another bioactive plant can give varied and unpredictable side effects. Several of the Betonys can be found tapping into *Thermopsis* (Mountain Pea or False Lupine), which contains anagyrine and N-methylcytisine (Caulophylline), active compounds that are mostly responsible for the effects of Blue Cohosh on the uterine muscles. I used to toss all my Betony together, since each batch and species seemed to differ in its effect. I would also consult with old friends and former students, although they had reached no more a consensus than I had concerning its constituents. Now that I know about the secondary constituent problem, I only gather from stands whose roots are free from attachments to a host. I *still* don't know which species are weaker or stronger in those native compounds that make Betony so useful.

COLLECTING Gather the plant in flower, and dry Method A or Method B, depending on the height and amount of basal leaf growth.

STABILITY The dried herb is stable for at least twelve months, with the larger varieties lasting up to eighteen months.

PREPARATION Standard Infusion, 4 to 8 fluid ounces, two or three times a day; the Dry Tincture, 1:5, 50% alcohol, 1 to 2 teaspoons, similarly.

MEDICINAL USES Much of the traditional use of Betony (not to be confused with Wood Betony, or *Stachys betonica*, of Europe) is derived from its uptake constituents, as in the case of its use as an expectorating cough remedy (coniferous aromatics), and as a treatment for diarrhea (tannins from host Oaks). By itself, it is one of our safest and most effective skeletal muscle relaxants. It takes tight, adrenalin-stressed muscles and decreases their tone and rigidity. If you have played too much tennis or moved too many boxes, drink some of the tea and relax. Also give Betony tea in reduced doses to children who can't relax after going to a scary movie, or have played so many video games that their hands, clenched around a 25-watt bulb, would light it dimly.

I have helped long-distance runners who can't relax at night after overtraining, and computer junkies whose necks seem permanently frozen at monitor-level. Massage therapists and rolfers might consider giving some Betony to their tougher clients. Body therapy adjustments to habitual stress problems seem to last longer if the patient has a bit of tea or tincture in the evening, dulling some of the structural patterning caused by muscle hypertonicity. Although I tend to take a minimalist approach to using herbs during delivery, several midwives have mentioned that it helps the mother relax better if she has some tea before and just after birthing. It may also have a salutary effect for those who have trouble relaxing and giving in to physical intimacy ("The kids are asleep, the alarm is set, and if we don't take more than thirty minutes doing it, we can get a full seven hours of sleep before getting up in the morning, unless Devon has another nightmare . . . although if we hurry too much, we both may lie awake for at least an hour, pondering what's wrong between us," and so forth.) If muscle twitches jolt you awake when you are trying to sleep, try Betony.

Bidens

Bidens frondosa, B. pilosa, B. pinnata   (Compositae)
OTHER NAMES   Burr Marigold, Beggar Ticks, Spanish Needles, Stick-Tight; *Aceitilla, Te de Coral*

APPEARANCE *Bidens frondosa* is usually called Beggar Ticks, and is one of those weeds, native to the U.S., that has crossed the Atlantic and become an introduced plant in Eurasia. It is an erect, often multibranched annual with long-petioled opposite leaves, pinnately compound; usually it has three, but sometimes five, narrow, toothed leaflets. The axils may give rise to other leaves, stems, or, particularly towards the top, flowers or flowering stems. The flowers are round, flattened composites, with yellow, scruffy little blossoms and extended, leaflike outer bracts. These mature into little flat, barbed achenes, with two hornlike awns that stick ticklike to clothes. *Bidens pilosa,* often a little taller (3 to 4 feet high), has fatter pinnate leaflets, also three or five, and sometimes a few white, scruffy ray flowers around the edge of the scruffy, yellow center flowers, and no extended leafy bracts. The seeds are similar, but four-sided, and sometimes with four horns. They also stick ticklike to clothing. Spanish Needles (*B. pinnata*) is an increasingly common weed along the coast, with pinnate, almost parsleylike opposite leaves and a tall, scrawny, and sparsely foliaged habit. The flowers are all fertile, extended, with the petals at the end of tubes, maturing into long, skinny, four-sided "needles" that, in their sheer obstinance, put the other two to shame, covering pants, skirts, socks, coats, ponchos, and pets with dark brown achenes— like wild rice from hell. There are other Bidens in our area, with cheerful little yellow sunflowers, but these are the three used medicinally, and I don't know the others well enough to recommend them.

HABITAT All three are widespread, but usually occur in lower altitudes, preferring moist riverbanks, meadows, pastures, and vacant lots. Many a picnic or an impromptu clover-roll has ended with sessions of removing barbed seeds from blankets, clothing, underwear, or the pelts of Frisbee-catching dogs.

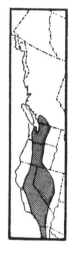

CONSTITUENTS Chalcone glucosides, volatile oils, gallic and oxalic acids, and some peculiar phenolic astringents.

COLLECTING Gather the whole plant in flower, dry Method A, and store as needed.

STABILITY Properly stored Bidens should be good for at least two years, although some of the expectorant effects, due to volatile oils, may not last much longer than a year.

PREPARATION Cold or Standard Infusion, 2 to 4 fluid ounces, up to four times a day; Dry Plant Tincture, 1:5, 40% to 50% alcohol, 45 to 90 drops, in a cup of water, also up to four times a day.

MEDICINAL USES Bidens, a hated, vilified (and vile) weed, is probably the best herbal therapy we have for irritation, inflammation, pain, and bleeding of the urinary tract mucosa. Although Shepherd's Purse may stop the hematuria quicker, and Mallow may stop the pain quicker, Bidens promotes healing of the membranes as well. For urethritis and cystitis that has had several closely spaced occurrences, with antibiotics helping briefly but with the irritation returning shortly after the finish of the regimen, try several days of the tea or tincture. If the pain goes away (it

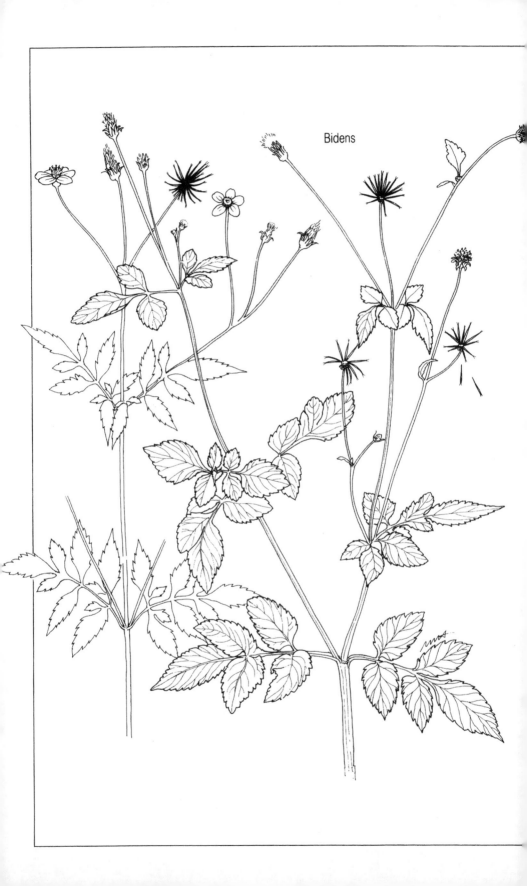

Bidens

usually will), continue the tea for a few more days to finish up the membrane healing. Although nothing is perfect, this treatment will usually stop the sequence. *Then* you might have to figure out a little better diet, find ways of binging other than on food, or have a long talk with your lover. Bidens may be our best herb for benign prostatic hypertrophy, usually decreasing the membrane irritability both in the urinary tract and the rectum, and often, over a few weeks of use, noticeably shrinking the prostate and giving its connective tissue better tone. For this purpose, it combines well with equal parts of White Sage.

For elevated uric acid in the blood and a history of gout or urate kidney gravel, Bidens will increase the efficiency of the kidney's excretion of uric acid from the blood (decreasing the likelihood of a gout attack); it will also act as a diuretic to dilute the urine (decreasing the likelihood of more urate stone precipitation in the pelvis of the kidneys). Unlike Devil's Club, Ginseng, Burdock Root, or Puncture Vine (*Tribulus terrestris*), it has no effect on the production of uric acid by the body; and if you eat shellfish and liver and spirulina, you still have the same dietary sources as always, but it does help the excretion in urine. The mechanism for stimulating the excretion is different from that of Shepherd's Purse, so the two can be combined for increased effects, in addition to watching your diet and taking metabolic modifying herbs such as those mentioned above. The herb is active against staph infections, and can be used as a wash, sitz bath, and eyewash. Its astringency helps take away the inflammation and pain as well.

Its astringency and anti-inflammatory effects on the mucus membranes help act as a tonic and preventative for gastritis and ulcers, and diarrhea and ulcerative colitis.

For respiratory infections or irritated membranes due to shouting, smoking, or dust, the tea or tincture acts to soothe the membranes, increase mucus secretions and expectoration, and decrease edema and swelling. For some asthma aggravated or induced by infection, it may be enough to turn the problem around, with the advantage of no drug effects. The tea will often help hay fever and sinus headaches from allergies, infections, or pollution.

For mucus discharges, use the tea two or three times a day for a week. This includes cloudy urine, vaginal discharges, mucus colitis, mucoid conjunctivitis, and chronic throat and nasal discharges. This common, drab, and irritating plant is, it turns out, a nifty medicine. Of our herbs, only Yerba Mansa and California Bayberry also have this ability to tighten, shrink, and tonify the structural cells of the mucus membranes, thereby preventing congestion and edema, while simultaneously increasing the circulation, metabolism, and healing energy of the functional cells of those tissues.

Bittersweet

Solanum dulcamara   (Solanaceae)

OTHER NAMES   Bittersweet Nightshade, Woody Nightshade;
Dulcamara

APPEARANCE Bittersweet is a scraggly, weak-stemmed vine, woody towards the base, and forming many irregular green branches. If it is growing in Willows and streamside growth, it can end up 6 or 8 feet high; if growing without much support, it can form an open, disorganized bush-vine-weed. The leaves vary, with a large, heart-shaped, pointed leaf and one or two lower leaflets, sometimes none. The flowers are tomatolike, purple, reflexed stars with a pointed center, maturing into bunches of tiny fruit that look like miniature cherry tomatoes. The dark green, unripe fruits are often mixed with blood red ripe ones on the same bunch, and the fruit may remain on the stems long after the leaves are dead or fallen.

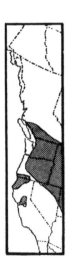

HABITAT A European weed, Bittersweet is now found in some abundance in Montana, Idaho, Washington, western Canada, and occasionally in northern California along the coast and in the Sacramento Valley. I have nearly always found it along slow streams and irrigation ditches, but it is good to avoid serious agribusiness drainage when picking the plant. Chemical residues that may be allegedly permissible in short-lived crop annuals are likely to accumulate in perennial weeds.

CONSTITUENTS Solaniceine, dulcamarin, dulcamaric and dulcamaretic acids, beta-solamarine, and small and physiologically unimportant traces of various Nightshade-type alkaloid and steroid variations.

COLLECTING Gather the green stems, all the way down to the overt wooden bark, when the leaves have started to wither in the fall. Sow the berries nearby, discard the leaves, and dry the stems, or tincture them fresh.

STABILITY The dried stems are good for at least two years if you leave them whole until needed.

PREPARATION Fresh Tincture, 1:2, Dry Tincture, 1:5, 50% alcohol, both forms 10 to 20 drops twice a day; Strong Decoction, 2 to 3 fluid ounces twice a day; 1 to 2 #00 capsules twice a day; Strong Decoction (½ ounce Bittersweet, ½ ounce California Bayberry bark), 1 quart in a bath.

MEDICINAL USES Bittersweet makes a lot of folks nervous, as there is no doubt that, like so many plants of the Nightshade family, it can be toxic in excess. In reality—in proper doses, in the right circumstances—it is perfectly safe. Bittersweet is an alterative and tonic, with little specific

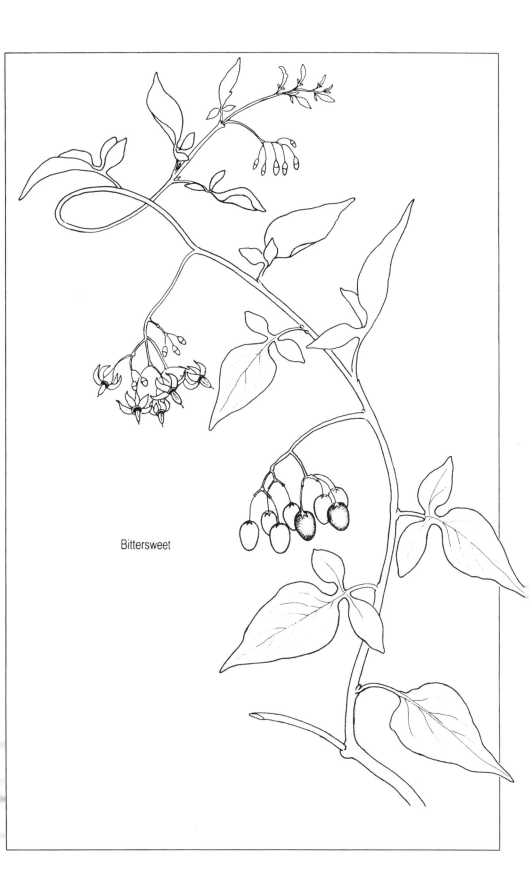

Bittersweet

use for particular disorders. The conditions are less important; the constitution is the indicator: it is appropriate for the person who has dry skin, often with eczema or psoriasis, has a chilly nature and likes dry hot weather best, and sometimes has a tendency for joint pain in cold and damp weather.

Generally, you will get good results using Bittersweet to support a chronic problem, while something else is used for the main problem. For long-standing scaly skin problems, especially eczema and psoriasis, when the problem has gotten gradually better but you are going through an acute episode, try some Bittersweet. If you tend to have these problems and you have aching joints or an externally derived skin infection such as heat rash or a tinea, try a Bittersweet/Bayberry bath in the evenings for a few days.

CONTRAINDICATIONS Don't use Bittersweet with kidney disease, and only use it externally if you are taking any medications. If you have arthritis or skin allergies that have been shown to be aggravated by members of the Nightshade family, don't use Bittersweet. It stimulates cutaneous and mucosal circulation and is not appropriate during pregnancy.

Black Cohosh

Cimicifuga elata   (Ranunculaceae)
OTHER NAMES   Western Bugbane, Tall Bugbane

APPEARANCE Black Cohosh is a big, handsome, forest-primeval plant, with large, expansive, bi- and triternate-toothed leaves, spreading out from the dark and tuberous rhizome somewhat like a fern or large carrot, without the scent, and with glandular swellings where the major leaflets and stems join. The foliage is larger and downy-hairy, but otherwise it resembles its smooth and smaller relative, Baneberry. A further difference is the 3- to 6-foot-tall flowering stem, covered in tiny white blossoms that mature into flat little seed capsules. Baneberry has a short, wide spike of white flowers that mature into red or white berries which stick out from the stem on peduncles. The roots of both plants resemble each other, and young Black Cohosh plants may be no larger than the smaller Baneberry; so look for the tall spike or its remnants (Black Cohosh) or the berries (Baneberry). Unless there are one or more plants in bloom in a stand, it is difficult to identify the plants by the foliage alone.

If you were to compare Black Cohosh and Baneberry side by side (even if not in bloom), the differences would be obvious. Black Cohosh is the larger plant, with broader foliage distinctly sandpaper-hairy on top, smooth

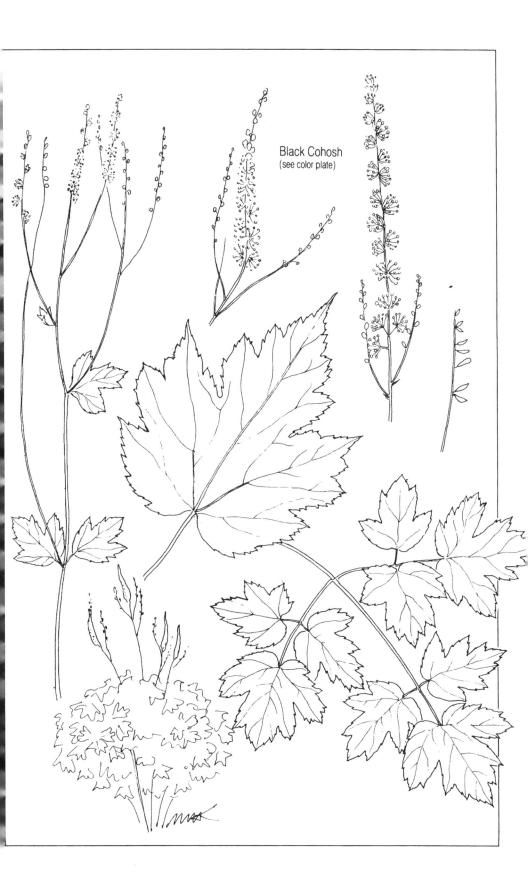

Black Cohosh
(see color plate)

below; Baneberry is smaller, less densely tropical in its leafing, and smooth both above and below. Several Black Cohosh plants in a shady, moist notch can completely fill the space with their large, overlapping leaves, whereas a stand of Baneberry plants forms a pleasant, closely knit, but somewhat sparser patch. All things considered, there are large variations in the size and panache of the two plants. Baneberry is the much more common plant and is found throughout the forests of North America. *Cimicifuga elata* is a less common plant, endemic to the low forests of the Pacific Northwest. As both plants only bloom in moist years, unless you know the latter's specific localities from previous hikes, when you discover stands of broad-leaved, deep-forest, Cimicifuga-like herbs with rather large, dark-skinned rhizomes bearing many leaf-scars—and without any flower, fruit, or seed stalks to tell you its name—the stands are almost always the more common Baneberry. Check a university herbarium for localities if you must; otherwise use Baneberry for its specific functions and buy some eastern Black Cohosh (*Cimicifuga racemosa*) for your herb use until you find our variety in bloom and reliably identifiable.

The roots of our western Black Cohosh are smaller than the official eastern species, which can be massive and broad in favored locations in the Northeast, but they still can be substantial. Dark grey on the outside, cream-white on the inside, as soon as you start to break them up they darken on contact with the air; the inner cream color turns reddish brown or dark grey and loses nearly 90% of its weight when dry.

Cimicifuga laciniata, a sparser plant with shorter and less elaborately divided basal leaves, is found only around the base of Mount Hood in Oregon and across the Columbia River Gorge in Washington. It is found at much higher elevations, and with decades of extensive logging, has been reduced to a few stands in wilderness areas. It is a threatened plant and should *not* be picked.

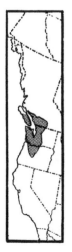

HABITAT Black Cohosh is found in lower forests from the northern half of Oregon, through Washington, to the southern third of British Columbia. It is found on the west side of the Cascades, the lower wetlands of the river basins, and the coastal forests of Washington and British Columbia. It needs old-growth or once-cut forests, with much species diversity, a lot of wildlife, rotting nurse trees around it—Devil's Club, Trillium . . . that kind of place. Look for it along hiking trails 2 miles from the nearest road or in little stream notches draining into scenic rivers, surrounded by old-growth forest too steep to cut or allowed to remain to form a cosmetic corridor for the public, with clear-cut forest boneyards hidden from the delicate sensibilities of the Sunday driver. *Cimicifuga* has a complex system of insect pollination and needs a complete forest to live in.

CONSTITUENTS Isoferulic acids, resins containing 15% to 20% cimici-fugin, including cimigenol, and the usual tannins, sugars, and so forth. Although these are the accepted contents of *Cimicifuga racemosa,* we are lacking any specific constituent analysis for our species. I feel the subjective effects are the same, and have found the resinoid contents from the dried root tinctures of both plants to be about equal and physically identical. The leaf and root have similar anti-inflammatory and sedative effects; the root seems to contain more of the estrogenoid effect.

COLLECTING Gather the fresh leaves from June through August; collect the roots for fresh or dried use from late July through September, and if in a flowering year, only in the fall, after the seeds have matured and self-sown from their little flat capsules. With large roots, it would be moral to remove the foliage and replant one or two root crowns in the hole. Our Black Cohosh is not endangered, unlike *Cimicifuga laciniata* and the southwestern *Cimicifuga arizonica,* but it grows in a fragile, complex, and vanishing ecological niche. It needs help and respect; if you live in the Northwest, it wouldn't hurt to bring some root crowns back to your garden, or tuck some in a city park or botanical garden. In the coastal Northwest, it is probable that the necessary insects will be present for pollination; elsewhere, it can be grown for root proliferation.

STABILITY The herb deteriorates quickly and needs to be tinctured fresh. The root is stable for several years in the dry state, although the same single root will create more therapeutic bounce for the ounce if tinctured fresh. As with so many herbs, the bioactivity of a square inch of the fresh root is rather greater than the same square inch if it were dehydrated. This drives some of my friends in the herb industry to teeth-clinching frustration, trying to establish some formula to equate dry and fresh strength. Generic preparations are just the processing of various plants in similar ways. Ten ounces of fresh Black Cohosh root may supply 60 full doses as a fresh root tincture. Ten fresh ounces will dry down to slightly over an ounce of root, which may only produce 20 full doses. By dried mass calculation, a 1:2 fresh tincture has not even a third the strength of the dry 1:5 tincture. In bioactivity, the fresh and dried tinctures are nearly the same strength.

For many plant remedies, we are so accustomed to using the commercially available dry plant that we forget how much stronger a fresh plant preparation can be. In North America, with many ecologies under siege, and less biomass morally available for our use, we need to consider how to get the most from the least. True, the threatened plant American Ginseng is provided little benefit by using fresh over dried plant, as the strength is little affected by drying. Goldenseal, however, another medicinal plant under siege due to overpicking, is much stronger as a fresh plant, with the fresh herb being equal to the dried root. Commerce needs dry botanicals. *We,* however, can hoard our marginal resources by making use of some plants in the fresh form. Like *Cimicifuga elata.*

PREPARATION Fresh Herb Tincture, 1:2, 30 to 40 drops, up to four times a day; Fresh Root Tincture, 1:2, 20 to 30 drops, up to four times a day; Dry Root Tincture, 1:5, 80% alcohol, 15 to 25 drops, also up to four times a day.

MEDICINAL USES This is one of our most useful medicinal plants. Its functions can be defined as anti-inflammatory, peripheral vasodilating, antispasmodic, sedative, and estrogenic. The root has all these functions; the leaf has all but the estrogenic.

Anti-inflammatory. Black Cohosh will help dull, aching, and congested tissues, muscles with a rheumatoid or myalgia-type distress, and the sense of heaviness and aching weakness. "My legs feel like lead this morning," saith the Black Cohosh person. This effect is most noticeable in the legs, hips, abdominal muscles, and neck. Remember that the characteristic for using *Cimicifuga* is a dull ache, not sharp pain. It works best for congestive, venous inflammation, not hot, red, and arterial inflammation.

Peripheral vasodilating. Black Cohosh helps to disperse blood out to the surface and will produce increased membrane secretions, ranging from the skin, to the kidneys, to the lungs, and to the intestinal mucosa. This effect is better in small, frequent doses and is most appropriate for adrenalin-stress people. By decreasing the constrictions of the peripheral blood vessels, it takes some of the back-pressure off of the arterial push, and will slow and strengthen the pulse and slightly lessen blood pressure. This is helpful for those with early symptoms of labile hypertension—the type of folks who get pissed off, red in the face, and look as if they are going to "throw a fit." It also helps people who get so uptight about seeing a medical person that their agitation spikes up their pressure when they see the arm cuff. These are all early symptoms in emotionally controlled adrenalin folks. Black Cohosh is for the early, functional imbalanced, subclinical person and has little or no place in treating folks who have developed pheochromocytomas or have early symptoms of kidney failure. This is an herb to help lower the thermostat (functional imbalance), not to rebuild the furnace (organic disease).

Antispasmodic. The antispasmodic effects of Black Cohosh help ease regular, spasmodic cramps in the tube muscles, and many women will attest to its value for uterine and fallopian cramps. With its effect on skin vasodilation helping to increase the organizing secretions of menstruation—those fluids that add volume, prevent coagulation, and inhibit bacteria—Black Cohosh is especially helpful for cramps that accompany a slow, spotty-clotty menstruation. It helps pain in the seminal vesicles in males, and can lessen or stop the pain of orchitis and the cramps that can arise from ejaculation or extended arousal (the near-mythic, seldom-encountered, but oft-claimed "blue balls"). Cramps in the belly from over-eating or eating under emotional tension will usually respond to Black Cohosh, and it can also help the sleeplessness caused by gallbladder or urinary bladder pain.

Sedative. The sedative effects of Black Cohosh are most reliable when you can't sleep because of cramps, aches and pains, or headache. It combines well with Valerian. The latter, besides being a central nervous system sedative, stimulates circulation and respiration when both are sedated by Black Cohosh. Together, they are a better sedative than either separately.

Estrogenic. The estrogenic compounds of the root are not the type that have an effect on the uterus or the breast tissue, but rather they are perceived by the hypothalamus of the brain as an estrogen metabolite and tend to lessen the pituitary surges of luteinizing hormone (LH) in the absence of ovarian estrogens. This makes it useful for women who are in menopause and have hot flashes. These are associated with decreased ovarian estrogen and the LH surges from a pituitary that is attempting to induce increased ovarian function—not possible, of course, since the whole point in menopause is to learn to do fine, thank you, without ovarian hormones.

CONTRAINDICATIONS Black Cohosh is not appropriate during pregnancy, and, in general, is best used in cold, deficient, and congested states.

It is not always a predictable plant, and some particularly sensitive individuals may need to be aware of the side effects that large quantities will induce in anyone. In excess amounts it will cause a frontal headache, often behind the eyes, that ceases after you stop using the herb. Further, it may slow the pulse and lower the blood pressure in hypotensive or bradycardic persons. Persons with elevated fluid pressure in the eyes should be careful with Black Cohosh, as it may sometimes dilate the pupils and cause a short-term elevation in interocular pressure. It is not so much that Black Cohosh is a particularly toxic plant—more that it is so helpful an herb that some people tend to overuse it, or presume to try to treat overt disease with it. It is not a "little drug," to substitute for proper medication; it is an effective herbal therapy for subacute, subclinical, commonplace problems that most folks would grab an over-the-counter pill for. End of lecture.

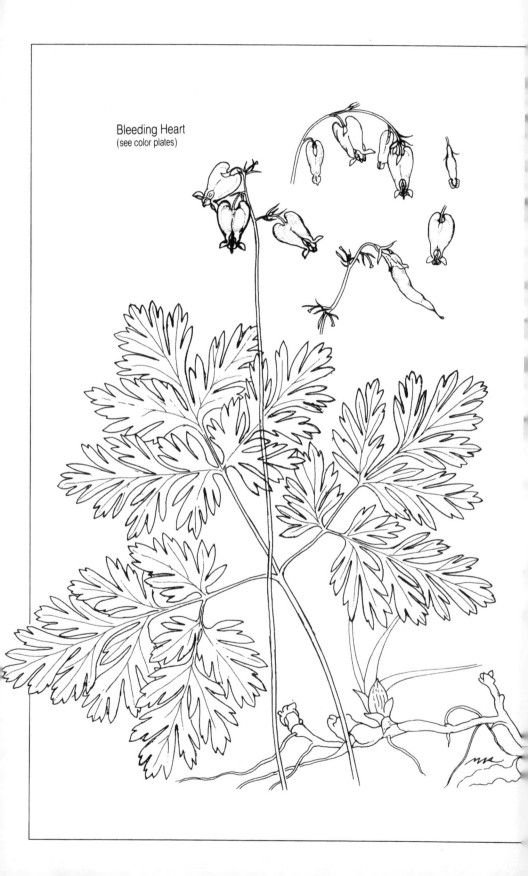

Bleeding Heart
(see color plates)

Bleeding Heart

Dicentra formosa   (Fumariaceae/Papaveraceae)

OTHER NAMES   Western Bleeding Heart, Pacific Bleeding Heart; *Corydalis formosa, Fumaria formosa*

APPEARANCE This is a pretty plant, with long-stemmed, blue-green basal leaves that are elaborately pinnate, resembling a fern or a parsley. From this attractive leaf mass the plant grows a long, scapelike stem that bears lovely little ¾-inch-long flowers that nod down in loose pink clusters, heart-shaped, inflated, and delightful. The root is a long, succulent rhizome, usually fairly close to the surface, unlike some of the *Dicentra* genus that have tubers or corms.

HABITAT Bleeding Heart grows in moist thickets and lower forests, from southwestern British Columbia to Santa Cruz County in California; across the Klamath Mountains; along the Sierra Nevada crest from Fresno County northwards (a more finely divided leaved variety); and west of the Cascades in Oregon and Washington. It is found sporadically in Idaho, Alberta, and northwest Montana.

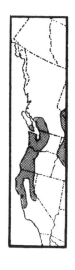

CONSTITUENTS Protopine, corydine, isocorydine, bulbocapnine, dicentrine, and other isoquinoline alkaloids.

COLLECTING Gather the roots in summer and fall, up until the leaves start to turn; collect the foliage in summer after the seedpods are matured and can be resown. Dry them separately, the roots Method B, the leaves Method A.

STABILITY The dried roots should be used within a year, the leaves should be used within several months.

PREPARATION Fresh Root Tincture, 1:2, 10 to 20 drops or applied topically; Dry Root Tincture, 1:5, 50% alcohol, 15 to 30 drops; Dry Herb Tincture, 1:5, 50% alcohol, 25 to 50 drops; all up to three times a day when needed.

MEDICINAL USES Bleeding Heart, like its eastern relative Turkey Corn (*Dicentra canadensis*), is both a tonic, suitable for helping some individuals strengthen and heal, and a general narcotic-analgesic for pain and central nervous system disorders, usable on occasion by anyone. The root is the strongest part, and either root tinctures (fresh or dry) can be used on a sore tooth, lost filling, or mouth trauma. It won't replace a dentist, but it will keep you sane until your appointment. It affects deeper nerve sensibilities, and can be followed by an application of Angelica seed, Cow Parsnip seed, or Yarrow root tinctures, which affect more superficial nerves. Any form of the plant can be applied locally to painful sprains, bruises, or contusions, although it will take a while to deaden the pain; a hot, moist towel with a little tincture underneath will speed up the process. It can be combined with Henbane or Yerba del Lobo tincture to broaden the analgesia (they affect different nerve sensitivities); and taking some California Poppy, Betony, or Skullcap internally will increase the pain relief.

Internally, the tincture will help calm down and center you if you are shaky, nervous, frightened, or uncontrollably angry as an aftermath of physical violence, an accident, rushing someone to the hospital, landing at LAX with one engine out—or taking a trip to the Department of Motor Vehicles to change title on a car, but without a notarized bill of sale and with only four hours off from work within which to get it accomplished.

Bleeding Heart is a tonic alterative that, a century ago, was widely used to strengthen people with long-standing syphilis. It increases appetite, stimulates liver metabolism, and generally helps anabolic functions in folks who have been sick for a while, are getting over a long down cycle, or generally have the punies, with cold sensitivities, nonorganic weight loss, shakiness when tired, and dry skin with eczematous patches. In this tonic use, it is comparable to Pipsissewa (*Chimaphila* spp.) and Bittersweet, but Pipsissewa is for those with impaired kidney function and a mild tendency to edema, and Bittersweet is for those who have joint pain and hate cold, damp weather. Bleeding Heart is for similar skin and metabolic weaknesses, but with shakiness and nervous tiredness.

CONTRAINDICATIONS Not for use during pregnancy, for overt neuropathies, or with prescription medications. It may induce a false positive in urine testing for opiates.

Blueberry

Vaccinium spp.   (Ericaceae)
OTHER NAMES Huckleberry (Red, Black, Dwarf, Western, Bog), Bilberry (Red, Dwarf, Low, Tall), Grouseberry, Whortleberry, Grouse Whortleberry, etc.

APPEARANCE Where do I start? Well, our *Vacciniums* can be loosely bunched into sizes: large (waist high or taller), small (around your knees), and dwarf (crawl on your hands and knees). The larger *Vacciniums* are universally open, spreading shrubs, with ridged branches and with light blue-green foliage, neat oval leaves that crisscross, hovering parallel to the ground. This growth habit allows the various types of berries to be available to birds, squirrels, and bears, all of whom help to spread the seeds in their droppings. The berries have a little depressed, round scar on them, the "vaccination." The only connection between "vaccination" and *Vaccinium* is the cows (Latin: *vacca*) that were supposed to browse the plant, and the first vaccine, using cowpox (*Vaccinia*) virus against smallpox. The small *Vacciniums* (*V. myrtillus* and the delightful *V. scoparium*) are little dwarf bushes with many green, intertwined branchlets, the latter (Grouse Whortleberry) sometimes covered with zillions of little light red berries, the first having sparse blue-grey berries. They both have a paucity of leaves.

HABITAT All the *Vacciniums* grow in acidic soil, usually moist and shady ground beneath trees. The smaller ones may form vast colonies beneath old-growth trees; some of the larger ones can become dominant plants after logging or fires have wiped out larger plant species. Get into the trees, up into the mountains, down in coastal bogs; look for Spruce, Red Cedar, Redwoods, Sequoias. The only major exception is *V. ovatum* (California Huckleberry), with its longer, pointed and serrated, dark green leaves; it is found in coastal thickets further north, in shady coastal canyons and on slopes in the south, growing all the way to San Luis Obispo and even Santa Barbara counties. Much of *Vaccinium*'s former range in central California has been built on, but large stands can still be found between cities and developments. There are some fine stands south of Big Sur in the Santa Lucia Mountains. From Oregon northwards, just ask anybody where the Huckleberries and Blueberries are growing. If they don't know, go to the nearest national forest and ask the ranger.

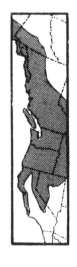

CONSTITUENTS Ericolin, arbutin, beta-amyrin, nonacosane, and a number of anthocyanosides, including myrtocyan.

COLLECTING Gather the leaves in the summer and early fall while still green, about the time the berries are ready. Dry in bundles, strip off leaves and small twigs, discarding large, woody stems. The strength and constituents vary greatly within the same species, depending on the local ecologies. Always chew some of the fresh leaves first. Good plants for therapeutic use have a tart, blueberry aftertaste. If you don't taste that, go further to another colony until you find a bunch that tastes right. My rule of thumb is the more berries in a stand, the better the foliage. I have found stands whose leaves even *smell* like their berries; other stands of the same species have barely managed the taste of day-old grass clippings. Besides, if you find *Vacciniums* with lots of berries and good-tasting leaves, you can browse while you collect until your fingers and mouth are stained red-blue-purple.

STABILITY No more than a year as dried tea.

PREPARATION Standard Infusion, 3 to 4 fluid ounces, up to three times a day.

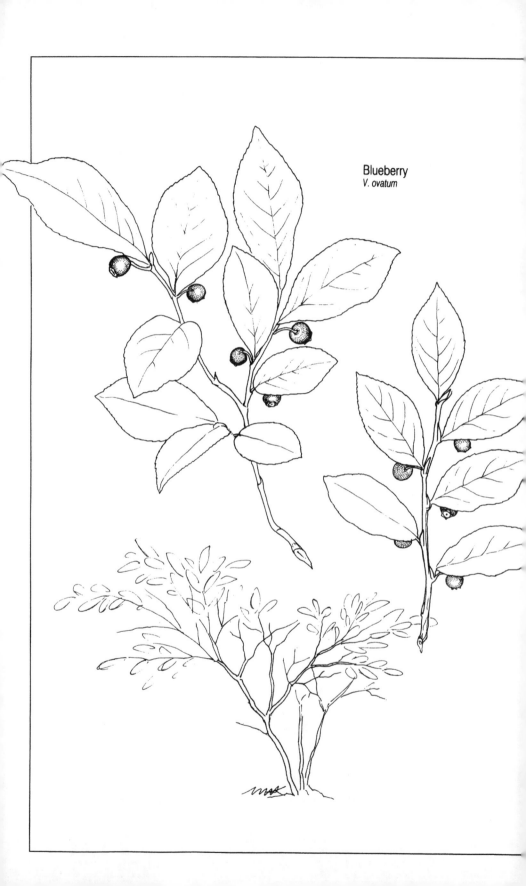

Blueberry
V. ovatum

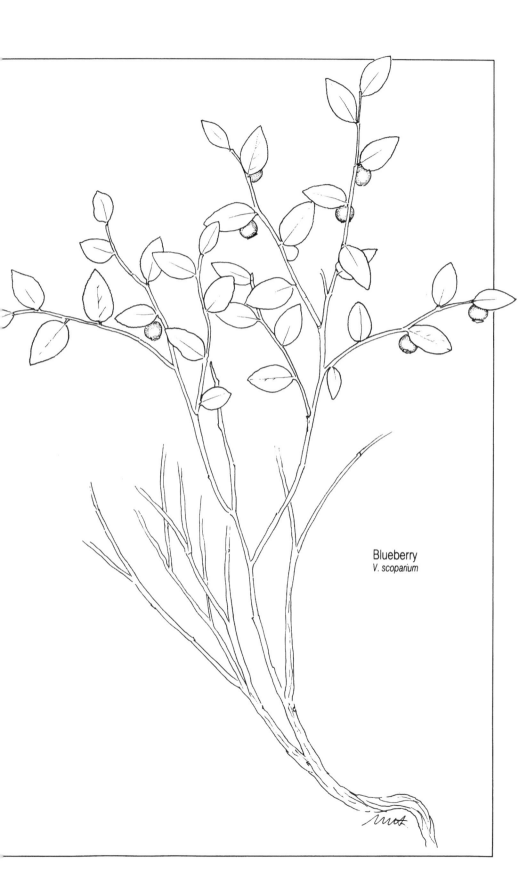

Blueberry
V. scoparium

MEDICINAL USES First off, the tea is quite useful for treating alkaline pH cystitis. As urine is normally slightly acid (pH 6.0 to 6.5), changes in diet or binging on sweets, greens, or fruit decrease the dietary intake of potential hydrogen ions. The result is that the urine excretes less acid and it gets alkaline. This creates a more ideal media for bacterial growth (usually colon bacteria), and you have your garden variety cystitis/urethritis. Men have a somewhat more anabolic metabolism, create more acids, and, if they have urethritis at all, it tends to result from more specific organisms that are adapted to acid urine. Women have a week or two after menses when they are less anabolic, produce less nitrogenous acid metabolites, and are more likely to have an alkaline urine infection. Rule of thumb: if cranberry juice helps (it acidifies the urine), then the infection has an alkaline basis. Try taking the tea three or four times, then start adding the juice the next day, along with the tea. Ericoline and arbutin, found in the leaves, are excreted as disinfecting quinones in alkaline urine. After the urine returns to normal acidity, the tea is no longer active, so a couple of days is more than enough. Then, add some beans, fish, yogurt, or cheese to the diet, and the urine will retain its normal acidity.

Practically speaking, any regular healthy diet results in acid urine. If you eat a lot of protein (high in acids), you need more stomach acid to digest it, and the surplus acid left over for the urine keeps it slightly acidic. If you have a diet high in fruits, vegetables, or cooked grains (macrobiotic, vegan-veggie, and the like), you ingest less acid, need less in the stomach, and you *still* have enough surplus hydrogen ions to keep the urine slightly acidic. It's binging that does it.

The other main use for *Vaccinium* tea is to help modify blood sugar elevations in juvenile onset, insulin-dependent diabetes (Type I diabetes). This is the disorder, manifested early in life (usually by adolescence), caused by too little insulin being made by the pancreas and results in dependence on periodic insulin injections. Most diabetes is adult onset (usually after age forty); in this type there is enough insulin being made, but the person is usually overweight, and cells, stuffed with stored fuel, become insulin resistant. For these folks Devil's Club is often useful, along with changes in diet and lifestyle. For Type I diabetes, however, a 3- to 4-ounce dose of the standard infusion of Blueberry leaves should be taken to extend the hypoglycemic effects of the most problematic injection during the day; this is usually best done in late afternoon. Blueberry infusions will never replace the need for injections—just help to decrease the number needed during the day or the units needed in each injection. I have been told by some folks with insulin-dependent diabetes (IDDM) who have experimented with the tea that it can help the early morning "dawn phenomenon"—waking up with hyperglycemia that keeps them from going back to sleep. Several of them have used the tea in the late afternoon, a couple of hours before their evening injection;

because they reduced their morning dose they had less hypoglycemia in the early afternoon, but started to get the blood sugar creep a couple of hours before dinner.

A warning: some hyperglycemia is really the adrenalin discharge in response to a dangerous drop in blood sugar that occurs a few hours after a meal and while the long-lasting insulin fractions are still active (but the food is gone). This is that oh-so-familiar effect in diabetics: sweating palms, nervousness, white face. Eat something. The use of *Vaccinium* tea for hyperglycemia with the insulin-dependent diabetic is this: you want to decrease your morning dose, you have less hypoglycemia in the early afternoon, but the insulin wears off a bit, and your blood sugar level starts to rise before your evening injection and dinner. Take some tea. I used to be reluctant to suggest anything to these folks. In the old days you monitored your urine sugar with strips. That shows hyperglycemia but not the more dangerous hypoglycemia. These days, with direct blood sugar monitoring, sensible Type I diabetics can safely experiment a bit.

Some folks with allergies and the tendency for skin hyperactivity may find that the tea decreases their inflammatory responses, as the anthocyanosides in the leaves have been shown to decrease platelet aggregation and stomach ulceration. Those with viscous blood from elevated blood fats may find fewer frontal headaches occurring, especially when *Vaccinium* is combined with Red Root.

OTHER USES Oh, those berries! The berries are also hypoglycemic for some people. You eat a whole lot and two or three hours later you get cranky, shaky, sweaty-palmed. Eat something right away. The hormones secreted by the stomach lining in the presence of food will stimulate insulin and soothe the adrenalin discharge and the blood sugar rush that the hypoglycemia induced.

Brook Mint

Mentha arvensis   (Labiatae)
OTHER NAMES   Field Mint; *Poleo*; *Mentha canadensis*

APPEARANCE Brook Mint is a medium-sized plant, the size and shape of Peppermint and with the axillary flowers of Pennyroyal. The leaves are from 1 to 2½ inches long, oval, and taper into a short petiole; the flowers range from light pink to light purple; and the whole plant is tomentose to some degree. Plants in open sun have many secondary branches and are overtly fuzzy; plants in shade and growing in thickets are taller, with few if any branches, and nearly smooth. Brook Mint resembles Peppermint, Spearmint, and Bergamot Mint in size and habitat, but with lighter colored foliage and axillary, not terminal, flowers. It can be confused with Pennyroyal, but it has leaves twice the size, and they are lateral, not reflexed. It can be confused with Bugleweed, which grows in similar localities, has the same axillary flowers, and sometimes similar shaped leaves; but the latter has no scent, white flowers, and usually strongly serrated leaves. Further, Brook Mint can be confused with Marsh Skullcap (*Scutellaria galericulata*), which has narrower leaves, no scent, and pairs of blue flowers in the axils.

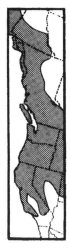

HABITAT Our only native true Mint, Brook Mint (called *Poleo* in New Mexico) is found in nearly every watershed in the West, preferring clean, fast-moving waterways and growing on sandbars, in thickets, and behind embankments in swampy areas from Ventura County, California, to Alaska; from there, Brook Mint is circumboreal.

CONSTITUENTS Volatile oils, with variable constituents, depending on chemical strains, but mostly containing menthol, menthone, pulegone, methyl acetate.

COLLECTING Gather in late summer, dry Method A; for tea, process in small sections, including stems. Plants gathered on stream banks above low watermark and in sun have a higher oil content; plants gathered in shaded thickets and with fewer stems (and taller) make a better-tasting tea. I have on occasion encountered a tall, stemmy variety (and this species forms many variations) that can be 4 to 5 feet tall, with lower stems too woody to utilize, so use your judgment.

STABILITY Usually Brook Mint, stored well, remains full strength for a year, with aromatics deteriorating selectively, until after two years the Peppermintlike aromatics have noticeably dissipated and the lesser terpenes, including pulegone, have become dominant. I would suggest replacing the herb every year.

PREPARATION The Standard Infusion or a simple tea to taste.

MEDICINAL USES Brook Mint, with its high levels of menthol, can be used in all of the ways that Peppermint tea is used, especially for stomach distress. In addition, it is a useful diaphoretic, especially when combined with Elder flowers. Because of its pulegone content, it is similar to, though more feeble than, Pennyroyal, and can be used as a better-tasting, gentler-tasting substitute for it.

The main characteristic of Brook Mint is its unparalleled lovely taste; it combines delightfully with Lemon Balm, Catnip, Peppermint, and many other herbs.

CONTRAINDICATIONS Although not high in pulegone, it would be inappropriate to use much Brook Mint during pregnancy or heavy menses.

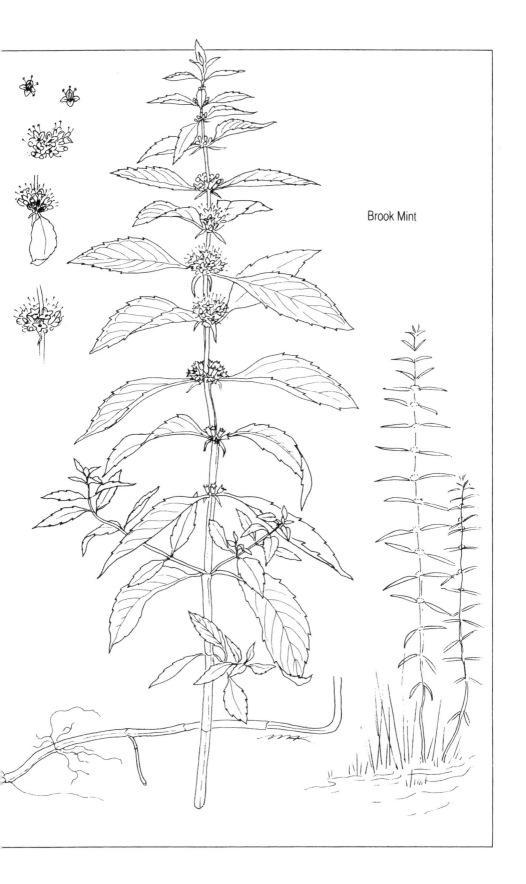

Brook Mint

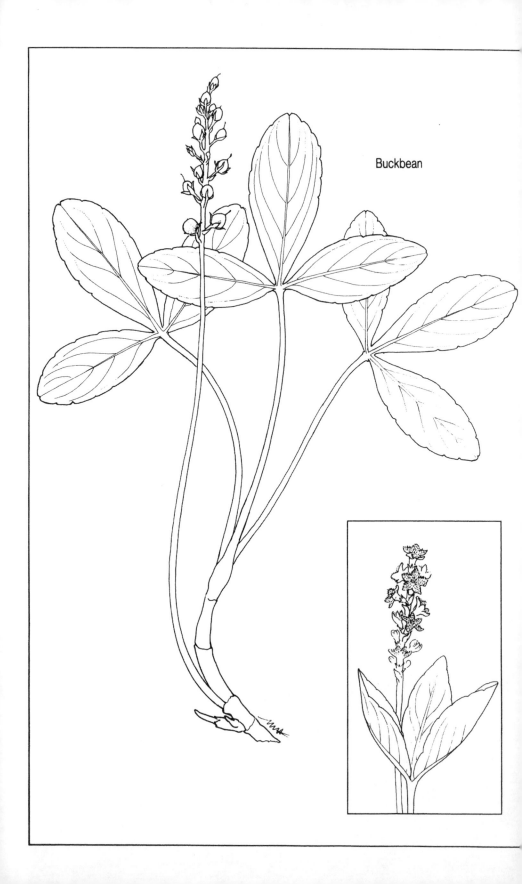

Buckbean

Buckbean

Menyanthes trifoliata   (Menyanthaceae/Gentianaceae)
OTHER NAMES   Bogbean, Marsh Trefoil

APPEARANCE Buckbean grows in colonies of many interconnected plants, with their rhizomes buried in water and mire. The leaves are all basal, on long stalks, and waxy green. They are made up of three elongated leaflets, slightly toothed and succulent; and the two side leaflets tend to form right angles from the main stem. The flower stalk is about a foot high; the plant blooms in late spring and forms a chunky little cone of small, star-shaped flowers; the petals are fuzzy on top, and the color varies from white to light pink, occasionally with a yellow tinge. The rhizomes are black and slimy, with joint scars from previous growth, and the leaf stalks have long stipules, often underwater. The plants look somewhat beanlike, hence the name Bogbean. Plants predominately out of water, as in summer sphagnum bogs, may be short, with irregularly curled leaves, and seldom bloom. The further north you go, the more expansive the foliage becomes until, in British Columbia and Alaska, the leaves and flowers may become large, open, almost luxuriant. Accustomed to the high-mountain glacier lake–lily-pond habitat and growth of Buckbeans I had encountered in Colorado, Oregon, and northern California, I was ill-prepared for the three-leaved "Lilies" on Vancouver Island—large, happy, an acre of bright green giants with upturned, sun-soaking leaves.

HABITAT A circumboreal plant in the Northern Hemisphere, it can be found along the Pacific Coast, across the northern inland ranges, and down the Rockies, usually up near the snowfields in the high mountains. It grows in natural lakes and ponds and their marshes, from 8,000 to 10,000 feet in northern California, to 3,500 feet in northern Washington, and lower still further north.

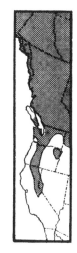

CONSTITUENTS Primarily menyanthin, with dihydrofoliamenthin, menthiafolin, loganin, saponins, amorphous bitter principles, and small amounts of a volatile oil containing hexanals, pentenols, and terpene aromatics.

COLLECTING Gather the leaves in the summer, reaching down far enough to get the full stem. Although the rhizomes are often recommended, the leaf is completely adequate. Contrary to much literature which recommends the dried plant only, the fresh plant tincture, in the small recommended doses, is the best medicine. With drainage of wetlands and acid rain, such pristine-environment plants as Buckbean are under great pressure. The dried herb loses much of its potency in just a few months; gathering the more stable root may damage small colonies; and the fresh leaf tincture, like that of Lobelia, performs all of its necessary effects in doses of a few drops, with the least amount of damage to this lovely plant.

STABILITY As mentioned above, the dried leaf deteriorates rapidly. If you prefer the dried herb for tea, keep it in airtight bags in the refrigerator or freezer when not being used. In this fashion, the dried leaves may be still active for up to two years; otherwise, six months is as long as you can expect Buckbean to retain its broad range of effects. After that, it is just another simple bitter tonic.

PREPARATION Fresh Plant Tincture, 1:2, Dry Plant Tincture (recently gathered plant), 1:5, 50% alcohol, both 10 to 30 drops. Cold Infusion, 1 to 2 fluid ounces. Use three times a day; as a bitter tonic, use 10 drops of tincture fifteen minutes before meals.

MEDICINAL USES Buckbean is for cold, deficient, achy conditions. It is not for hot, inflamed, or excess states. It is a widely used bitter tonic, particularly in Europe, but it is not for indigestion, dyspepsia, or acid indigestion when the throat is red, the tip of the tongue inflamed, and the mouth hypersecreting. Rather, it is for indigestion with a dry mouth, a heavy sensation in the stomach, poor digestion of proteins and fats, and a tendency for hemorrhoids and pelvic congestion. This is an herb for a lot of folks who need to eat carefully or combine foods to avoid intestinal problems, or who eat the wrong kinds of foods and develop a bit of rectal aching (if not an overt hemorrhoid flare-up) followed by constipation; Buckbean, by itself or with Yellow Dock, taken just before meals (or before lunch, dinner, and retiring) will distinctly aid this condition.

Those with arthritis or chronic allergies aggravated by food will find Buckbean particularly useful. It combines well with Baneberry or Black Cohosh for use when you have aching of joints, or with Figwort when you have swollen joints. If the skin is dry and/or scaly, or there is eczema or psoriasis combined with the arthritis, add a little Bittersweet or Oregon Grape root to the Buckbean. Give the herbs at least a couple of weeks to work.

CONTRAINDICATIONS Do not use for active intestinal inflammations.

Buckwheat Bush

Eriogonum spp.   (Polygonaceae)
OTHER NAMES   Wild Buckwheat, Sulphur Plant, Telegraph Weed

APPEARANCE   The *Eriogonums* are an immense genus, with over one hundred species in California alone, thinning out in numbers and diversity from Oregon northwards. Buckwheat Bush is a misleading name, as they bear little resemblance to their relative Buckwheat (*Fagopyron esculentum*). Our common species can be lumped crudely into three types. The bushes (*E. fasciculatum* and *E. wrightii*), both in the southern part of our area, are woody towards the base. The first type, 2 to 4 feet in height, having tight little bundles of green, Rosemarylike leaves up and down the stems; the pink-white flowers form compound umbels on skinny stems above the leaves. The second type has short, foot-long, woody, branching stems, with downy thin leaves and white flowers. Like most *Eriogonums*, these two take on a red-brown color in the stems, flowers, and leaves as the season progresses. Another type of *Eriogonum* is the Skeleton Weed (*E. deflexum* and others), with a few basal leaves and intricate, lacy branches with sometimes hundreds of little inconspicuous pink flowers. These are annuals that can cover the edges of roads and mesas with their filagreed remnants in the fall. They are mostly found in the eastern parts of the coastal states, on the dry sides of the ranges. The third type, characterized by Sulphur Flower (*E. umbellatum*), has many lower basal rosettes, with long, usually leafless flowering stalks covered in white, pink, or yellow umbels of pom-poms, sometimes appearing one umbel per stem, sometimes from secondary umbels, and sometimes up the stems, spike-style. These types of *Eriogonum* are nearly always silver-, grey-, or copper-leaved. Most of the *Eriogonums* have fuzzy leaves.

HABITAT   The bush types are found in foothills and chaparral of California, from Monterey County and Inyo County south to Baja California and east to Nevada and Arizona. The second, filigree-type annuals, are found everywhere in the desert, east of the Sierras and Cascades, and even east of the coastal ranges in the south. The third type, characterized by the most common species, *E. umbellatum*, can be found throughout the West, generally in foothills and mountains with a predominance of native flora.

CONSTITUENTS   Beta-sitosterol, gallic acid, quercetin, europetin, and myricetins flavonoids. *Eriogonums* are phosphorus concentrators, and high in that mineral.

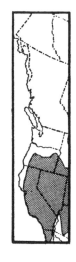

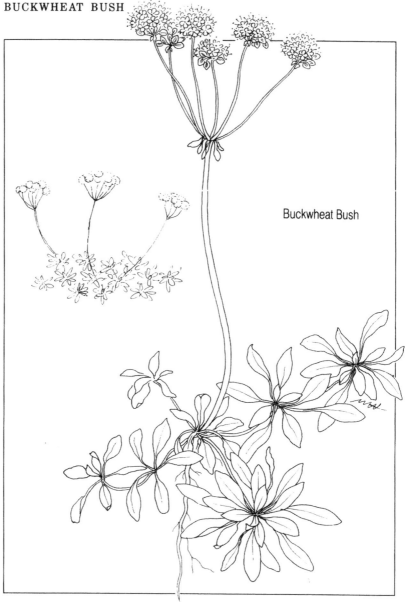

Buckwheat Bush

COLLECTING Gather the whole plant, in bloom—leaves, stems, and flowers. Dry Method A, Method B, or in paper bags, depending on the size of the plants or your mood.

STABILITY The herb should be stable and usable for at least two years.

PREPARATION Standard or Cold Infusion, as needed.

MEDICINAL USES Our information on the uses of the *Eriogonums* is completely the result of Native American and Mexican herbal traditions.

Buckwheat Bush is water soluble, without any toxicity, and can be taken as often as needed. It shrinks and soothes membranes that are inflamed, and slows secretions from irritated membranes. The isotonic tea is a good eyewash, and a number of California Indians have used the tea for washing newborn babies. Although not particularly heroic and glitzy, the tea is a soothing douche, gargle, and enema, as well as a good sitz bath. The dried flowers (not so much the foliage) make a simple diuretic, increasing the volume of urine, lowering the specific gravity, without irritating the kidneys. Because it makes the urine astringent, it is also useful for decreasing the mucus irritation of simple cystitis and urethritis. Its diuretic effects aid in premenstrual water retention, and its lack of any toxicity makes it safe to use for water retention in the last month or two of pregnancy.

The tea is a mild hemostatic; it will decrease spotting towards the end of menstruation; in addition, it can also be used internally for excessive postpartum bleeding *and* as a postpartum sitz bath. The Cahuillas use the tea for dull, nagging back and hip pain in the last trimester. Sick headaches, accompanied by coated tongue and pain predominately around the eyes, will sometimes respond to the hot tea, especially when it is the result of consuming too much booze or too much fried pork rind and (bleh) generic lite beer while watching Monday night (nite?) football. "Go Raiders! (Belch)."

Bunchberry

Cornus canadensis   (Cornaceae)

OTHER NAMES   Dwarf Dogwood, Dwarf Cornel, Pigeonberry

APPEARANCE Bunchberry is a cheerful forest-floor plant, usually around 6 inches tall, with at least one whorl of pointed overlapping oval leaves, usually from four to six in number, with occasional paired leaflets below, or even a second whorl. The leaves are bright green on top, lighter underneath, with seemingly parallel veins (Lilylike) that branch and network to a certain degree. This never occurs with the Lily family. If you grasp a leaf in both hands and carefully pull it apart a bit, you will find the signature of the Dogwoods: the veins contain a latex that connects, threadlike, between the separated halves. Dogwoods are big bushes and trees— except for Bunchberry. There is a single flower in the spring, with a light green center and four snow-white petals made out of modified leaves. By late summer these mature into bright red berries, from one to ten in number, that are edible but bland.

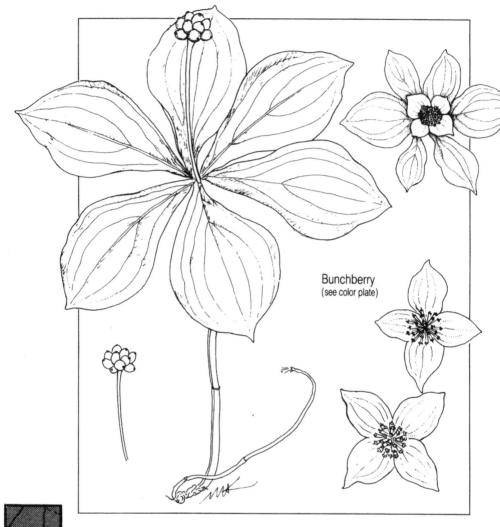

Bunchberry
(see color plate)

HABITAT Bunchberry grows in woods, period. Look for it in old- or second-growth forest, with duff, shade, and an established, diverse panache. Although found in northern coastal California, it is a plant of the coast ranges and Cascades, from Oregon north through Alaska and the Yukon; south through Alberta to the forests of Idaho and Montana; and east through Canada to the Atlantic.

CONSTITUENTS Cornine, cornic acid, quercetin, phenylethylamine, tannins, and at least eight flavonoids.

COLLECTING Gather the whole plants from summer to early fall, dry either Method A or, if all the plants are small and munchkin, simply dry Method B or in a paper bag. You can separate the ripe red berries for food or preserves, or let them dry up with the herb. Try to include an inch or two of the creeping root. I have no idea which part of the Bunchberry contains which constituents, so gather a bit of all.

STABILITY The dried plant is good for a year, probably two.

PREPARATION Standard Infusion, 3 to 4 fluid ounces, or 3 to 4 grams for a cup of tea, up to four times a day.

MEDICINAL USES Bunchberry has a mild, aspirinlike effect; it decreases inflammation, fever, and pain but does not cause stomach irritability or allergic reaction in those with negative responses to salicylates. Although not as strong or predictable as the aspirin relatives, it holds up under extended use, and for people with clammy headaches (slightly nauseating and causing a dampness of the neck and back), Bunchberry tea is useful. For fevers that are chilling, with goose bumps and shivering, Bunchberry is more reliable and less nauseating than other herbs I have tried, such as the bark of Dogwoods and Magnolia, and works well when salicylate plants like Poplar, Aspen, Willow, Wintergreen, and Meadowsweet cause undesirable, aspirinlike effects. The anti-inflammatory effects of both the cornine and the flavonoids, coupled with the astringency of the tannins, makes it a mild and predictable herb for colitis, dysentery, diarrhea, and chronic gastritis. Although not an antispasmodic like Angelica or Silk Tassel, it will often aid the heat and irritability of the lower ileum and ascending colon that causes abdominal gas cramps or mild colitis, lasting for several days after eating undercooked legumes, grains, or over-the-hill pepperoni sticks you bought at a convenience store before you noticed the sell-by date was two months expired.

OTHER USES In her delightful book *Discovering Wild Plants,* Janice Schofield has the following recipe for Bunchberry-Raspberry Syrup:
   2 cups bunchberries
   2 cups raspberries
   4 tablespoons water
   ¼ cup honey
Place fruits in a small saucepan with water and honey. Cook until soft, about ten minutes. Press cooked fruit through a colander or food mill. Use on pancakes or crepes. Store remainder in the refrigerator or root cellar.

California Bay

Umbellularia californica (Lauraceae)

OTHER NAMES California Laurel, Oregon Myrtle, Pepperwood, Mountain Laurel, California Pepper; *Oreodaphne californica*

APPEARANCE This well-known tree has the same size variation as its eastern relative, Sassafras. It may form a small, scraggly bush of only several branches or reach 100 feet in height. The leaves, whether growing on a baby shrub or mama tree, are the same size: 3 to 5 inches long, oblong, and pointed (like a Bay leaf), borne on a short petiole. The leafing branches may be long, often divided, and slender, of the same light and bright green color as the leaves, giving the appearance of long leaf stems; but the actual petiole is short. The leaf and stems are shiny-smooth, and the central vein is pronounced. The leaves are completely flat. The flowers form little lateral umbels in April, usually light yellow-green in color, and produce two or three oval seeds, green at first, and turning brittle and brown when mature.

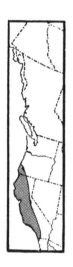

HABITAT California Bay grows from Coos County, Oregon, south to San Diego County, California. It is a plant of canyon walls, shaded slopes, and the remnants of our alluvial coastal plains; it sometimes even grows up on high, rocky knolls where vertical strata permit the roots of larger trees to strike deep for water. It basically follows deep or shallow moisture and is most fond of steep canyons with running water and gravelly creek deposits, where it can attain its greatest age and size. It can also be found in more modest numbers in lower canyons of the Sierra Nevada, following the inland ranges up across the Klamath and Siskiyou Mountains, and south across the Tehachapi and the Transverse ranges—in other words, the lower, wetter reaches of larger ranges west of the Mojave and Colorado deserts, and west of the Central Valley in California.

CONSTITUENTS Primarily the aromatic oil which contains camphene, pinene, and some other terpenoids, as well as domesticine, nordomesticine, isoboldine, and bufotenine.

COLLECTING Gather the healthy green leaves from April to late summer and dry in a paper bag. Fall and winter leaves may be fine for a cooking spice, but there seems to be some degradation of the oil constituents. It is possible to stuff a quart jar with 10 ounces of the fresh leaves in order to make a proper 1:2 tincture, but you will need a stick or piece of broom handle to do it, as they are very bulky for their weight.

STABILITY If kept in a closed bag in a cool place, the whole leaves will stay strong for about a year. They fade and chemically deteriorate if exposed to light for a prolonged time.

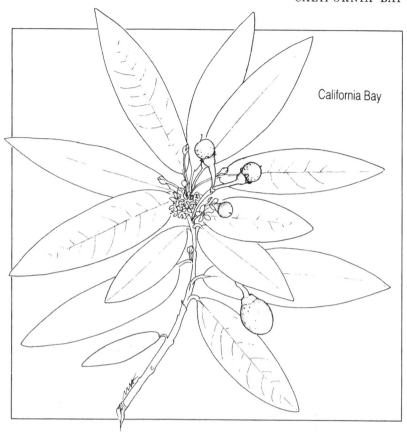

California Bay

PREPARATION Fresh Leaf Tincture, 1:2, or Recent Dry Leaf Tincture, 1:5, 65% alcohol, 15 to 30 drops in warm water or the tincture inhaled from a saturated cotton ball.

MEDICINAL USES The crushed leaf or the inhaled tincture acts as an effective "smelling salt" for someone who is dizzy or faint. Too much inhalation gives you a sharp sinus headache, which passes in a few minutes. Oddly enough the tincture is sometimes an effective therapy for frontal headaches or migraines that center around the forehead or behind the eyes. In general, the crushed leaves for tea or the tincture in a little hot water is a surprisingly useful anodyne and antispasmodic for headaches from muscle stress or neuralgia, and will help diarrhea or intestinal cramps that are the result of being tied up in emotional knots.

The diluted tincture or strong tea can be used as an antimicrobial skin wash or as a mild antifungal for tineas, athlete's foot, and general jungle rot in moist places. The herb causes a mild tingling at first, followed by a decrease in the itching. For joint pains and general arthritis, the tincture can be applied to the area, or a bath can be taken with the tea from a dozen crushed leaves added to the water. You may find that the bath makes your skin warm and prickly, but a good body rub with a towel will disperse the sensation and leave the joints looser and less painful.

OTHER USES The leaves can be used as a substitute for Bay Laurel leaves in cooking. The two trees are closely related, but Bay leaves from the Mediterranean region are usually old tree-dropped leaves, with much less fragrance than they should normally have; our leaves are (hopefully) fresh and strong, and you will need to use a third or half as much as your recipe calls for. Further, the taste is a bit different, although in the scheme of a 1-gallon barley soup batch there isn't a problem.

California Bayberry

Myrica californica   (Myricaceae)

OTHER NAMES   Pacific Wax Myrtle, California Wax Myrtle, Pacific Bayberry

APPEARANCE California Bayberry is a tall, spreading shrub or small tree, with several or many tall trunks (or thick stems) from 6 to 20 feet in height, forming a rounded crown. If it is growing by windy coastal strands, the shape may be lopsided in the direction away from the ocean gusts.

The bark is light grey to brown, with silver and green mottling, often covered with lichens and moss. The trunks divide into slender branches, fuzzy and green when new, gradually turning the same color as the larger trunks. The whole plant, especially around the sunlit edges, is densely covered in shiny green leaves, 2 to 4 inches long, with a few teeth along the edges, and broader above the middle. The foliage is somewhat sticky, and spicy-aromatic when crushed, evoking memories of old fraternal lodges, polished brass and leather, and clean-shaven, ancient white men wearing burgundy sashes. In the spring the junctures of the alternate leaves sport male and female flowers, stubby little spikes of different sexes, the males usually lower on the branches. The females mature by early fall into mauve or brown clustered berries, pitted like golf balls ⅛ inch around, and spicy-waxy tasting. The roots are woody, irregular, and thick barked, with reddish brown color that sometimes permeates the wood as well.

Plants that have fallen, been injured, or damaged by weather have the most red pigment, and I usually ignore the big, verdant bushes, looking instead for partially uprooted or weather-damaged plants with some live branches and some dead growth. Roots partially exposed by erosion are strongest, and the surviving trunks will have stronger bark as well.

HABITAT California Bayberry is a plant that grows within coastal breezes,

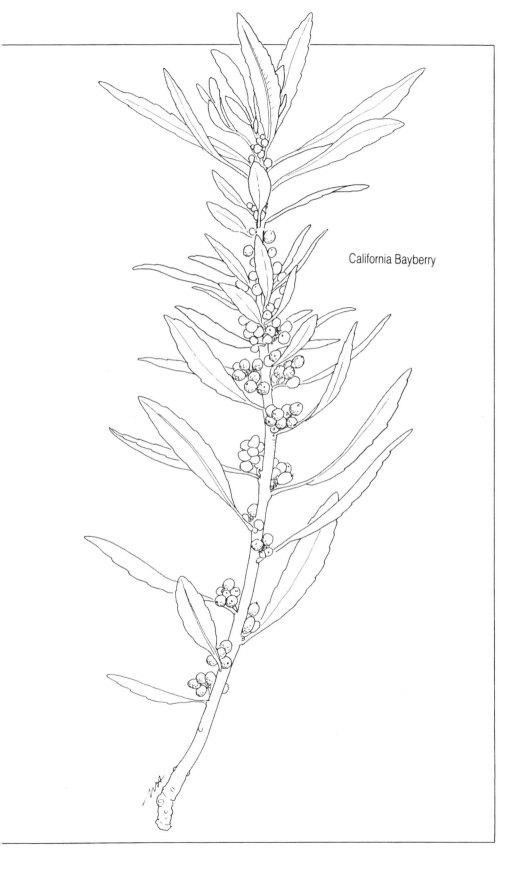

California Bayberry

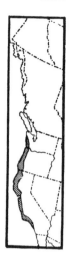

from the Ventura–Los Angeles County line north almost to the Olympic Peninsula of Washington, usually within sight of the ocean and below 500 feet. I have found stands 50 miles inland on the west slopes of coastal mountains, but if you see some Bayberry you can nearly always still hear seagulls . . . if not be engulfed in fog or splashed by seawater.

CONSTITUENTS Myricinic acid (an astringent resin) accounts for much of the effect of the herb, along with the flavonoid myricitin, several triterpenes, myricic acid, tannic and mallic acids, and, in the leaves, myricic and gallic acids and volatile oil.

COLLECTING Gather the leaves in the spring or early summer, and the root bark, lower trunk bark, and usable root wood in late summer through late fall. As mentioned, stressed plants will often have the root and even trunk wood permeated with the red resins that signal strength. That being the case, keep the roots, stems, and root crown pieces covered in wet cloth while you strip off the bark and gradually hack down the root wood. It is a tough-rooted plant and takes a lot of work to dig; and that is why I like to cheat. I find a semidowned grove of bushes, cut off some exposed roots, exposed crowns, high-grade a stunted trunk or two, and leave the rest. If you don't break down the pieces into manageable chips while fresh, it is a lost cause, so when your hand gives out, store the roots with your vegetables in the refrigerator for a day or two. If you simply aren't able to work the wood, or the wood is lacking in the red resin, just use the bark of the root and trunks. If you do not wish to damage the bushes, or if it is inappropriate to dig, then clip an older central trunk or two from the center of a grove, and just use the trunk and mature branch bark. It won't be as potent, but it works just fine. Simply use a little more tincture or tea. If you need the root as a powder, you will have to use the bark; you will powder your blender blade before the wood chips are any more than blunted.

STABILITY The dried leaves, left whole, are still tasty after eighteen months. The dried bark and wood are strong for at least a year, both in heating and astringent aspects. After that, the vasodilating resins deteriorate, with the astringent acids becoming more dominant. *Myrica cerifera*, the "official" herb (formerly the drug plant), is higher in myricinic acid resin when recently gathered (and more heating) than our plant. I have picked *M. cerifera* in Louisiana, and it is overwhelmingly peppery; I drooled into my beard for hours. If, however, you have purchased Bayberry from the trade, you will find it more astringent and less stimulating than the Pacific plant you picked a year ago. What does *that* tell you, kids?

PREPARATION Fresh Root Tincture, 1:2, Dried Root Bark Tincture, 1:5, both 20 to 60 drops, or diluted for topical use or as a mouthwash.

The powdered bark is used to make the Thomsonian Composition Powder: bark 60%, dried Ginger Root 30%, Capsicum (African Cayenne) 5%, and Cloves 5%. The best method is to combine the four herbs coarsely chopped, grinding them together, straining them, and regrinding the coarser pieces until they are all reduced to a consistent particle size. Store in a closed container in a cool dark place. Dose, ½ to 1 teaspoon in a cup of hot water, sipped slowly.

MEDICINAL USES The diluted tincture is a world-class treatment for puffy and sporadically inflamed gums; if you use it morning and evening, the gums will usually heal. Bayberry has two distinctive effects: it stimulates blood supply through vasodilation, and it shrinks connective tissue and surface membranes—hot *and* cold, if you will. When an inflammation occurs, it is usually the result of injury to the local tissues that triggers the release of substances such as histamines, meant to bring blood to the area and increase the permeability of capillaries. This brings fuel and building materials to the injury, and ideally speeds up the removal of the waste products by white blood cells and increases lymph drainage. Capillaries are able to withstand this drastic increase in their diameter, intentional leakage, and disruption of their blood protein-repelling membrane charge by constant movement of the white blood cells in the blood out through the gaps . . . for a while.

If the irritation that caused the inflammation does not cease, after a period of time the distended capillary cells start to lose their ability to keep the blood proteins inside, and they leak out. In most tissues, the cells outside the bloodstream are held in compact masses by a starch "Jell-O" that dehydrates water from them (a waste product of glucose combustion), maintains a constant stream of blood serum across their surface, and sends the blood serum either back into the exiting capillaries or out into the lymph capillaries. Too much blood protein dissolves this "Jell-O" and, with increased rates of combustion and metabolism made possible by the increased blood supply, and with increased waste products from healing, the loss of the "Jell-O" results in fluid stagnation between the cells. This postinflammatory state brings edema to the injured tissues and also prevents lymph from draining away the dirty interstitial "mother ocean." The hot tissue gets puffy and congested. This is very obvious in a burn on your hand, with hot followed by edema, the edema then organized into a fluid cyst (blister). In the general scheme of things, cells can store extra fuel, either as lipids or glycogen, and they don't starve easily. Cells *cannot* store their waste products; they are supposed to be removed from the "Jell-O" surrounding them by exiting blood or by the lymph, and they are far more damaged by stagnant fluids than lack of fuels and oxygen. When a tissue is congested in this fashion, it needs to have its structure tightened and its waste products removed by being bathed by moving fluids. Bayberry is tightening and astringent to the connective tissue cells that are the skeleton to any group of cells, and it dilates the blood vessels that go through the tissue. If you have a sore throat, gargle the herb, particularly if you have had it a while. If you have been sick, with poor digestion, constipation, and a general sensation of coldness, use the herb internally in some hot water. If you have some slowly healing skin abrasions or minor ulcers, use the diluted tincture or the powdered bark for several days. Further, if you have a skin fungus, or tinea, mix the tincture with equal parts of Red Cedar (*Thuja plicata*) tincture, and paint it on the sores.

Finally, the composition powder, an old remedy of Samuel Thomson, will abort a simple viral cold, if taken at the first signs: dry throat and sinuses, crankiness, and recent exposure to someone else with a cold, or recent exhausting physical or emotional trauma. Just use ½ to 1 teaspoon of the powder, suspended in a cup of boiling hot water that has cooled a bit, and sip it slowly. For sinus allergies, it will cause rapid short-term drooling and running, but it will leave you with open sinuses . . . for a few hours.

The leaf tea tastes spicy and tart, and can be used alone for a nice warming tea (vasodilating to the surface) or added to other more conventional herbs simply for its pleasant aftertaste.

California Buckeye

Aesculus californica   (Hippocastanaceae)
OTHER NAMES   California Horse Chestnut

APPEARANCE This is a handsome deciduous shrub-tree, with a branching, spreading appearance, vaguely resembling a wild fruit tree. The typical Buckeye/Horse Chestnut leaves are palmate, with five or seven leaflets, the leaflets strongly central-veined, and the lateral sides folded upwards from the vein forming a "V" in cross-section. In late May or early June, especially with good early spring rains, the 10- to 30-foot-tall shrub sends out white flowering spikes. These spikes are covered in four- or five-petaled flowers with long stamens. A pleasant, subdued bush otherwise, these spikes make it startling in appearance. By early fall the single capsule that forms from the spike starts to split, showing a single reddish, pear-shaped nut inside.

HABITAT The coastal and inner coastal ranges of California, and the southwestern foothills of the Sierra Nevada range, from Trinity and Mendocino counties, south to Ventura, Kern, and even northern Los Angeles County. Look for it where the Oaks meet the Pines, from almost sea level to (usually) 2,000 to 4,000 feet.

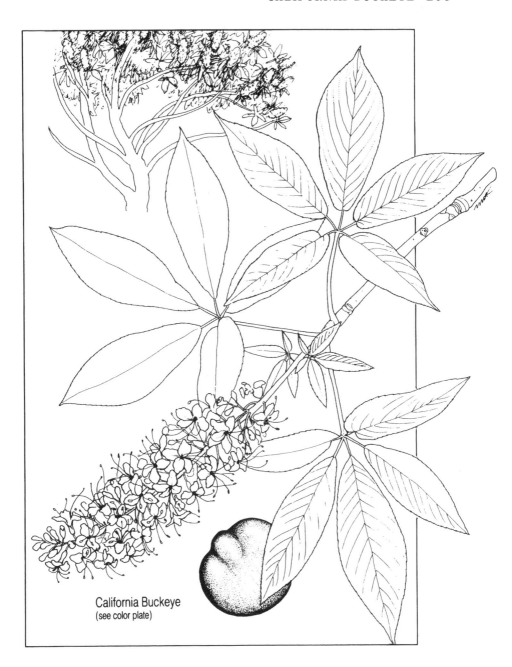

California Buckeye
(see color plate)

CONSTITUENTS Aesculin (esculin), aescin, hydroquinone, (-)-epica-techin, and several other assorted flavonoids.

COLLECTING The nearly ripe to ripe seeds (the husk beginning to sep-arate from the seed or already split from it), sliced while still fresh, and dried, Method B. The leaves (summer), dried on the branch.

STABILITY Not pertinent.

PREPARATION Dry Fruit Tincture, 1:5, 50% alcohol; Leaf Salve, Method A.

MEDICINAL USES This, like its other relatives, is a tough one for the medical profession to understand. Its drug effects are scary and would seem to point to using it as a pharmaceutical, not an herb. Its strychninelike stimulus of motor functions, with increased firing of both halves of the autonomics, makes it a typical weasel-drug perfect for pharmacologic and medical study. In fact, the whole genus has been studied extensively and relegated to the toxicologists. The drug effects are simply poisonous, and indeed it is consumed accidentally by enough kids and ignorant adults that poison control centers get calls every year from people who have ingested it and gotten sick. *Our* use is ten levels below the toxic effects, and has nothing to do with its drug properties. In the proper adult doses of 5 to 15 drops of the tincture, morning and evening, it acts to strengthen the capillaries, decreasing their permeability, and lessening edema. This is most noticeable in the intestinal tract (hemorrhoids) and the portal system that drains the intestinal blood into the liver (subclinical portal congestion). If you have hemorrhoids, varicose veins in the inner thigh, dull ache on urination, or dull pain in the prostate or uterus, try this approach, adding some citrus flavonoids, rutin, and a quercetrin source, such as White Oak bark. Short-term food-related congestion is handled better by Ocotillo (*Fouquieria splendens*); California Buckeye works better for the chronic, congested, and vascular-weak person. For varicose veins, apply the salve at night (covered with gauze), and take the tincture twice a day. For spiderweb varicosities, use the salve alone at night, wash off in the morning. For general portal congestion, with all the above pelvic symptoms, combine the California Buckeye tincture with Red Root and use 60 drops of the tincture, twice a day.

California Mugwort

Artemesia vulgaris, var. *Douglasiana*   (Compositae)
OTHER NAMES   Douglas Mugwort; *A. Douglasiana, A. californica*

APPEARANCE California Mugwort is a colony plant, forming stands of several to hundreds of individuals, all interconnected by underground rootstalks. In the full growth of late summer, the plants are from 3 to 7 feet tall. The leaves are lance-shaped, the lower ones variously cleft and the upper ones smaller and entire. They are dark green above and sil-

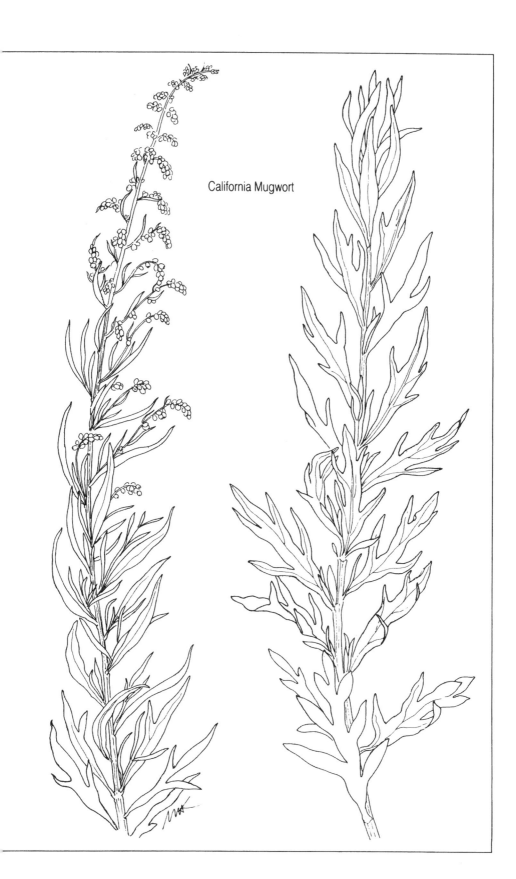

California Mugwort

very underneath, fading variously by fall to mottled silvery brown and red on the lower leaves. The flowers, in many and extended small-stemmed spikes, may extend to a foot or more in height, and emerge from leaf axils. They are the typical tiny blah-buttons of the Wormwood genus. The stems are ridged for strength: the taller the plant, the more pronounced the ridges. The whole plant is strongly and pleasantly aromatic, Sagelike, and quite bitter to the taste.

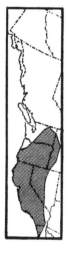

HABITAT California Mugwort is found from northern Baja California, northwards through nearly all of California; in western Nevada, Oregon, and California, mostly west of the Cascades; and east through Idaho, into Montana and the Rockies. This is not a clearly defined variety, especially in the north and east of its range; from Oregon southwards it is a clear biotype; elsewhere it intergrades with var. *lindleyana* and var. *ludoviciana,* which some botanists class as separate species. The *Artemisia ludoviciana* type is furry on top of the leaf as well, and tends to a semireclined shape under normal growth conditions. This is of more than passing importance, since the constituents of the typical California Mugwort are rather different than those of the typical *A. ludoviciana.* California Mugwort is most common in lower moist valleys and near lower mountain streams, although it may occur up to 6,000 feet in California. It is most common on the west slopes of inland foothills and along the coast.

CONSTITUENTS Caffeoylquinic acids, chlorogenic acid, and at least twenty-two related guaianolide sesquiterpene lactones, including dihydroleucodin, a cytoprotectant.

COLLECTING Gather in summer and fall, discarding discolored leaves, and dry Method A. When dry, strip foliage and floral parts from the larger stems, and, in order to retain the aromatics, store in a whole herb form, in a way that avoids crushing.

STABILITY Stored properly, the herb should be usable for up to two years.

PREPARATION The Cold Infusion, 2 to 3 fluid ounces. This is the basic form for stomach and liver uses. For sweating, expectoration, and sinuses, use the Standard Infusion, 2 to 3 fluid ounces every three to four hours, as needed. For external use, the tea (either form) or a 1:5 tincture using apple cider vinegar as the menstruum are the best methods.

MEDICINAL USES First of all, the tea is very effective for chronic gastritis and gastric ulcers. It acts to decrease secretions when taken as a cold infusion, and several of the constituents act to decrease degradation of the cells of the stomach and esophagus mucosa, protecting them both from degeneration and from the excess secretion of the proteolytic acids that cause the irritation. The tea is best taken an hour before dinner and just before retiring at night. When things are in a painful, acute phase, make up a pint of the tea at night to have for the next day, and take a few sips when the pain occurs (as well as the evening doses) until the pain subsides.

California Mugwort is also an antioxidant for cooling fat metabolism, especially in the liver. If you wake up in the morning with a grey sheet over your psyche, your head hurts in the front, your mouth tastes like a three-day-old Greek salad, your hemorrhoids are aching, and you crave things like pizza, potato chips, or fry bread, take the cold infusion once at night for a couple of weeks. Usually the craving for fats will lessen, the chylomicrons (fat globules) in the blood will lessen, and the fat overload on digestion will improve. Everyone knows sugar cravings, but some people have the same feelings about fats, overload their diet with them (the sleazier the better), snack on them at night, wake up with what old docs called "biliousness," and never make the connection. Elevated blood fats lower the colloid charge of both the blood and the vessel linings. The blood tends to stack up, clump, and move less gracefully through the capillaries, causing headaches, exciting inflammatory responses, backing up the blood into the liver from the portal system, and causing pelvic congestion. Take the tea at night . . . trust me.

The hot tea is an effective diaphoretic with which to break fevers and is sometimes a very effective stimulant to the discharge of mucus in the sinuses and the lungs. Try combining the tea with Yerba Mansa. For sinus pain, with red eyes and frontal headache, use the hot tea with a couple of squirts of Feverfew or Oxeye Daisy tinctures. California Mugwort, especially drunk hot, will tend to stimulate uterine secretions and may help shake loose a cold, slow, and crampy period; conversely, at the wrong time it may overstimulate a normal menstruation, so bear that in mind when using it.

The tea or acetum (vinegar) tincture can be used as a liniment or fomentation for sprains, hyperextensions, and bruises, as it is a mild counterirritant, a topical anesthetic, and somewhat anti-inflammatory. Use it on the forehead for sick headaches, headaches from the sun, and nausea.

The tea is antifungal and antimicrobial, and can be used for a variety of first aid purposes. The flowers especially can be used in making a first aid salve, using either Method A or Method B.

CONTRAINDICATIONS Since California Mugwort stimulates the uterine lining, it is inappropriate to use during pregnancy.

OTHER USES The spring plants, about ½ to 1 feet tall and growing in sandy riverside soil, can be gathered, dried Method A, the leaves stripped from the stems, and rolled up to use for moxibustion in Traditional Chinese Medicine.

California Poppy

Eschscholzia californica   (Papaveraceae)
OTHER NAMES   Gold Poppy; *Amapola Amarilla, Dormidera; E. mexicana, E. arizonica*

APPEARANCE California Poppy, in good localities, has many lime green basal leaves, divided into blunt-lacy succulent leaves, and forming orange, bowl-shaped, four-petaled flowers on leafless stems. It has the color of a double-dip lime and orange sherbet cone. The flowers mature into succulent, horned capsules with a round ring around the base. The plant is usually an annual, but in warm, moist areas it may become a short-lived perennial with a juicy taproot. The plant usually flowers in the spring, but may bloom until fall, with consistent rains, or die back and blossom again with late summer rains. Patches of yellow-flowered plants in an orange-flowered stand, or areas with only yellow flowers, signify a patch of heavily mineralized soil, containing anything from arsenic to selenium to copper. This phenomenon has been used with some reliability as a copper signifier by miners, both in the U.S. and Mexico. Considering this, it is probably not a good idea to gather yellow-flowered plants, thereby avoiding the potentiality of unwanted metals in the dried herb. It is known to concentrate them when they occur.

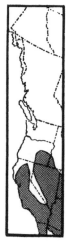

HABITAT With good spring rains, it grows in abundance throughout the lower altitudes of California, Oregon, Nevada, and Arizona. Those glorious wildflower displays after March rains in California are composed of Lupine, Indian Warrior, California Poppy, and one of several yellow flowers, airbrushed in Day-Glo paint across hillsides in a most improbable mixture of yellow, orange, blue, and purple. In the northwest and the colder mountains of the south, California Poppy escapes gleefully from gardens and may form wild populations that last for several years. In Baja California and Sonora it interbreeds with (or becomes) *E. mexicana,* a marginally distinct form with smaller leaves and a flowering stalk usually under a foot in height. There is no difference between any of the varieties, at least in terms of their medicinal use.

CONSTITUENTS Protopine, cryptopine, chelidonine, sanguinarine, macarpine, chelerythrine, chelirubine, and other isoquinoline alkaloids; rutin and other flavone glycosides.

COLLECTING Gather orange-flowered plants in full bloom, root and all; remove dead basal leaves, and dry Method A (if tall enough), Method B, or in a paper bag.

STABILITY The dried herb should be good for at least eighteen months. California Poppy is a delicate plant, easily degraded by sunlight, so store it in a dark, airtight container.

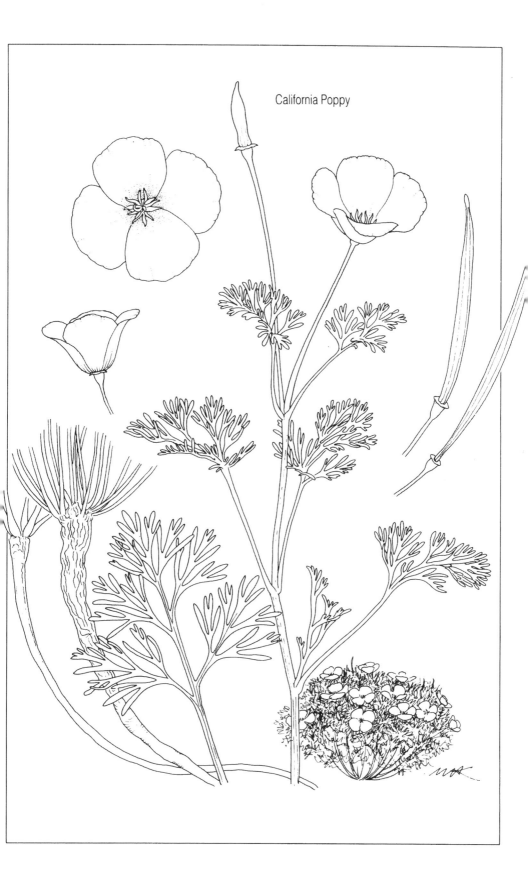

California Poppy

PREPARATION Dried Plant Tincture, 1:5, 50% alcohol, Fresh Plant Tincture, 1:2, both 30 to 60 drops, up to four times a day; Standard Infusion, 2 to 4 fluid ounces, up to four times a day (although the tea tastes ghastly).

MEDICINAL USES The therapeutics for California Poppy can be divided into an antianxiety and sedative use, and an analgesic use.

To begin with, it is a surprisingly effective herb for use with anxieties, jittery nervousness—a sort of controlled heebie jeebies, with skin hypersensitivity and peripatetic movements. It isn't as subtle and etheric as Hypericum or Western Pasque Flower (although it can be combined with them), as nerve-oriented as Skullcap, as overtly sedative as Valerian (although California Poppy modifies Valerian's tendency to overstimulate cardiovascular and digestive functions when used together); nor is it as sedative to the skeletal muscles as Betony (although it, too, combines well to amplify any analgesic effects needed). When used as a sedative, California Poppy causes relaxation and a genial lethargy, most pronounced in the fresh plant tincture, but present in preparations of the dried plant. Be aware that the higher, sedative dose can interfere with such activities as driving, operating a drill press, or working as a flight controller. The lower, antianxiety doses should not induce this, but everyone's different. It is safe, however, and a little tincture helps hyperactive, bright-eyed, can't-fall-asleep children—if you can get them to put up with the nasty taste.

For pain relief, such as stomach cramps, bruised muscles, a toothache the night before seeing the dentist, take enough to deaden the pain a bit. It ain't opium, and it will only have a certain degree of analgesic effect, but it always helps, especially when the pain is keeping you awake. Combine it with Valerian for added effect.

CONTRAINDICATIONS Do not take with prescription medications; the alkaloids are present in safe quantities, but undesirable synergies are always possible. Although it does not contain the same alkaloids as the opiates, they are chemically similar enough to cause a possible false positive in urine testing for opiates. It is probably inappropriate to use during pregnancy, although I don't know any specific reason to worry.

California Snakeroot

Aristolochia californica   (Aristolochiaceae)

OTHER NAMES   Dutchman's Pipe, California Pipe Vine

APPEARANCE This is a large and substantial vine, with large alternate, silky leaves, bigger on the lower stems, smaller towards the ends. In most localities it is velvet-smooth. In dry localities the leaves may be rough and fairly thick. They are from 2 to 4 inches long, with a somewhat rounded, triangular shape, and bitter-tasting. The stems are thick, succulent-tough, often woody towards the base, and arise from a thick, grey-brown root, often traveling below the ground for many feet like a buried cable. The flowers hang from long stems at the end of the vine—large, pendulous, inflated, green-purple, peculiar looking, and from 1 to 1½ inches long. They mature into thick, six-winged, football-shaped pods, usually around two inches long. This plant seems to bear a closer resemblance to the Pacific *Aristolochias* of Mexico than to the eastern North American species.

HABITAT It is found from Monterey County in California, north on both sides of the north coastal range; east to the northern foothills of the Sierra Nevada; and down on the lower western sides as far south as Tulare. It seems most common in the foothills of the northern Sacramento Valley and the north coastal range in Sonoma and Mendocino counties. It is fairly abundant in general, but hard to locate (as are most of its relatives). It climbs up shrubs and into trees, across and into Raspberry and Blackberry thickets; and on open, sandy riversides, it may even send up stubby, erect stems of 2 or 3 feet in height, with large alternate leaves, widely spaced and horizontal to the ground. It may be easiest to ask a local botanist where it can be found or check for specimen collection localities at your nearest college herbarium. It does not occur outside of northern California, although it would be an interesting plant to grow from a root section with the crown.

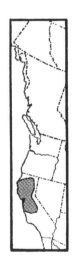

CONSTITUENTS Aristolochic acid, aristolactone, and probably the alkaloid aristolochine. This striking plant, from a well-studied genus, seems to have had no natural products chemistry research.

COLLECTING It's best to gather the roots and main stems (removing the leaves) from late July to late September, after it has seeded and is in its photosynthesizing, root storage stage. If there aren't too many individuals where you gather, feel in the soil around the crown to find which way the roots grow, and dig the roots from a foot away, distal to the stem. Trim the stem back to the lowest couple of leaves, keep the rest of the main stem, and then (as always) cover the trench back up. This will allow the deciduous plant to regenerate the next year.

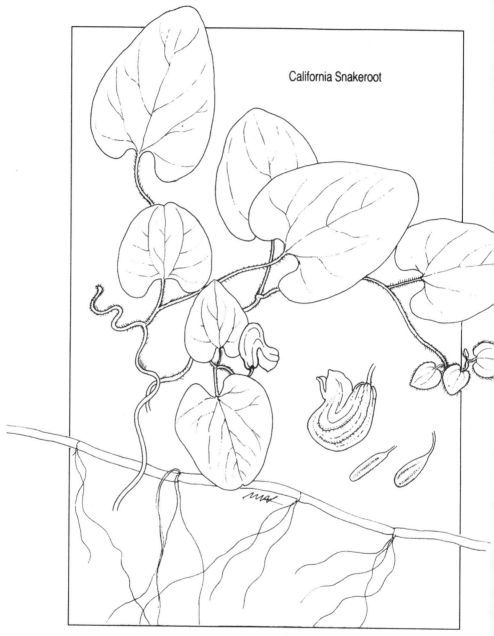

California Snakeroot

STABILITY Not pertinent.

PREPARATION Fresh Root and Stem Tincture, 1:2. Dry Root Tincture (no stem), 1:5, 70% alcohol. Dose: 5 to 20 drops, up to four times a day.

MEDICINAL USES There are few equals to the North American *Aristolochias* as simple bitter tonics. Like the Gentians, the bitterness of California Snakeroot is primarily derived from an acid (aristolochic acid), and traditionally that is the ideal characteristic of the best vegetable bitter tonics.

Much of the ability to digest, absorb, and excrete your food depends on an orderly sequence in the upper intestinal tract. You salivate in the presence of food (beginning complex carbohydrate digestion from saliva enzymes), trigger stomach secretions and relaxation of the esophagus, then acidify the food in the stomach in small, consecutive, ½-cup amounts. These are sent into the duodenum, where hormones secreted by the stomach have stimulated the gallbladder and pancreas juices, and the acidified stomach bolus is inoculated by alkaline, fat emulsifying mixed duodenal secretions. The rest of the small intestine has absorption sites and juices that further break down and methodically absorb the progressively digested foods. When upper GI functions are impaired, the usual cause is adrenergic stress, although heavy drinking can also contribute. If you just have a dry gut, with indigestion and symptoms of achlorhydria, probably your best bet will be a bitter that has little physiologic or drug effect, such as Gentian. If you also have poor fat digestion, dry skin, frequent low-grade infections, and a thick, broad tongue, California Snakeroot would be a preferable bitter, as it has the added effects of stimulating liver protein metabolism and white blood cell (innate immunity) scavenging.

During recuperation from an illness, the tincture helps improve appetite and restore nitrogen metabolism. Aristolochic acid is tumor-inhibiting, and the refined substance was screened thoroughly in the 1970s as a potential cancer treatment. Unfortunately, by itself, in anti-tumor doses, it is highly toxic. In the process of researching, the whole plant extracts of a number of *Aristolochias* were found to have strong stimulant effects on cultured white blood cells (neutrophils and macrophages in the tests), increasing their rebound and scavenging after being chemically depressed. In real people of reasonable vital signs, and without serious disease, there is little doubt that a little tincture, together with sensible treatment in general, helps to speed up both resistance and recovery. The big macrophages are resident in many organs and tissues, and cleanse and protect their turf. They act as intermediates between the basic cleansing, healing, and scavenging resistance (innate immunity), and the resistance that can program, remember, and learn specific disease-causing agents (acquired immunity). Both California Snakeroot and *Astragalus* stimulate macrophages and would reasonably aid both general and specific immunity. Further, the liver, spleen, and lungs are very dependent on their macrophages to function smoothly, and it would also be reasonable to use this plant to support them under stressful circumstances. Of course, this is not a panacea; excessive use can overstimulate the intestinal tract and overheat the skin and mucosa from peripheral vasodilation. Use it for a few days if you feel sick, in small doses with other herbs, or for a change in lifestyle if you are using it tonically.

CONTRAINDICATIONS Avoid during pregnancy or for vascular or liver disease (except for early arteriosclerosis). As with most of the stronger *Aristolochias,* the effect of increasing liver metabolism and phagocytosis makes it inappropriate to use with medications, as their effects are carefully measured, in part based on normal liver catabolism. Medications may be metabolized too quickly or, often being liver irritants anyway, they may be synergistic with the Snakeroot and result in hepatic irritability.

California Spikenard

Aralia californica   (Araliaceae)

OTHER NAMES Western Aralia, Western Spikenard, California Ginseng

APPEARANCE The striking thing about this lovely plant is how *big* it is. It is the largest herbaceous North American Aralia, sometimes 10 feet tall. The leaves are large, too, and compound into three stems that pinnate into five or seven leaflets, all borne off of long stalks that terminate variously in panicles of yellow-green flowers (midsummer) that mature into blue-black juicy berries the size of peppercorns (early fall). The leaves vary in form, the flowers may come off of side branches, and there may be one to ten stems from a single root. With its tendency to form stands of individuals in ravines, on creeksides, and in shady notches, what you see is a big bunch of improbably large, green, succulent plants, nodding out from some shady dell, like Elderberries on growth hormone.

The crushed foliage is sweet-balsamic smelling, and the fresh berries taste, to this herbalist, like freshly dug American Ginseng from the Missouri Ozarks. The roots are brown on the outside and yellow-beige on the inside, with the thick outer bark honeycombed with resin glands. The roots are as gigantic as the foliage: thick, tumorous, with long, snakelike roots deeply embedded in rocks and humus, the crowns bearing steplike round scars from previous years' growth, Ginsenglike. The fleshy roots taste balsamic and bittersweet. Plants from the inland ranges have a stronger taste than the more common coastal plants and are probably a stronger medicine.

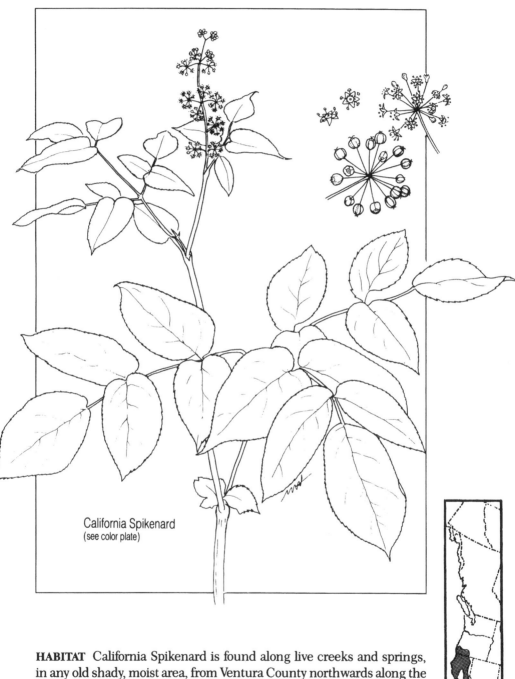

California Spikenard
(see color plate)

HABITAT California Spikenard is found along live creeks and springs, in any old shady, moist area, from Ventura County northwards along the coastal side of the coastal mountains; to southwestern Oregon; across the Klamath Mountains to the northern Sierra Nevada–southern Cascade Range junction; and down the western face of the Sierras to

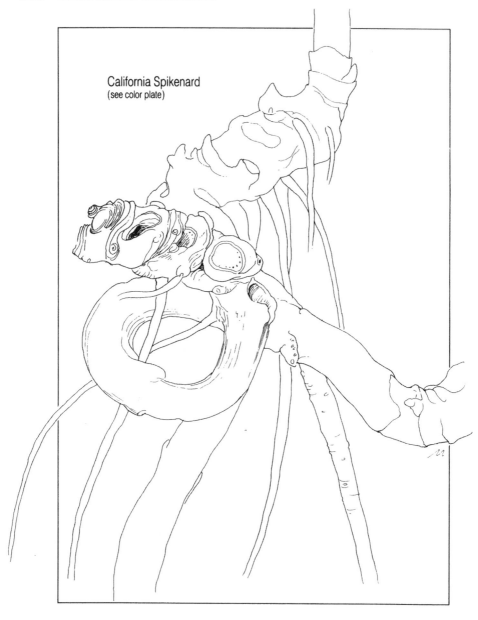

California Spikenard
(see color plate)

Mariposa County. I have seen it growing to almost 6,000 feet in Siskiyou County, California, but it usually likes much lower areas.

CONSTITUENTS The oleoresin seems to resist analysis; other constituents can be presumed to be choline, chlorogenic acid, ursolic acids, beta-sitosterol, araloside, oleanic acid glycosides, and some panaxosides.

COLLECTING The roots can be gathered at any time of the year, although spring roots make a better cough syrup and expectorant, and fall roots seem to have better tonic effects. Dry the roots whole or in large chunks, Method B, and keep them intact until you use them. They dry brittle-pulpy and are not particularly difficult to process when dry. The leaves are best gathered in summer and dried Method A. The berries are only around for a couple of weeks at the end of August and early September, so gather the umbels then and make fresh tincture.

STABILITY The dried root and leaves are surprisingly delicate and not much good after a year. The oils deteriorate rather rapidly for such a large root, and much of its respiratory effects are lost after a year. That's why I like the tincture or cough syrup.

PREPARATION Fresh Root Tincture, 1:2, Dry Root Tincture, 1:5, 60% alcohol, both types 30 to 90 drops, up to four times a day. The Cough Syrup, 1 teaspoon every couple of hours or as needed. The Fresh Berry Tincture, 1:2, ½ to 1 teaspoon when necessary. The Leaf Tea as needed. For the syrup, chop up 1 cup of the fresh root, add 4 cups of honey, bring to a *very* low boil, simmer for a couple of hours, remove from the heat, and allow the mixture to sit overnight. Warm it up enough the next morning to pour and strain. Measure the finished syrup; if the volume is greater than 4 cups, simmer it slowly to reduce the volume until it is back where it started. Juicy roots may add so much moisture to the honey (which dehydrates them) that the additional juices might cause fermentation. If it's the same or less, ignore me.

MEDICINAL USES California Spikenard, along with its better-known eastern relative *Aralia racemosa*, is an excellent tonic and soothing expectorant for people with chronic moist-lung problems—the person who responds to damp, coastal fog with morning hacking, or the binge smoker, usually a pack-a-day consumer who does up to two packs (plus borrowed ones) at a drunken brawl on Saturday night and breathes *carefully* all day Sunday. The cough syrup, tincture in hot water (toddylike), or the leaf tea is a good way to recuperate from some bronchitis or the winter lung-grunge. Older folks with a history of lung problems, mild emphysema, or who are recuperating from thirty years of cigarette use will find that the tincture or leaf tea in the morning and evening will improve respiration noticeably.

The syrup is also particularly helpful when you first start to get throat or pulmonary irritation, with sharp, dry, and percussive coughing, but without any mucus to expectorate. Between the physical soothing of the honey and the antimicrobial and anti-inflammatory effects of the fresh root constituents, it allays the pain and heat rather quickly; the aromatic resins help to stimulate throat and bronchial secretions by reflex excitation of the mucus glands, helping to reestablish normal moisture.

The tinctures, both of the root and berries, are similar to those of other

Araliaceae herbs, such as Ginseng, Siberian Ginseng, and Devil's Club; they act as tonics and modifiers both to the limbic system and to physical stress. If you are in finals week, have one of those mythic "reports" to get out, have to move both your household and business, are playing out the endgame of a long relationship, or going on a two-week Sierra crest hike with full 50-pound pack ("*How* did I let myself get talked into this thing, anyway?"), then taking some California Spikenard will help decrease some of the adverse stress responses. I have found that if you are a cold-blooded Sunbelt kind of person, the berry tincture helps keep you warm and cheerful while attending a family reunion in Coos Bay, Oregon, in November, or attending the myotherapy symposium in Victoria, B.C., in March, when the fog is so thick you walk blindly into the Japanese maples in the botanical garden that you visit on your free day.

The root is a useful topical anti-inflammatory, and the fresh pulp, a strong batch of the dry root tea, or the diluted tincture can be applied to shingles, herpes eruptions, rashes in moist skin folds, eczema, and contact dermatitis. Further, the dried herb helps both the flavor and function of electrolyte or alkalizing teas that contain Nettle, Red Clover, and/or Alfalfa. Further, an old hiker's manual from the Teddy Roosevelt–John Muir era (when everything was made from leather, cotton, canvas, and oilcloth) recommended chewing on the root to keep your mouth moist, your lungs clear, and your mind smack-dab on the hardy good fellowship of the wilderness (and off the bone bruise on your left heel, the strap rash under the pack, and the provisions, now reduced to coconut-pineapple-sunflower seed-and-weird-green-things trail mix and a package of freeze-dried turnip and leek soup). Anyway, it seems to help.

Desert Milkweed

Asclepias erosa, A. subulata, A. albicans   (Asclepiadaceae)
OTHER NAMES Lechona, Rush Milkweed, White-Stemmed Milkweed

APPEARANCE Although in the accepted botanically patronizing "Common Name" (taxonomy for the unwashed lay public) tradition only *Asclepias erosa* is called Desert Milkweed, the other two are only found in the desert, they are relatively common, and I have decided to lump them together.

Asclepias erosa is a xerophytic adaptation of the Common Milkweed theme: large opposite leaves, semiclasping around the stem and woolly-cobwebby in the spring, maturing to dusty, fuzzy, glabrous, 6-inch-long oval, pointed, and leathery leaves. The typical rounded Milkweed flowers, when blooming, are chartreuse to light yellow; the length of each flower's stem (pedicel) is longer than the length of the whole cluster's stem (peduncle) above the nearest stem-leaves. (Forgive me, but it is hard to say the pedicels exceed the peduncles with a straight face. Word-playing ex-musicians should not be allowed such straight lines . . . at least in print.) Distinct characteristics of this plant are the large Mintlike, strongly light-veined leaves, the thick, light-colored, and upright stems, the yellow-green flowers, and, when broken, the copious quantities of white latex that exude from wounds. The whole plant is usually 3 to 4 feet tall. The flowers mature into stubby, dusty, grey-green pods, filled with silky, fly-away parachuted seeds.

Asclepias albicans is white-mealy all over, with the flower stems being the fuzziest. The leaves are usually in whorls of three, grasslike, and are shed early in the year, leaving 3- to 6-foot-tall, slender, white waxy stems with few branches and terminal cream and brown flower clusters. The flowers bloom erratically during the year, and long, skinny seedpods may be present simultaneously with newly blossoming umbels. The whole plant as seen growing out of some arroyo rocks is a white-stemmed, naked shrub, with a dozen branches and little, starlike, drooping flowerheads and skinny, greenish white pods that look as if they are made of burnished leather.

Asclepias subulata is *truly* weird. It resembles a big bundle of smooth sticks—4 to 5 feet tall, succulent, light waxy green—stuck unceremoniously into the sand. One early spring day it had a few little thread leaves; the next day they were gone. The little cream-colored flower clusters stick out from the tips or near the tips of the stems, maturing into waxy, tapering pods (3 to 5 inches long) that shed little narrow seeds borne on silky, yellow-brown parachutes.

The roots of all three Desert Milkweeds are deep, gnarly, and light brown, and have many scars, breaks, and dead sections. The two leafless species have roots that drive you close to madness (use a backhoe . . . ?). Dig them in the late fall and winter, get what you can, leave a depression, pour a gallon of water into it, and they will regenerate easily from the remnant tuber/root. *A. erosa* is a bit smaller, but try to dig it in sand, not talus-rubble. It is a more common plant, with broader distribution, and probably doesn't need such careful treatment.

If the plants have maturing pods, always help them along by distributing the airborne seeds in other, similar localities; at the very least, put a pod in the hole you filled in. If they aren't quite mature, put them in a puffed-out paper bag, scrunch up the top, and save them for a friend with a green thumb who would like to grow one of these exotic lovelies.

HABITAT *Asclepias erosa* grows on dry slopes and in washes from the Sea of Cortez, north through the desert foothills to Kern and Inyo coun-

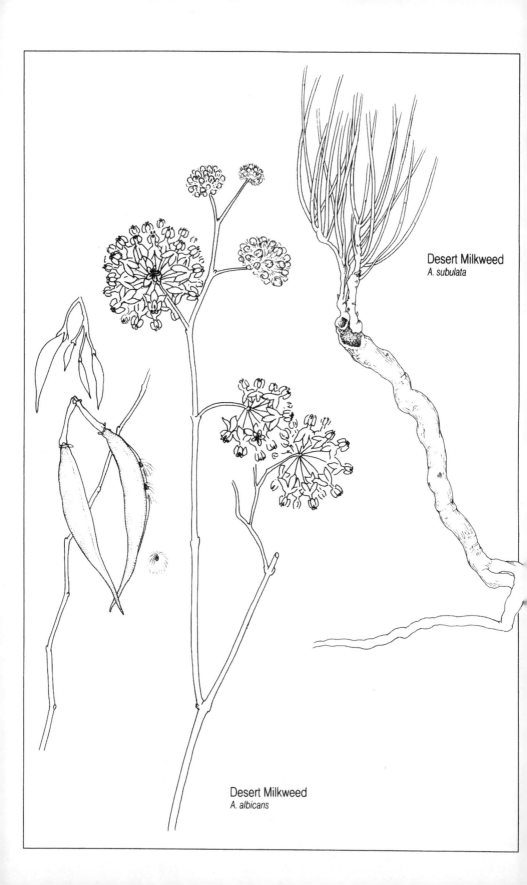

Desert Milkweed
A. subulata

Desert Milkweed
A. albicans

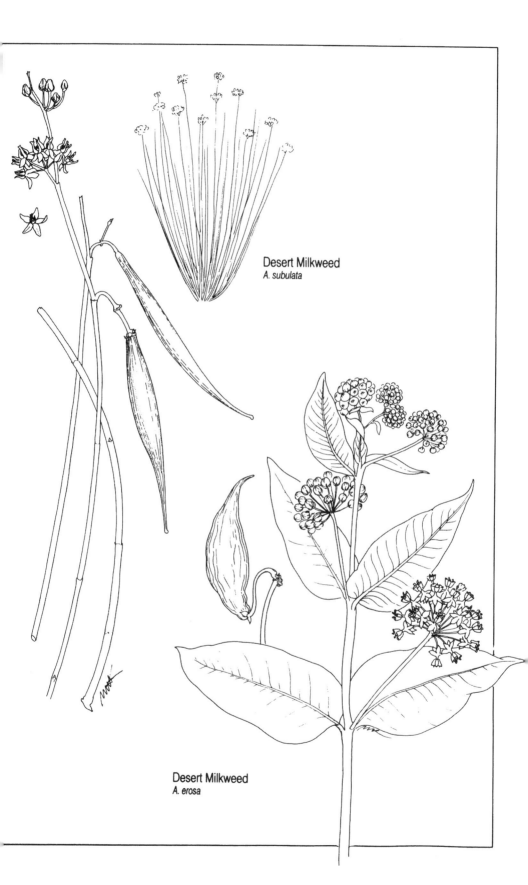

Desert Milkweed
A. subulata

Desert Milkweed
A. erosa

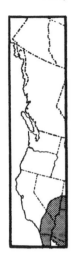

ties, west to San Diego County and northwestern Baja California; and in the Mojave Desert as far as the southern Great Basin foothills of Arizona, Nevada, and southwestern Utah. It usually grows between 2,000 and 3,000 feet, never much above 4,500 feet.

Asclepias albicans grows below 2,500 feet in talus and rocky arroyos in partial shade, in the Colorado Desert and lower Mojave Desert, south into Baja California, and east into the Arizona Desert.

Asclepias subulata grows in nearly frost-free dunes, washes, and depressions all up and down the Colorado River drainage (I mean *low* places!). It is found in southern Nevada and the Colorado Desert of Arizona, and on both sides of the Sea of Cortez in northwestern Mexico. If it is 95% humidity, 95 degrees in the shade, 6:00 P.M., early January, and you can almost see the riverside thickets and the first trailer parks on the Arizona side . . . you are in the right place to find our plant.

CONSTITUENTS *Asclepius subulata* roots contain at least thirteen cardenolide glycosides and one lignan glycoside; *A. albicans* and *A. erosa* contain similar glycosides, desglucosyrioside, and alpha amyrin; and the latex of *A. erosa* and probably the other two contains labriformin. The mild cardiac glycoside asclepiadin appears in *A. erosa* and undoubtedly (being nearly universal in North American Milkweeds) in the others as well.

COLLECTING Gather the roots as described above; wash them, split them, and remove dead sections by scraping with a knife or a wire brush. The latex is obtained by slicing sterile green stems just below the tips, catching the milky sap in a stainless steel or glass container, reslicing an inch lower when the higher wound seals, and continuing down a foot or so on several stems (leave most of the stems uncut). Whisk or stir the latex until it evaporates to dried rubber cement consistency.

STABILITY The dried roots remain strong for several years. The dried latex (depending on when it is gathered in relationship to the most recent rain) loses its rubbery qualities in a few months or sooner.

PREPARATION Dry Root Tincture, 1:5, 50% alcohol, 10 to 20 drops, up to four times a day. By and large, *A. subulata* is the stronger of the three (in terms of potential toxicity), but this low dosage seems to work well for all three.

MEDICINAL USES The root works well as an expectorant-diaphoretic when you are just getting sick, with a dry heat in the sinuses or across the chest, and the sense that your skin is not quite big enough to contain you—or, less fancifully, when you toss and turn, hot, fretful, and are not quite sure exactly *how* sick you are but know that you're coming down with something in your head and chest. The Desert Milkweeds work nicely to bring the heat out by stimulating secretions in the lungs, sinuses, digestive tract, and the skin. I would suggest drinking a lot of tea or electrolyte replacements, since all this secreting makes you thirsty. The tincture seems the best way to use the roots; cups of the boiled tea can upset the stomach, whereas the small amount of tincture doesn't. This is a simple medicine for acute disorders: take it every couple of hours (alternating with liquids) until you feel moister and more relaxed; then fall back on the usual, more prosaic therapies. Wild Ginger, Lomatium, Osha, Balsam Root—that type of tincture or tea is better for the following few days; I have found that even though they work for a day or two, they begin to irritate the mouth and stomach if used for too long a time.

The rubbery latex is a good chewing gum if you have a dry, irritative cough and impacted phlegm. Its bitter taste stimulates saliva, and the small amount of constituents, though safe, add to the expectoration.

CONTRAINDICATIONS Do not use during pregnancy or with confirmed heart disease.

Devil's Club

Oplopanax horridum   (Araliaceae)

OTHER NAMES *Echinopanax horridum* is the preferred name in Asia and Alaska, and some authorities have suggested realigning it with the related taxa of *Eleutherococcus*, *Acanthopanax*, and *Kalopanax* found in eastern and northeastern Asia.

APPEARANCE There is no mistaking Devil's Club. Large umbrella leaves sit on top of thick, spiny stems that range from 3 feet to well over 10 feet in height, growing up from spreading rootstocks. These roots are partially fallen-down stems from previous growth and partially true central roots and rhizomes. Rooted former stems retain the remnants of former spines, and the true roots have harder central pith and smooth reddish bark, somewhat succulent and without any trace of spines. The flowers bloom in greenish panicles in the spring and mature into flattened pyramids of bright red berries in the late summer. The whole plant is sweetly aromatic, sort of like a balsamic Ginseng, the roots strongest smelling, the leaves less strong.

HABITAT Devil's Club is found along both sides of the Cascades in the northern half of Oregon, throughout the Red Cedar forests of Washington, British Columbia, and Alaska, and sometimes forms impenetrable coastal thickets in the northern Pacific. It is found in western Alberta,

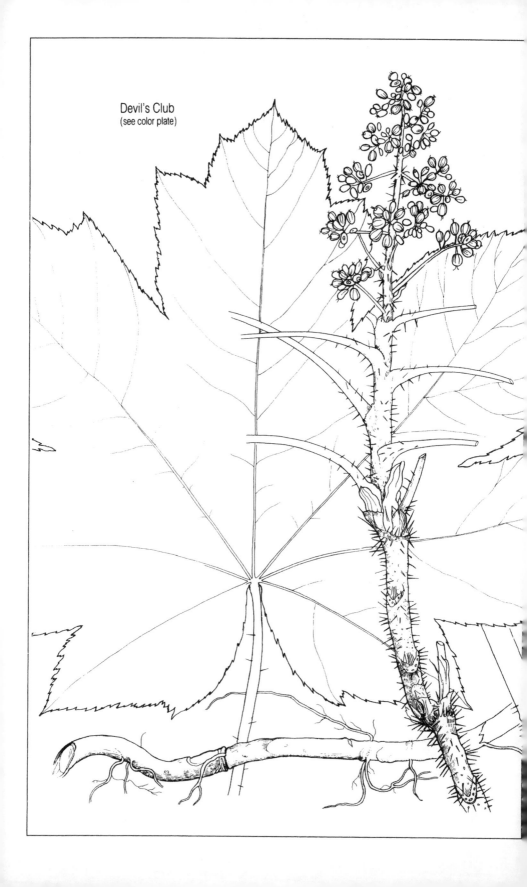

Devil's Club
(see color plate)

and sporadically in the forests of northern Idaho, Montana, and extreme western Wyoming. It then reappears in the forests around the northern and western edges of Lake Superior, where acid rain is decreasing its abundance. In the southern and eastern edges of its Pacific area growth, it is found in deep, wet, shady places, and is generally smaller in height than elsewhere. From central Washington northwards it may be found in full sun (or full fog) and in many more circumstances. In wet northern forests it may completely obscure the banks of creeks and rivers and completely fill the floors of hollows.

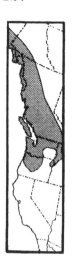

CONSTITUENTS The essential oil of the root contains nerolidol, torreyol, dodinene, bulnesol, dodecenol, cadenene, and cedrol (among others), as well as araliasides and panaxosides of varied and unspecified nature.

COLLECTING For fresh root preparations I prefer using the bark of the stem-roots together with the bark and the heartwood of the true roots. For dry tincture or tea, I prefer just the bark of both the stem-root and true root. Strip off the bark after washing the roots and after scrubbing with a stiff brush, dry Method B. The shorter plants in the southern edges of its biosphere grow slowly, often with greater potency, and you should consider using the bark of the upright stems as well. Just make sure that you wear good gloves whenever gathering Devil's Club, as the spines, although not specifically toxic, can break off under the skin and produce a surprisingly wicked and slow-healing abrasion.

In order to gather in a moral fashion, I suggest digging just the distal sections from a small stand (leaving the heart of the thicket untouched). In large stands with many rooted lateral rhizomes that are fixed and stable, I gather roots from the older, central section. This growth is heavy with the stronger true roots, but digging or pulling them up will not affect the independent growth that rings it. The roots are best gathered in late summer and early fall, when they are the strongest. Bark gathered in the spring can mold very quickly, and is lower in sterols and glycosides and presumably less useful. In a few areas with mild, foggy coastal climate (the Columbia River Gorge, the Olympic Peninsula, and the coastal strands from Vancouver north to the Alaska Panhandle), it can be gathered through late fall, but the winter roots are generally weaker. Conversely, some herbalists such as Terry Willard prefer a tincture of the spring bark, particularly in treating adult onset diabetes.

STABILITY The bark will stay strong in all aspects for at least a year. The lung-stimulating aromatics will dissipate after that, but the other properties will remain for another year at least.

PREPARATION The Fresh Tincture, 1:2, the Dry Tincture, 1:5, 60% alcohol, both 15 to 30 drops, up to three times a day; a Cold Infusion, 1 to 3 fluid ounces, also up to three times a day.

MEDICINAL USES First of all, and most simply, Devil's Club is a strong, reliable, and safe expectorant and respiratory stimulant, increasing the mucus secretions to initiate fruitful coughing and soften up hardened bronchial mucus that can occur later on in a chest cold.

The cold infusion, and to a lesser degree the fresh or dry tincture, is clearly helpful for rheumatoid arthritis and other autoimmune disorders, taken regularly and with sensible modifications in the diet. It is most helpful when taken during remissions and has little effect during active distress; its main value is in modifying extremes of metabolic stress and adding a little reserve to offset the person's internal cost of living. Many plants of the Aralia family, including Ginseng, contain glycosides that decrease the outside extremes of hypothalamus and pituitary stress responses, and Devil's Club is high in these constituents.

It has a long history of use by Native Americans for adult onset, insulin-resistant diabetes, and the several studies that were made of its use a few decades ago clearly showed its benefits. The studies only evaluated those already taking the herb, and made no attempt to evaluate its use under normally accepted clinical trials; but, as with a number of widely used folk treatments for diabetes (*Brickellia, Tecoma, Cacalia decomposita, Opuntia*, and *Vaccinium*), although unverified by control group trials, it is clearly helpful for diabetics of this type. My observations and those of some other herbalists and physicians have been that the herb, as a tea, works better for stocky, mesomorphic, anabolic-stress-type, middle-aged folks with elevated blood lipids, moderately high blood pressure, and early signs of adult onset, insulin-resistant diabetes. Furthermore, it seems to decrease the abject lust for sugars and binge food in those of this physical type who are trying to lose weight or deal with generally elevated blood fats and glucose. In general, Devil's Club seems to be an aid in times of body/mind stress and a means of increasing one's feeling of well-being.

European Pennyroyal

Mentha Pulegium   (Labiatae)
OTHER NAMES Pennyroyal, True Pennyroyal

APPEARANCE Pennyroyal is a small plant, from 1 to 1½ feet tall in bloom, with the usual square stems and opposite leaves of the family. The flowers of blooming branches are all in the axils of the leaves—small, puffy, and sometimes strikingly pink. The stems branch extensively; and most, if not all, have flowers. After blooming, and in moist areas during the entire growing season, roots put out long runners, and much of the plant's

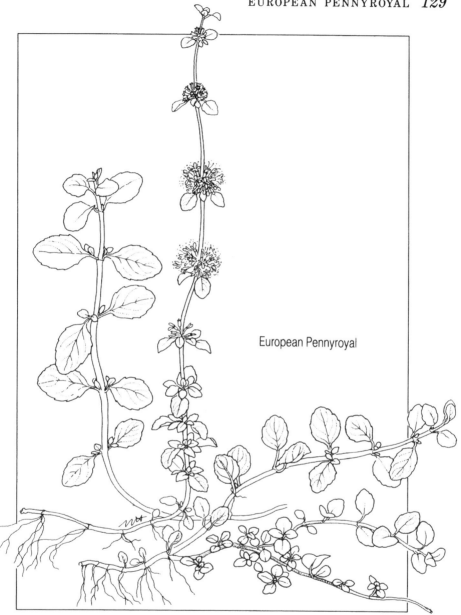

European Pennyroyal

growth in the fall and spring is predominantly basal and matlike. The leaves are small, oval, lightly serrated, fuzzy, and often so sharply down-turned that the axillary flowers stand out as far from the stem as the reflex leaves. The scent of the crushed foliage is strong and distinctive: minty, sweet, and a little camphorous.

HABITAT Pennyroyal, a garden escapee, can be found in moist locali-ties, along ditches and roadsides, and in shady localities along the coast

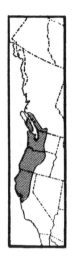

from San Francisco northwards, with a few stands southwards as far as Santa Barbara. There are large stands inland, from northern California lakes and rivers northwards, through Willamette Valley, and up through central Washington. It can occur almost anywhere, but occasional stands outside of these areas are usually short-lived or marginal.

CONSTITUENTS The volatile oils contain the active principles, primarily the ketonic monoterpene with small amounts of menthone and piperitone.

COLLECTING Gather the flowering tops, including stems, in summer, and dry Method A. Leave it as whole bundles until needed, in order to keep the aromatics as intact as possible. Those who have gathered their own Pennyroyal, either American (*Hedeoma* sp.) or European, will have trouble understanding the universally poor quality of the commercial herb.

STABILITY If left whole until used, and stored in an airtight container, the characteristic (and biologically active) aromatics may be present for at least two years. The older the herb, the more herb should be used in tea.

PREPARATION Fresh Tincture, 1:2, ½ to 1 teaspoon, Standard Infusion, 2 to 4 fluid ounces, both as needed.

MEDICINAL USES Pennyroyal has been a much maligned herb in recent years, partially because the essential oil has been used as a potential abortifacient (highly dangerous, with several deaths reported in the literature), partially because of the poor quality of the commercial herb. The tea or tincture has two basic uses. It is a safe and effective diaphoretic to induce sweating with fevers and sick headaches with nausea and red eyes. Further, in suppressed menses from sickness, infection, stress, or exhaustion, either in the current month or the previous month, the tea, taken on the first, second, or third day of normal menses, will stimulate uterine secretions and, in effect, stimulate uterine sweating. In my opinion, it is not an abortifacient. The oil is a hundredfold more toxic than the tea, but drinking large quantities of the tea can cause light-headedness and nausea.

CONTRAINDICATIONS It should not be used during pregnancy.

OTHER USES The essential oil is an effective insect repellent, but I have seen it cause rashes in humans and, when used to repel fleas in pets, cause convulsions. It's better in combination with such oils as Citronella, Lavender Spike, Cedarwood, and the like.

False Solomon's Seal

Smilacina racemosa   (Liliaceae)
OTHER NAMES   Branched Solomon's Seal; *Vagnera racemosa*

APPEARANCE False Solomon's Seal grows from creeping rhizomes, growing at or just below ground level, with descending, succulent rootlets. The aerial parts are simple, unbranching arched stems, with alternate, Lilylike, semiclasping leaves, usually 3 to 6 inches long, parallel-veined, and bright and cheerful green. There may be several stems from a rhizome, and the plants tend to form colonies. The flowers are creamy white terminals, clusters—branching, foamy affairs, often semipyramidal in shape. They mature into small terminal bunches of juicy berries, first creamy yellow, then green, then mottled, marbled red . . . then they get eaten by birds.

HABITAT False Solomon's Seal grows in moist, shady places, with rich soil, almost anywhere in our area, from the San Bernardino Mountains of southern California, northwards to the Alaska Panhandle, across into the Rocky Mountains, and east to the Atlantic Coast. In the same habitat, with a little more drought tolerance, and often growing in the same places, is the smaller *Smilacina stellata* (Starry Solomon's Seal), with narrower leaves and considerably smaller roots. Although less rewarding to gather, I have found that it serves the same purposes. Botanists sometimes separate some varieties of the *S. racemosa* in California into genetically different plants, but the differences (leaf sizes and such) are not clear and distinct enough to worry about.

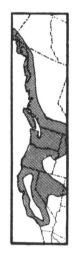

CONSTITUENTS Sitosterol, allantoin, asparagin, mucilage, and several saponins.

COLLECTING For cough syrup, the fall roots are best; for a poultice and a simple, soothing astringent, the root may be used anytime.

STABILITY The fresh roots can remain stable for a month in the refrigerator, the dried roots for a couple of years.

PREPARATION The Cough Syrup is made by adding 1 part by volume of fresh chopped root to 4 parts by volume of honey, bringing them to a slow simmer in a pot, cooking for a couple of hours, removing from the heat, rewarming the next morning, straining, and storing in jars. If you make sure that the finished product is the same volume as the original honey (or less), it will store at room temperature without fermenting. If the honey has picked up too much moisture from the roots, reduce the volume by slowly simmering. If you wish to add other herbs to the syrup, such as Balsam Root, Lomatium, Osha, Angelica, or California Spikenard root, just substitute some of the freshly chopped root for some

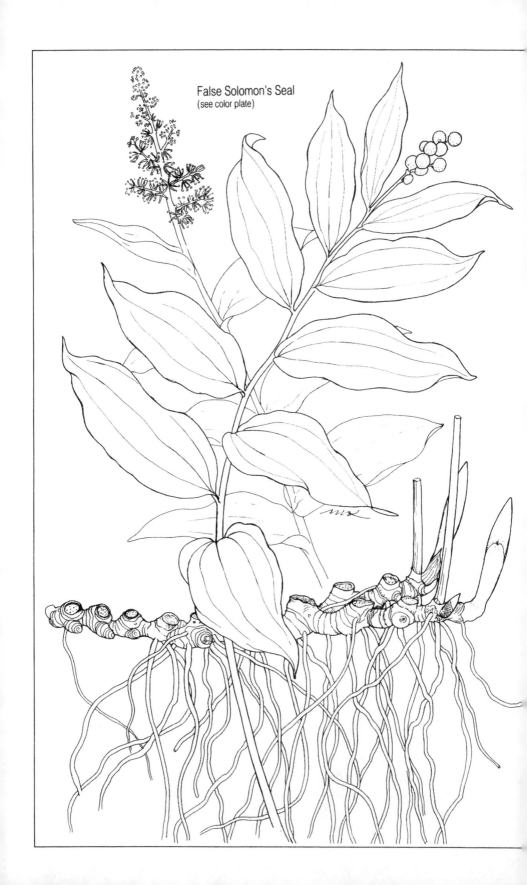

False Solomon's Seal
(see color plate)

False Solomon's Seal. You can make some incredibly tasty and effective honey syrups this way. For a poultice of the fresh root, just mash it up between two clean rocks and apply. The dry root makes a useful poultice if you grind it and mix it with enough hot water to paste up. The Dry Root Tea can be made by simply steeping a teaspoon of the ground root in a cup of tea.

MEDICINAL USES The syrup, tea, or a chunk of the fresh root, chewed, will soothe the throat, allay irritation, and decrease respiratory excitability in sore throats and chest colds. The root is mildly anti-inflammatory, both internally and topically, and the chewed root may help gum irritations, pharyngitis, and gastritis, especially when there is esophagus pain from frequent acid indigestion. The soothing, relaxing, and sedative effects on the lungs and bronchi can be synergized with Mullein, California Spikenard, Hypericum, Mallow, or Maidenhair Fern. For intestinal inflammation, it combines well with Angelica, Yellow Pond Lily root, Evening Primrose root, Yerba Mansa, or Yerba Reuma.

Topically, the fresh root, and to some degree the dry root, helps to decrease swellings and inflammations. This is useful for stings and bites as well, and it has a long history of use for small, localized Poison Oak rashes. If you have any handy, grind up some fresh Grindelia flowers along with the False Solomon's Seal for poulticing. In addition, with its allantoin content, the root further stimulates skin proliferation and regranulation from burns; and, again, this effect is increased by the use of Grindelia. The dry plants work as well; mix equal parts of them with enough hot water to form a paste and cover the poultice with hot, moist towels. Leave the poultice on for at least an hour, and repeat again the next day.

Figwort

Scrophularia californica, S. lanceolata   (Scrophulariaceae)
OTHER NAMES Carpenter's Square; *S. oregana*

APPEARANCE Figwort is a big, handsome plant that *looks* like a useful herb. It grows, in summer maturity, from 3 to 6 feet tall. The leaves are opposite, with short petioles that usually wrap around the square stem, and are variously notched, resembling Catnip or a large Sage. The flowers are borne on branched axillar and terminal peduncles, and when mature, still *look* immature. They are purple, mauve, or reddish brown, small, and tubular, with two distinct lobes to the upper hood, looking like small Penstemons. The plants are perennial, with variously lumpy and smooth rhizomes that may connect several plants. In their usual stand habitat, some will be tall and mature, some will be short, with only several tiers of large, 5-inch-long triangular leaves. If they aren't in bloom, they resemble a big mint, except when you crush the leaves, expecting a pleasant aromatic. Figwort smells rank. The genus seems to form many varieties; I have seen large plants with secondary ridges to supplant the four corners of the normal stem, and with lower leaves bearing secondary leaflets on the petioles, both characteristics of eastern species. The leaves and stems are always dark green and smooth.

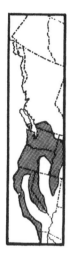

HABITAT *Scrophularia californica* (and its many varieties) is found along the coast, in moist and shady localities from nearly the shoreline up into the various coastal ranges; and from Baja California to British Columbia. In the inland ranges, it grows on both sides of the Sierra Nevada; into Nevada; and on the west side of the Cascades. In the eastern part of its range it mixes with *S. lanceolata,* a similar plant with longer leaves, found in Montana, Idaho, eastwards to Arkansas, and seemingly interbreeding with the other species in Washington, Oregon, Nevada, and Arizona. Some of these hybrids have been given their own names, so it gets confusing. Don't worry about it.

CONSTITUENTS A number of iridoid glycosides, including harpagosides, scrophularine, hesperitin, and some rather amorphous glycosides that sometimes have weak cardiotonic effects, which are more pronounced in the eastern and European species, *S. marilandica* and *S. nodosa.*

COLLECTING Gather the flowering herb preferably in late July and August, and dry Method A. Strip everything off the big central stem.

STABILITY The whole herb should last a year.

PREPARATION Standard Infusion, 2 to 4 fluid ounces, in evening. Salve, Method A.

MEDICINAL USES Figwort is a subtle and useful long-term anti-inflammatory for people with chronic low-grade skin and mucosa sores and irritations. If you get frequent cold sores, rectal aches, and have a tendency for sore throats, or if you have long-standing eczema with periodic acute episodes of redness and itching, try this plant and some Yellow Dock in the evening. For general arthritis, aggravated by cold and damp weather, and with an overall lassitude and bogginess more typical of a large amphibian, take some tea in the evening and add a couple of squirts of Devil's Club tincture. It takes a while, but there is nearly always some improvement with the skin and joint conditions.

The salve, the powdered herb mixed with water for a poultice, or the fresh leaves or roots crushed up into a green mud pie are *very* soothing for bruises, stings, and recent joint injuries. The salve or poultice, applied laterally from the armpit to the nipple, helps decrease the occa-

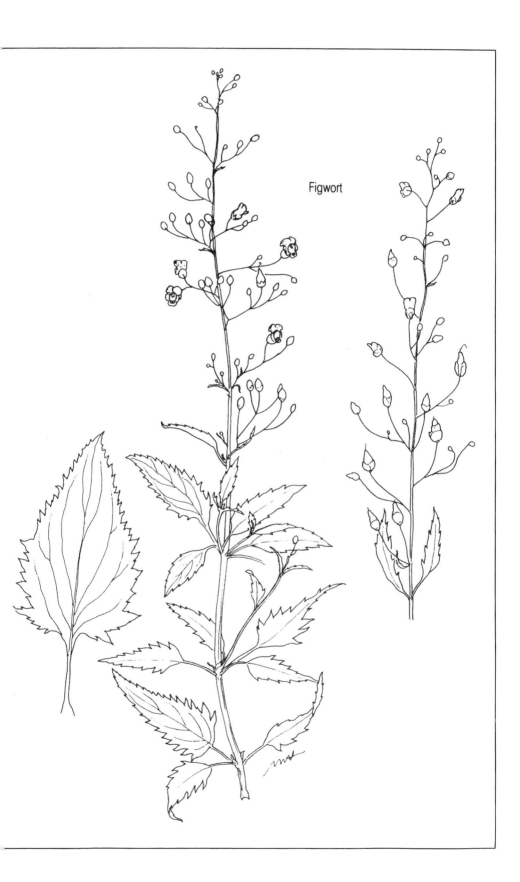

Figwort

sional episode of PMS breast pain; and the salve is soothing to hemorrhoids, vaginal irritations, cracked, weathered skin, and moist-fold redness such as diaper rash.

For the slow viruses (CFS, CMV, EBV, and HIV), with a tendency to somewhat enlarged lymph nodes, try the Figwort with Red Root mornings and evenings until the swelling decreases, then return to only an evening dose. This isn't for the infection itself, but to lessen the distal lymph node congestion.

CONTRAINDICATIONS I have no information about the levels of cardioglycoside in our native Figworts, and I have never observed any effects; but, to be on the safe side, avoid using with ventricular tachycardia or heart medications or during pregnancy.

Fireweed

Epilobium angustifolium   (Onagraceae)
OTHER NAMES Great Willow Herb, Rose Bay

APPEARANCE Fireweed is a perennial plant, usually growing in colonies connected by underground roots. The aboveground plants form tall, erect, and somewhat woody stems, from 2 to 6 or 7 feet tall, and crowded with long, narrow leaves that are alternate and from 3 to 6 inches long. The leaves are dark green above, and lighter, glabrous, almost silvery-downy below, with the central vein distinctly lighter than the rest of the surface, above and below—a typical characteristic of the Evening Primrose family.

The flowers are a bright, cheerful lavender to pink, sometimes an almost carmine-purple, with the showy flowers below the thin, succulent buds. Sometimes the flowering spikes form secondary branches, especially in isolated plants, but most of the time they are singular. The pods are long and narrow, and filled with feathery seeds that unfold and blow away. It can be disconcerting to go up into the mountains, bring back several bundles of bright, cheerful Fireweeds, leave them on the back seat or hang them from the inside of your vehicle, and arrive back home to find the whole inside of your car covered with seed-bearing fuzz, released by mature pods below the red flowers. To avoid this, pick them off the stem up in the mountains and toss them on a rock to disperse the fuzz in the air.

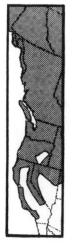

HABITAT Fireweed is found throughout the West and can be expected in any forested, logged, or burned mountain area. I have never been able to figure out if the common name Fireweed comes from its bright, pink-

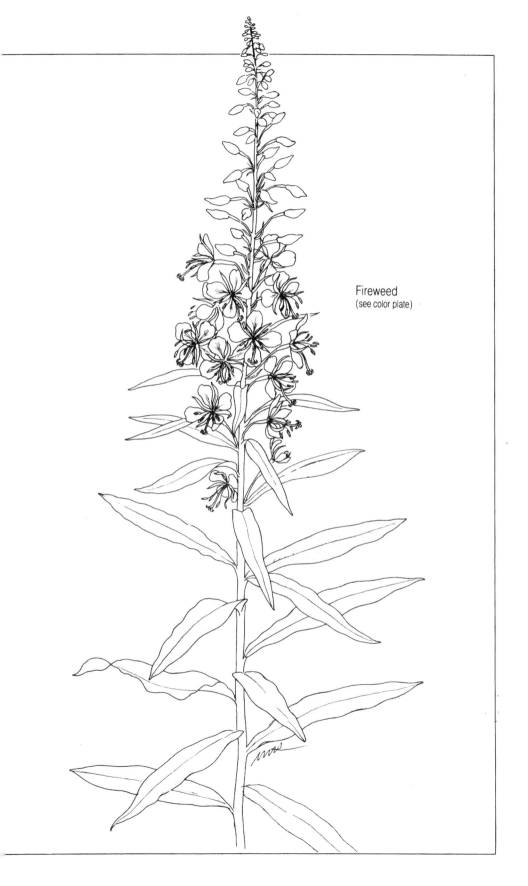

Fireweed
(see color plate)

purple flowers, or its tendency, because of efficient wind-dispersed seeds, to be one of the first big flowering plants to recolonize after a burn. Whatever.

CONSTITUENTS Myricetin 3-O-B-D-glucuronide and related flavonoids, tannin, and an antiphlogistine principle of unknown nature.

COLLECTING Gather in flower, picking as far down the stem as there are green, unwithered leaves; dry Method A. Strip, and discard the large, central stem.

STABILITY Fireweed, although seemingly delicate in structure, will last up to two years, if stored as whole leaves and flowers.

PREPARATION Standard Infusion as needed.

MEDICINAL USES The tea is safe, bland-tasty, and can be taken in a fair quantity. The single, specific indication for Fireweed is chronic, pasty diarrhea, without heat and fever, and green or yellow in color. This is a common complaint in the spring in the north country, due to changing from a meat and potatoes type of winter eating to a diet of green and red spring plants. Children and older folks are more likely to manifest this than the rest of us. In any case, it is the bout of noninfective green or yellow diarrhea that Fireweed is so useful for.

It is an anti-inflammatory herb—benign, gentle, but eventually effective—for mouth, throat, stomach, and intestinal inflammation. It helps piles and hemorrhoids that flare up for a few days after eating food that you are hypersensitive to—spicy foods like chili that leave you with that lingering "heat," along with rectal itching and aching that persists after a day or two. Some prescription drugs for ulcers, colitis, and arthritis can induce a lingering, low-level descending colon swelling and dryness, and, in men, a low-grade prostate heaviness; two or three cups of the tea each day for a week will help; and Fireweed has no contraindications with drugs. Oddly enough, by decreasing this boggy swelling that results from the unwanted but unavoidable side effects of some otherwise appropriate drugs, Fireweed can improve the colon tone and act as a laxative. The tea can be freely used for douches, enemas, and infant washes, where there is inflammation of the orifices and tender folds.

Externally, it cools, soothes, and helps to bring down swelling, but it is not as emphatic as such herbs as Arnica, Yerba del Lobo, or Henbane. On the other hand, it is without danger. If you are using an Arnica poultice for a sprain, you might want to drink a bunch of Fireweed tea.

Goldthread

Coptis laciniata, C. occidentalis   (Ranunculaceae)
OTHER NAMES Canker Root, Mouth Root, Yellow Root

APPEARANCE Coptis is a little evergreen plant, with several leaves on long, wiry stems. The leaves are shiny dark green, with three leaflets on petioles, the central one the longest. In *Coptis occidentalis,* the leaflets are sharply notched, giving the leaflets a three- or five-sectioned, bluntly rounded shape. *C. laciniata* looks similar, but the three leaflets are deeply and sharply lobed, with a more triangular shape. These are the two most common Goldthreads in the Pacific West, and they have thin, tough brown roots with a Day-Glo yellow or orange pith, which is intensely bitter to the taste. Both species may form several leaf groups from the same roots, Strawberry-style, but they are much less likely to form the interconnected root-leaf masses of other species in the genus. The flowers, easily overlooked in the spring, are small, greenish yellow, and starfish-shaped. In British Columbia and Alaska coastal areas, you find *C. asplenifolia,* with low-growing trifolated leaves, pinnately divided with a fernlike appearance, and *C. trifolia,* with three wedge-shaped leaflets, very short petioles, almost Strawberrylike in shape, and somewhat showy little flowers with white sepals that can be pink tinged.

HABITAT Goldthread is a deep-forest plant, growing in moist and shady areas, usually near creeks and river drainages. *Coptis laciniata* grows from the Redwood area of Mendocino County, California, north to the southern edge of the Olympic Mountains in Washington, and eastwards to the western slopes of the Cascades. *Coptis occidentalis* is found in northeastern Washington, across through the northern forests of Idaho and western Montana, and north to Alberta and southeastern British Columbia. The other two species are found in the coastal forests of British Columbia and Alaska, as far north as Anchorage. *C. asplenifolia* can be found as far south in Washington as the Mount Baker area.

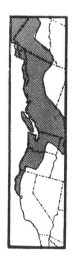

CONSTITUENTS The alkaloids berberine, coptisine, and others are responsible for the effects of the herb.

COLLECTING I prefer gathering the roots and leaves in late summer and fall, from August to October. They could be gathered in the winter, if you could find the evergreen leaves under two feet of snow. I use both the roots and leaves, since the same constituents are found in both.

STABILITY The plant is stable for several years.

PREPARATION Fresh Whole Plant Tincture, 1:2, Dry Whole Plant Tincture, 1:5, 50% alcohol, both 30 to 60 drops, up to three times a day (GI chronic inflammation), 10 drops fifteen minutes before meals (bitter

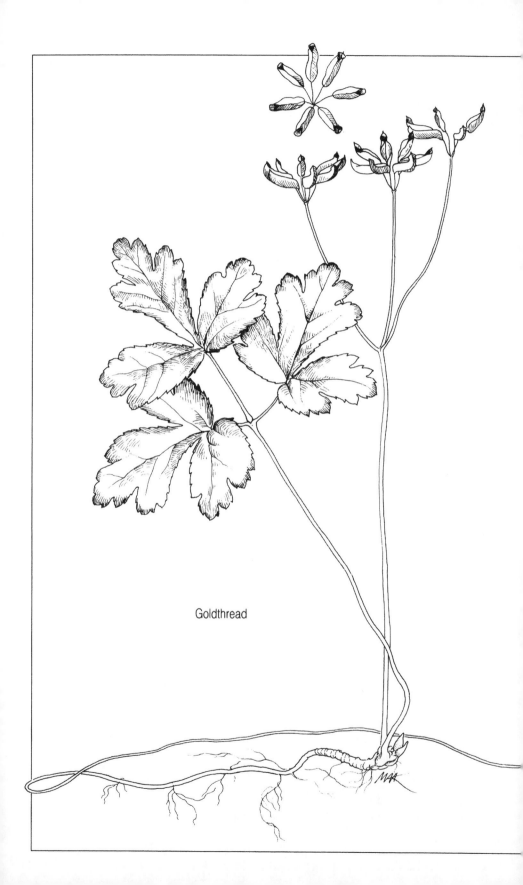

Goldthread

tonic); the leaves for a Method B Salve. The leaves are necessary for the salve, as the roots are poorly soluble in oil, even with the alcohol moistening step.

MEDICINAL USES First, Goldthread is a great bitter tonic, for upper intestinal tract deficient conditions, with dry mouth, gum problems, coated tongue, and sluggish gastric secretions. If you have gastric inflammation, with a moist mouth and pointed, red-tipped tongue, you should not use Goldthread (a mucus membrane stimulant).

For chronic intestinal congestion, with irritable bowel syndrome, constipation with hemorrhoids, and mucus colitis, the internal use is recommended. If you find that it stimulates the appetite too much, use half as much (say, 15 drops) and add Yerba Mansa tincture (say, 30 drops). They both work similarly on the mucosa and are probably more effective in combination than separately.

Goldthread is also called Canker Root and Mouth Root, because of its excellent effects on cold sores, herpes sores, and aphthous stomatitis; apply the tincture directly to the sore, straight or diluted, and use the diluted tincture as a mouthwash several times a day during acute episodes. The herb is antimicrobial, and the salve can be used as a dressing on skin abrasions, as well as for herpes sores and ulcerations of the vagina or anus.

Berberine, the yellow alkaloid, is very water soluble, unlike coptisine, and the tea can be used for a cleansing wash, sitz bath, douche, enema, or eyewash, where bacterial infection is a possibility.

Hawthorn

Crataegus Douglasii, C. columbiana   (Rosaceae)
OTHER NAMES Black Hawthorn, Western Black Haw, Douglas Hawthorn, Columbia Hawthorn, River Hawthorn; *C. rivularis, C. brevispina*

APPEARANCE *Crataegus Douglasii* is a tall shrub, from 10 to 15 feet in height under good conditions. It is a Willowlike thicket tree, with few large trunks, mostly composed of robust stems and branches, covered in rough, grey-brown bark (older growth) or reddish brown bark (younger branches). The leaves are small, uniform, bright green, and from 1 to 2 inches long. They are fan-shaped and widest towards the toothed tip. The flowers bloom in open bunches, white little roses growing in leaf axils and side branches. These mature in early fall to red and finally black little apples in irregular clusters. The stems and branches are armed with short, slightly curved thorns, usually less than an inch long.

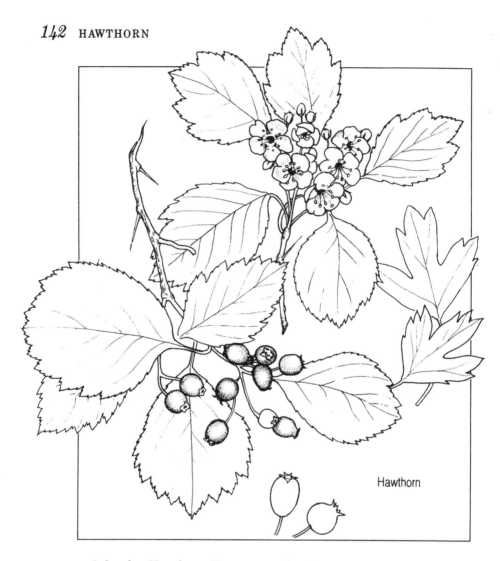

Hawthorn

Columbia Hawthorn (*Crataegus columbiana*) is shorter, but usually with greater lateral growth, and tends to form trunks within the many branches. The bark is nearly all reddish brown, with newer branches covered in light, mealy hair. The leaves are the same size, but more ovate, and less fan-shaped, with the leaf notches more along the sides and less completely terminal. The fruit is smaller and forms showy, less diffuse bright red or sometimes somewhat purplish masses. The thorns are much more formidable than the previous type, sometimes even 3 or 4 inches long. Two European cultivated Hawthorns are sometimes encountered growing wild; they have deeply cleft leaves, often so deep as to form nearly compound leaflets, three to seven in number. These two types are often distinctly treelike. The fruit is yellow to red and one-seeded (*Crataegus monogyna*) or two-seeded (*C. oxyacantha*). Our two native species usually have three or more seeds.

HABITAT Both native species are found along rivers, in moist canyons, and in thickets around the edges of natural meadows. *C. Douglasii,* the more widespread plant, is found from Sonoma County in California north along the Pacific to the Fraser River in British Columbia; east through Modoc County in California; into Nevada, Utah, and Montana; and north through Alberta, Canada, reappearing sporadically as far east as Michigan. *C. columbiana* is found east of the Cascades from northern Oregon to British Columbia and eastwards to Idaho, western Montana, and southwestern Alberta. The two European escapees are plants of urban northwestern coastal areas and the valleys west of the Cascades.

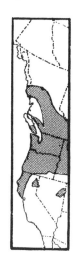

CONSTITUENTS Flavonoids, including vitexin 4'-xyloside and other C-glycosyl flavones, oligomeric procyanidins, including 1-epicatechol, triterpene acids (oleanolic, ursolic, crataegolic), purines, choline, acetylcholine, trimethylamine, chlorogenic acid and the usual ascorbic acid, sugars, rutin, and the like associated with Rose family fruit. One of the maddening things for European pharmaceutical manufacturers has been that none of this stuff is singularly responsible for Hawthorn's heart effects, nothing can be relied upon to test singly for the drug potency, and nothing seems to facilitate standardization of strength. All widely used Hawthorn preparations in Europe use the whole plant; they only try to standardize the cultivation and harvesting.

COLLECTING Gather the flowering branches in the spring, drying carefully Method A, or loosely in paper bags for tea, dry tincture, or a fresh herb tincture. For the fresh tincture, I like using all the flowering branch—leaves, spines, small twigs, and floral parts. For the dried herb, I follow the German method (if anyone knows Hawthorn, it is the heart-crazed Teutons): dry on the terminal branches and remove the leaves and flowers, discarding the twigs. The other time to collect is in the early fall, when the berries are ripe. *Crataegus Douglasii* berries should be collected when they are fully purple-black, but before the first major frost. With *C. columbiana,* the fruit is ripe when fully dark red and also before the first frost. Unlike their relative Roses, whose hips need heavy frost to turn them the proper stable, transparent red, Hawthorn berries start to ferment and get squishy after freezing. The birds like the red berries when they are overripe and generally ignore the black ones altogether; but by that time the berries are over the hill for medicinal use. They (and their naturalized relatives) may be tinctured fresh or dried quickly for tea or syrup. After following various tips about the alleged differences in the effects of the flowering tops as opposed to the fruit, I have given up any subtle presumptions and combine the fresh flowering tops tincture with the fresh berry tincture, calling it fresh Hawthorn tincture, and use it as is.

STABILITY The dried flowers and leaves are not stable too long but will last for a year or more if stored in a Ziploc bag or closed jar and frozen between uses. The dried berries are good for several years and have the advantage of deteriorating the least (which is why they are the part found in commerce) but the disadvantage of having the least potency. The fresh and dried tinctures are stable for years.

PREPARATION Fresh Plant Tincture (flowering tops or berries or both), 1:2, 15 to 30 drops; Dry Herb Tincture (flowering tops, berries, or both), 1:5, 50% alcohol, 10 to 20 drops; Simple Infusion, a well-rounded teaspoon of the flowers and leaves or a scant teaspoon of the crushed berries in a cup of hot water, steeped for thirty minutes. All the above preparations should be taken three times a day, decreased to twice a day morning and evening after a few weeks.

MEDICINAL USES Hawthorn is a heart tonic—period. In the past it has been confused in value with such drug plants as *Digitalis* and *Strophanthus*, but it is slow, gentle (even feeble), acts to strengthen weak functions or to decrease excessive functions, and has no part in overt heart disease. First of all, it is a mild coronary vasodilator, increasing the blood supply to the heart muscles and lessening the potential for spasms, angina, and shortness of breath in the middle-aged or older individual with stage 1 impairment (symptom-free at rest) or stage 2 impairment (difficulty with moderate effort). Further, I have seen it help the middle-aged mesomorph, with moderate essential hypertension, whose pulse and pressure are slow to return to normal after moderate exertion, and whose long, tiring days leave the pulse rapid in the evening. It will gradually help to lower the diastolic pressure and quiet the pulse; it combines well with Passion Flower for such individuals. As with all uses of Hawthorn, the benefits take weeks or even months to be felt, but are well maintained, not temporary.

It is useful for arrhythmias or extrasystoles of a functional nature and not from overt heart disease, and for disturbing but not dangerous episodes of rapid heartbeat (tachycardia). The German Ministry of Health recommends Hawthorn for mild bradycardia (slow pulse) and for bradycardiac arrhythmias of a functional nature; but frankly, the only ill effect I ever observed was with an older woman with bradycardia and occasional palpitations who found Hawthorn made her faint and dizzy within several days of beginning the herb. The symptoms ceased after she stopped the tea. Since then, I don't like recommending Hawthorn for a slow pulse but instead for the above types of early cardiac imbalance. Use it to prevent degenerative disorders, as it is slow, safe (except as mentioned), and gradual. It is not useful in real heart disease—period.

In recent years the berries have been used increasingly in syrup or tea for strengthening connective tissue that has been weakened by excessive inflammation. The high level of flavonoids, particularly in the darker-colored species, makes this sensible. Flavonoids have often been shown to aid in chronic inflammations. I would suggest that the berries be made as a decoction, as the majority of cardiotonic constituents are heat-sensitive and are probably broken down by boiling. Personally, I consider Hawthorn a heart medicine and have mixed feelings about using it for its nutritional constituents. You decide.

Hedge Nettle

Stacys rigida, etc.   (Labiatae)
OTHER NAMES Woundwort

APPEARANCE *Stachys rigida* is the most common of the genus in the Pacific Coast region, and the other species resemble it greatly. Hedge Nettle tends to grow in stands; find one and you will find more nearby. Mature plants are usually 2 to 3 feet tall and bloom in mid- to late summer. The whole plant is prickly-hairy, with stiff, four-cornered stems, and large, petioled lower leaves. They are crenelated, opposite, and stand out straight from the stem, larger and closer towards the ground, smaller and more dispersed towards the top. The flowers are borne on terminal spikes, with the pink to purple flowers subtended by small leaves towards the bottom. The flowers form beadlike whorls, spaced apart towards the bottom of the spike, merging together as the buds are forming at the top. The plants have a minty, rhubarblike scent, sometimes verging on the unpleasant.

Hedge Nettle resembles Nettle somewhat, with the same prickly foliage, opposite leaves, and similar habitat, but Nettle has long strands of seeds, not whorled terminal spikes. Hedge Nettle resembles Figwort, especially earlier in the year, but it seldom branches, and Figwort's leaves are smooth and rank-scented. One Hedge Nettle, *Stachys albens,* is atypical in appearance. It is downy white and tends to form a more reclining, basal-leaved growth; the stems are thick, succulent, and soft-hollow. It has the typical scent of Hedge Nettle. California Hedge Nettle has distinct right-angled leaves and spiny calyx teeth. The latter plants are only found in California, primarily along the coast. Both, and other species as well, have the same scent and use, although S. *rigida* is the most typical and most common.

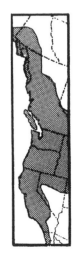

HABITAT Found in all the coastal areas in moist conditions, from bottomlands to shady canyons, and, to a lesser degree, the inner ranges as well; *Stachys palustris* grows east to the Atlantic and occurs in bottomlands in Nevada and Idaho eastwards.

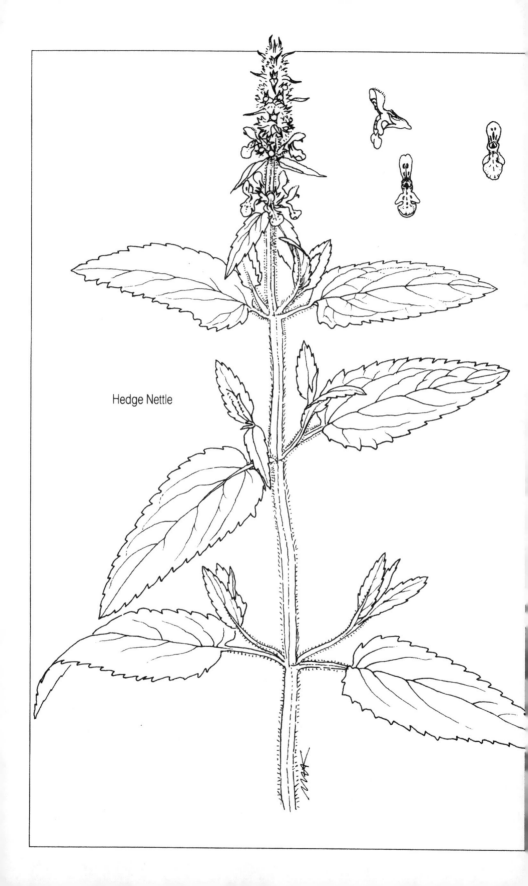

Hedge Nettle

CONSTITUENTS Stachydrine, stachyosides, phenethyl alcohol glycosides, at least one iridoid glycoside, and a high level of tannins.

COLLECTING Gather in summer to mid-fall for tincturing or tea; use anytime for fresh poultice of foliage or root.

STABILITY The herb is good for probably eighteen months, especially if stored in the whole form. The tincture is good indefinitely; fresh roots may be stored for several weeks in the refrigerator.

PREPARATION Fresh Plant Tincture, 1:2, Dry Plant Tincture, 1:5, 50% alcohol, both ½ to 1 teaspoon, up to four times a day. The tea may be drunk as an infusion, as needed. For topical use, make a fresh plant tincture by chopping up the moistened, fresh plant (1 part by weight), adding 1 part of menstruum, by volume (made up of ⅔ glycerin and ⅓ alcohol), pureeing them together, and storing for two weeks in a covered jar. Press out the tincture if you wish, using the fluid topically, or store it all intact, stirring up the mush and applying it to the injury as needed.

MEDICINAL USES The tea and the standard tinctures are useful for painful internal inflammation. Hedge Nettle helps migraine and hangover headaches, headaches from eyestrain, with the eyes inflamed and sore, and lessens the pain of simple urethritis and cystitis. For sprains and joint inflammation, take the herb internally and use the herb externally. A poultice made from mashed roots is the most effective topical form, but the tea, tinctures, or topical glycerin tincture are all useful. For headaches, try the herb, in any form, topically on the forehead. For sore throats, the fresh root can be chewed on or the tincture gargled. The glycerin tincture is a very effective first aid when applied to abrasions, contusions, sprains, and cuts. It is hemostatic, astringent, disinfectant, and, most importantly, lessens the inflammation and pain. The tea or tincture may be combined with Lemon Balm or Scullcap for nervousness, irritability, and insomnia with sensory hypersensitivity.

Horehound

Marrubium vulgare   (Labiatae)

OTHER NAMES Common Horehound, White Horehound; *Marrubio* (common Spanish name), *Mastranzo*

APPEARANCE This is a perennial, growing from a short, irregular knobby root, and with several to dozens of square stems. The stems, at maturity, are 1½ to 2 feet tall. The leaves are opposite, crinkly like Sage, with each pair of leaves at right angles to the ones below, and with many balls of flowers along the ends of the stems, subtended by paired leaves. The flowers are insignificant white blossoms inside of ten-toothed, bristly calices. These grow into the nasty stick-to-your-clothes burrs that, by summer, make stands irritating and maddening to walk through. The stems are woolly and the leaves variously fuzzy, dark green in shaded areas (with fewer hairs), and light green in the sun (with many hairs). Plants in colder climates have a sharp, acrid scent when crushed, those in the southern part of our range have little scent. The constituents, including aromatics, are highest just before full bloom, which can be May in southern California and July in Washington. The taste of the leaves is intensely bitter.

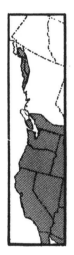

HABITAT This European plant might be found *anywhere*. The worse the soil, the more overgrazed the flora, the happier the Horehound. It is uncommon north of southern British Columbia and only occasional in Alaska, but it can be expected to grow everywhere else. Cattle do not graze it, but they carry the burr seeds, and the plant is most common around them, as well as around greenbelts in cities and rural slums.

CONSTITUENTS Marrubiin, marrubiol, marrubenol, peregrinol, and vulgerol (diterpenes); the lactoyl flavonoids luteolin and apigenin; the flavonoids vicenin II, vitexin, luteolin 7-glucoside, apigenin 7-glucoside, and chrysoeriol; betonicine, choline, volatile oils, tannins, and so forth.

COLLECTING Gather the stems, just as they begin to bloom, bundle them, and dry Method A; process the stems, leaves, and flowers, storing them in the shade.

STABILITY Although some of the expectoration effects start to deteriorate after a year, all other effects are still intact for at least two years. One of the things that amazes me about even well-intentioned commercial herb teas is their weakness, resulting from what I call the "inverted pyramid syndrome." I can gather Horehound in late summer, from the window of a speeding car, let it dry on the floor in the front room, curse it in Yiddish and Tewa, store it in open paper bags over the oven, and it still remains a usable medicine. Commercial Horehound is one of those herbs that is junk right out of the bag; I imagine the processing of it in terms of long conveyer belts that pass the herb under an inverted pyramid, sucking the life forces out, and into things like macadamia nuts and mock apple pie made from stale crackers. There are green herbs that, no matter how you process them, are delicate and short-lived—Shepherd's Purse, Skullcap, Spearmint. Such herbs just don't stay strong too long, and it is understandable when the commercial herb is feeble; they would be weak if you picked them yourself six months earlier. But with Horehound that old "inverted pyramid syndrome" applies.

PREPARATION Cold Infusion, 2 to 4 fluid ounces, up to three times a

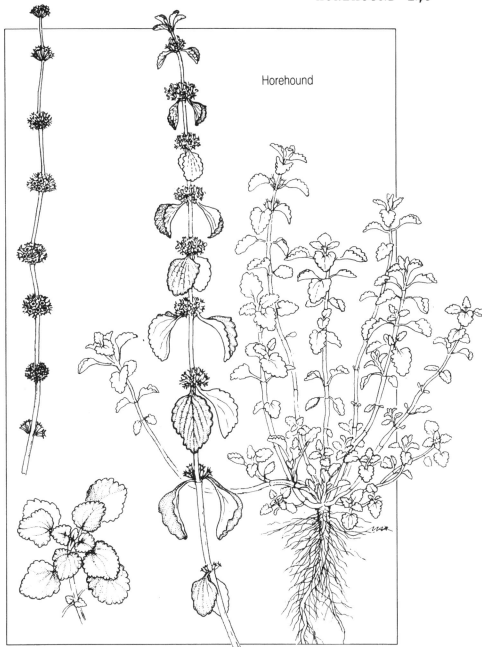

Horehound

day, Fresh Plant Tincture, 1:2, or Dry Plant Tincture, 1:5, 50% alcohol, both 30 to 90 drops, up to four times a day; 2 to 3 #00 capsules, up to three times a day.

MEDICINAL USES Horehound is mostly known for its expectorant effects, and any preparations will be helpful for moist, humid, hot bronchitis, flu, and your basic lung cold. It helps asthma that is moist and humid, particularly when there is an allergic basis to the acute episodes. Like most herbs that help asthma, Horehound will have little benefit for people taking daily medication and/or using inhalers every day. The anti-inflammatories, bronchial dilators, and decongestant drugs that some people depend on are so strong that not only would herbs have little effect next to such emphatic agents, but the withdrawal from them would make the symptoms worse. For others, with less dependence on asthma medications, or a less severe problem, taking four capsules of Horehound a day as a preventative is sound. I have found that a combination of *Echinacea angustifolia,* Passion Flower, and Horehound is the most effective regimen for preventing asthma of an allergic nature.

Further, Horehound is mildly stimulating to cardiopulmonary function, mucus membrane secretions in the lungs and intestinal tract, and bile secretions from the gallbladder. This makes it useful for those who have a little shortness of breath, a little too much recent increase in belly fat, tend to binge or eat large meals, and who suffer from palpitations and hiatus hernia heart-racing.

Horehound tastes rasty, but can be made into a nice cough syrup by brewing strong tea, evaporating it down, and adding honey.

Hummingbird Sage

Salvia spathacea   (Labiatae/Lamiaceae)
OTHER NAMES   Scarlet Sage, Pitcher Sage

APPEARANCE This is a strange and striking Sage. To begin with, it never branches but lives in its creeping roots, sending up one or several pyramidal annual plants with only a single flowering stalk. Instead of the pleasant, rough-textured Sage leaves (or smooth, as in White Sage), it puts out huge triangular or arrow-shaped leaves around the base of the annual stems. The lower leaves may be 6 or 8 inches long, on petioles half again as long, that bask around the base of the plants in an exotic, reptilian fashion—we're talking *big* leaves. Further up the stem, the leaves get smaller and narrower. The whole plant is sweetly aromatic-sticky, even gooier than Yerba Santa, and the leaves are dark and oily green on top, with a crenulated, wavy, iguana-skin surface, and fuzzy and whitish below, with a strongly swollen central vein. The spring flowers are a shocking scarlet, well over an inch long, with well-extended stamens. These form several large whorls of five or six flowers each, with a purplish or mauve ring of leafy bracts. The whole plant, in all its blooming glory, rises from 1½ to 3 feet in height, and there are usually several plants rising from the same root system. The foliage, when crushed, has a sweet, piney, sage-mint smell, like nothing you have smelled before. Why this lovely plant isn't the rage of native plant gardeners, I don't know.

HABITAT Hummingbird Sage grows in shady, rich-soiled places, often with Oak and usually where there is a fair amount of moist, rotting leaf mulch. It likes some slope to the terrain, although nothing too extreme, and you may need to walk up a small, shady notch until you find a colony growing in a fairy ring of Oaks. I am not implying it *only* grows with Oaks, but that is where I always find it. Hummingbird Sage is found only in the coastal ranges and usually only on the ridges immediately in from the ocean. Look for that typical chaparral-grassland–Oak-forest habitat that peeks out from behind the concrete, that ancient coastal grass-woodland undercoat upon which we have built our cities. It is found from Mount Diablo in the East Bay all along the California coast to Orange County but is most prolific from Big Sur down to Malibu.

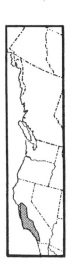

CONSTITUENTS I have *no* idea, although you could presume volatile oils (it smells), resins (it is sticky), and ursolic and oleanolic acids (most other Sages have them on their leaf surface).

COLLECTING Gather several of the large, healthy basal leaves, petiole and all, from each plant, preferably from May through July. Otherwise be careful of the plant; it isn't rare, and it isn't delicate, but it is so lovely and a group of plants help to hold a whole little mulchy biosphere together. This is the kind of place that supports the Columbia Lily and Fritillaries, and our plants are major players in a diminishing life circumstance.

STABILITY You can usually keep whole dried leaves for two years, although the sweet taste will be diminished somewhat.

PREPARATION Very simply, make a cup of the tea from a healthy pinch of leaf. Only crush the herb when ready to use so it stays as aromatic as possible.

MEDICINAL USES As a therapeutic agent, Hummingbird Sage will act as a decongestant expectorant, helping to stimulate secretions when you have had a cold or chest cold and are having difficulty in expectoration. The tea seems mildly antimicrobial and can be gargled and swallowed for sore throats; the Pomos of central California used a plug of the dried leaf as a vaginal bolus for vaginosis and as a leaf cud, chewed on hot days to lessen thirst, and for sore throats.

The main use, as far as I am concerned, is as a delicious tea. I have brewed it with Lemon Mint and Spearmint, and made a sweetened iced tea with lemon juice, Lemon Mint, or Sumach berries. It has a strong, musky, sweet taste that is never bitter but which can be overwhelming if you don't like strong teas . . . and just perfect if you do. When I had my herb store in Topanga, California, I liked to brew up some Lapsang

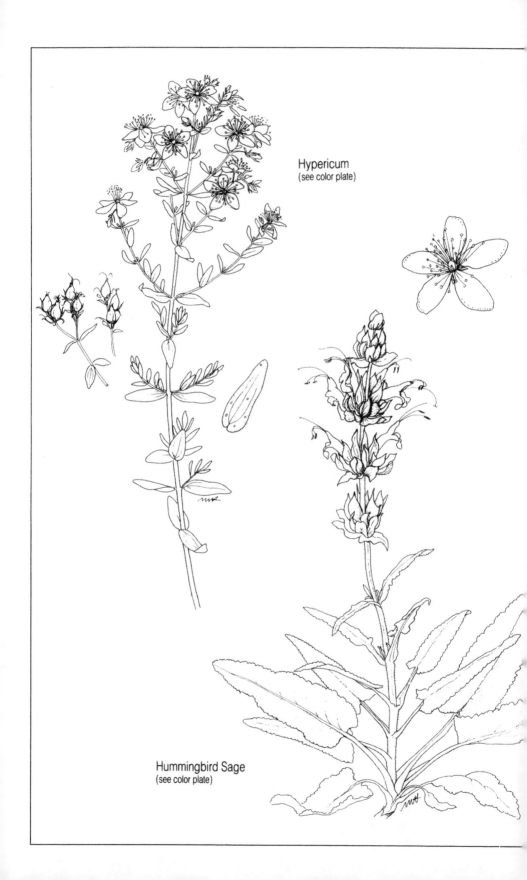

Hypericum
(see color plate)

Hummingbird Sage
(see color plate)

Souchang and some Hummingbird Sage for those cold, clammy February mornings, when the coastal dampness held no pleasure and I would drive to North Hollywood just to get warm.

OTHER USES Like White Sage, you can make an incense or smudge stick from the leaves. Let them wilt a day, roll them up into a cone, wind them around with thread, and let them dry in this form. Light the tip, blow out the flame, and let the embers smoke.

Hypericum

Hypericum perforatum   (Hypericaceae/Guttiferae/Clusiaceae)
OTHER NAMES   St. John's Wort, Klamath Weed

APPEARANCE Hypericum is an introduced European plant that now grows all over the Pacific West. It is a perennial plant, reproducing by seeds and rootstocks. Individual plants may actually be connected to the same creeping root mass. The aboveground part is usually 2 or 3 feet in height, and each plant has one or several main two-edged stems, which are bright green and tough. These stems branch extensively into smaller paired stems, with larger leaves at the junction of branches and smaller leaves along the length of the stem. The leaves are opposite, oval, and bear pellucid, transparent dots along their bright to dark green surfaces. The flowers are numerous, piled in profusion along all the tips of the many stems. They are bright golden yellow, five-petaled, and have many yellow Roselike stamens in the center. The buds are light yellow, and the seedpods are orange to red; if you crush the flowers, they stain your fingers purple. The plants are found in stands, sometimes very extensive ones, and when you find them, you start to see them everywhere.

One native species is common and useful—*Hypericum formosum*, also called *H. Scouleri*. It is a perennial plant, from 1 to 3 feet tall, with round opposite green leaves, and with single stems that only branch towards the top. The leaves have fewer transparent dots, usually only around the edges, and the flowers are also terminal at the ends of the branches. With fewer branches, there are fewer flowers. The constituents are the same, but the plant is only about half the strength of *H. perforatum,* so you may need to use twice as much.

HABITAT *Hypericum perforatum* is found from Monterey and Fresno counties, California, all the way north to British Columbia; and east through Idaho and western Montana, and the high, wet country of west-central Nevada. It is a spreading weed, and I have found stands, although small ones, in Utah, Arizona, and New Mexico. There is no clear habitat; it just requires moisture and people: it follows the plow and the tim-

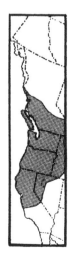

ber cutter, the cattle and the RV parks. *Hypericum formosum* likes cool, shady, and moist places, from coastal creeks to mountain meadows. It is most predictably found in streams that foster some Mints. It occurs in all of our states but can be maddening to locate. It can be found (with luck) in the moist areas of southern California—it isn't rare, just hard to see. Basically, the main species follows habitation (and roads); the native one is common in wild, moist places. If you find it at the top of a mountain, it will occur sporadically all down the waterway, at least until you reach that suburban mall at the bottom. (Don't they know they built right over a floodplain?)

CONSTITUENTS The red pigment hypericin is the main active constituent, but there are also bioactive oils, resins, antimicrobial rottlerin-type compounds, hypericum xanthones, and procyanidins that all contribute to its effects. Hypericin and Hypericum complexes are widely used in European medicine, both as over-the-counter and prescription pharmaceuticals. It isn't aggressive enough (or patentable enough) for American drug use. This is another safe plant drug that the FDA says doesn't work. I guess American patients are genetically different from French or German patients.

COLLECTING Gather the flowering tips (including a few leaves) from June through late August. This is a longer stretch than most sources acknowledge, but I have picked fresh blooms as late as the first week in September. True, it was at the top of St. Mary's Peak (4,000 feet) near Corvallis, Oregon, and in little, sheltered canyons up from the Lochsa River in northern Idaho; still, if you need it, it can be found. Stuff those quart jars full to the top with yellow and green tips, include some seeds if they are there, jam some more in, and cover with grain alcohol—it will be a perfect 1:2 Fresh Flower Tincture. If you are going to make an oil, let the flowering tips set loosely in an open paper bag for a day, then pack the oil. The bugs will leave, and the flowers will lose some of their water and synthesize a bit more hypericin and aromatics. Some folks like to dry their Hypericum. Believe me, the fresh preparations are so superior, I won't even mention drying.

STABILITY Both the tincture and the oil are stable for years. And, as I promised, I won't even talk about the dry herb.

PREPARATION The Fresh Herb Tincture, 1:2, 20 to 30 drops, up to three times a day. Hypericum Oil is best made by grinding the wilted flowering tips and covering them with olive oil. Jam your jar full to the top, remove them and grind, return them to the jar, and fill it to the top with the oil. Placing a coffee filter on top of the herb before adding the oil will assure that the herb stays below the level of the oil. Store this out of light in a warm place for two or three weeks and express the oil by wringing in a cloth or using a press. If there is any remainder of water-soluble juices in the oil, allow them to settle overnight and decant off the bright red oil. Water dregs left in the steeped oil can eventually induce fermentation or mold. The oil can be used externally, or a teaspoon taken internally, three times a day.

MEDICINAL USES Hypericum is one of our best herbal therapies for depression and numbing frustration. It seems to work best for those people, especially men, who find things falling apart but who really have little life experience with failure or loss of confidence. This is all very subjective on my part, but I think of using Hypericum when someone whose circumstances have changed is unable to alter his ways of acting and responding. Such people follow the previously reliable responses and strategies, but their life needs new approaches; they are stuck in a rut, spinning their wheels, and feeling growing frustration and depression with their problems. Hypericum has little or no value in bipolar depressions or depressive states with a clear pathology. It is for normal folks whose strategies have failed and who are temporarily adrift. I realize this is an almost impossibly broad description, but you can narrow it down a bit, since there are usually transitory and ill-defined physical symptoms that further define Hypericum as appropriate. Old physical problems or nervous habits may have returned, such as nail biting, breathing problems, sexual dysfunction, constipation, or skin disorders—signs that there are underlying physical frustrations and unresolved nervous agitation as fellow travelers to feeling frustrated. Of course, this is also the time to check your diet, do some walking, go to church, throw the I Ching, or read some of the 1,200 pounds of books on emotional self-help to be found in the bookstore at your local mall. I will add Hypericum as a useful herb to these self-help strategies. Think of it for the friend who is out of work, the overwhelmed postgrad student, the woman who feels graceless and unprepared for menopause, or the self-appointed saviour of (younger) women with his third tuck, bad prostate, and scared, haunted look behind the (tinted contacts) eyes. Some will find quick help from the tincture; others will find it takes a week or two to start feeling more focused and alert.

The oil is recommended in European medicine as a healing agent for chronic gastritis and stomach ulcers; Weiss recommends a teaspoon on an empty stomach first thing in the morning and last thing at night. The oil is useful for any abrasions, skin ulcerations, or moderate burns, as it stimulates granulation and capillary regeneration, as well as having substantial antibacterial effects. Christopher Hobbs, quoting a German study, says that first-degree burns healed in forty-eight hours when treated with an Hypericum ointment. It is very effective for gradually lessening the pain and can be used during the day, while applying a Prickly Poppy seed butter ointment (if you made any) at night.

The oil should be used topically when there is muscle or nerve pain that is distinct from joint or tissue inflammation, myalgia, and neuralgia. It is also good for such things as sciatica, back spasms, and neck cramps that continue after the structural problem has, if possible, been dealt with. It combines well with Arnica and Poplar Bud oils as an all-purpose ache and pain reliever. Use 2 parts Hypericum with 1 part each of Arnica and Poplar Bud oils. For temporomandibular problems, with stress headaches and neck pain, rub the mixed oil into the jaw several times a day.

There are conflicting reports about the antiviral effects of Hypericum; some reports have even claimed it to be effective against the HIV virus. I would take that with a large boulder of salt, but there is no question that it helps the depression and agitation which accompany both HIV and chronic fatigue syndrome infections, and it has great value strictly on the basis of its nontoxic, antidepressive effects.

CONTRAINDICATIONS Hypericum has MAO type A inhibition effects, although moderate, and should be avoided wherever pharmaceutically appropriate. Although it has a reputation for causing potential photo-sensitization, with skin eruptions and hives being possible side effects when coming in contact with lots of sunlight, this problem is largely sham. I have encountered one person with a sun/skin reaction—a man with very white skin, and jet black hair, what's called Black Irish in some quarters. He took too much of the tincture—a compulsive amount, actually. Moreover, he had a long history of depression, really needed medical counseling and treatment, not Hypericum, and spent a week fly-fishing at 9,000 feet while gargling the tincture. And in spite of all this, he only had a moderate and short-lived skin reaction.

The FDA and the antiquack brigades from the right wing of the medical establishment have tried from time to time to prevent sales of Hypericum preparations, since the plant, eaten in large quantities by cattle with white albino patches, has caused them to get skin lesions. German physicians, when using hypericin injections, are told to keep the patient out of direct sunlight as a precaution, but there is no evidence that human reactions have occurred; the precautions are based on the indications of grazing animals.

Inside-Out Flower

Vancouveria hexandra, etc.   (Berberidaceae)
OTHER NAMES Duckfoot, Redwood Ivy

APPEARANCE The three species of *Vancouveria* are only found in the Pacific West. They are little plants, usually about a foot high, and have wiry stems and roots. The leaflets are arranged a little like Clematis,

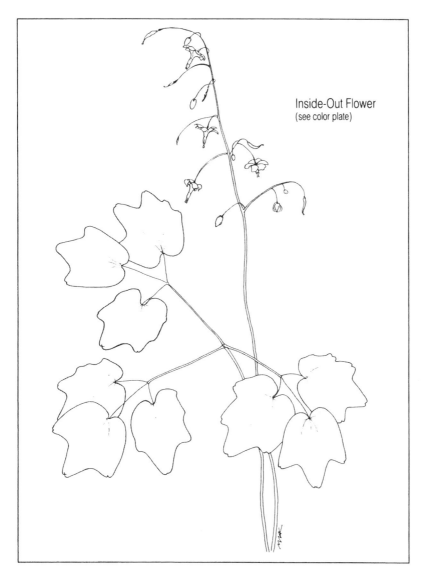

Inside-Out Flower
(see color plate)

with usually a lower pair of opposite petioled compound leaves, most often three in number, and a central compound leaf, also made up of three leaflets. Technically this is called biternate, but just think three sets of three, and that will describe the main form of these compound basal leaves. These leaflets are peculiar and distinctive in shape, being bluntly triangular or quadrangular, usually with three points, webbed between (hence the common name Duckfoot), and superficially resembling the leaflets of Maidenhair Fern, Rue, Meadow Rue, or Blue Cohosh (an eastern relative). The flowers arise loosely from a long, nodding, wiry stem and are white or cream-colored, with a peculiar swept-back form, somewhat parachutelike, resembling tiny versions of the well-known mountain wildflower Shooting Star (*Dodecatheon* sp.).

The two white-flowered species, *Vancouveria hexandra* and *V. planipetala* (*V. parviflora*), are the most common and the ones I prefer to see gathered. The third species, *V. chrysantha,* has yellow flowers, and the petioles and pedicels are covered with reddish fur; the leaflets are nearly round and somewhat downy underneath. It seems only to be found in sporadic stands in northwest California and southwest Oregon, and should not be picked. To locate the other two, find the right kind of forest, and they will predictably be there.

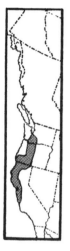

HABITAT *Vancouveria hexandra* is the most widespread, found in deep forest and shade, with old-growth or second-growth conifers, from the west side of the Cascades, a little below Seattle, to the north coastal range of California, as far south as Mendocino County, and into the Klamath Cascade interface in Siskiyou County. *V. planipetala* grows in a little drier environment, within the coastal fogs and the current or former range of the Redwoods, from Santa Cruz north into Curry County in southwestern Oregon. Inside-Out Flower is often associated with Vanilla Leaf, Wild Ginger, Goldthread, Pipsissewa, and Pyrola.

CONSTITUENTS Two anhydroicaritins (flavonol glycosides), a berberine-type alkaloid, and, according to an older, dubious report, hydrastine.

COLLECTING Gather the whole plant, roots and all, during the heat of late summer and early autumn. *V. hexandra* loses its leaves by autumn, and *V. planipetala* is an evergreen; but July through early September is the best time to gather either plant. Dry Method B or in paper bags.

STABILITY The dry plant should be good for at least a year and a half, the root for several years.

PREPARATION The Dry Plant Tincture, 1:5, 50% alcohol, 30 drops, up to four times a day. The ground whole plant, Standard Infusion, 1 fluid ounce, up to four times a day; or 1 gram in tea, up to four times a day.

MEDICINAL USES Inside-Out Flower seems to be particularly useful for boggy, edematous, and congested mucosa. The most predictable uses are for sinus congestion, chronic rhinitis, and hay fever; for stuffy sinuses in the evening; and after meals (in which case check for food hypersensitivities). It combines well with Yerba Mansa, California Bayberry, and Bidens for this purpose; and Hawthorn berry syrup will provide additional capillary-strengthening flavonoids for all of the uses of Inside-Out Flower. Further, it can be used for extended, noninfectious bloodshot eyes, and should be combined with Yerba Mansa (for internal use) and some Yerba Reuma or *Eriogonum* for an eyewash. It works well, in general, for dull, aching, and boggy tissues in any of the orifices, including the throat, esophagus, rectum, or vagina. It is not strong and needs another herb to affect the problem more specifically, such as Shepherd's Purse or Mallow for the urethra or bladder, California Buckeye or Figwort for the rectum, and so forth.

CONTRAINDICATIONS I really have no idea about the hydrastine alkaloid presence in this plant, so I do not feel secure recommending it for use during pregnancy, since hydrastine, like its normal source Goldenseal, is not particularly safe during pregnancy.

Labrador Tea

Ledum glandulosum, L. groenlandicum (Ericaceae)
OTHER NAMES Trapper's Tea

APPEARANCE The various varieties of *Ledum* may or may not be distinct species; they may interbreed; and different stands of the same variety growing in divergent environments may look far more distinct from each other than supposedly different species growing in similar environments. Labrador Tea is a low-growing bush, with stubby, woody, and widely spaced branches having grey, dark tan, and, towards the tips, reddish brown bark. The leaves are oval to lance-shaped (depending on habitat and variety), alternate, and cluster densely around the ends of the stems. Like other relatives in the family, such as Madrone and Rhododendron, the lowest leaves in a bunch will often be reddish brown, particularly in late summer and fall.

The northern species, *L. groenlandicum* (really a variety of the circumboreal species *L. palustre*), has leaves that are turned under at the margins, usually with fuzzy red undersides but sometimes nearly white. *L. glandulosum* usually has leaves that are less rolled or almost flat, and the underside fuzz is white, although it may be reddish as well. The flowers bloom in May or June, are showy, flat terminal clusters, usually between five and ten in number, and snow-white to cream in color. They have five petals and five to ten well-extended stamens. The five-sided greenish brown capsules open up from the base to the tip, discharging minute seeds.

Ledum can be confused with Mountain Laurel (*Kalmia*), which is similar in habitat, but is smaller and has pinkish flowers that are more round in outline than five-petaled and none of the strong spicy smell when crushed. Bog Rosemary (*Andromeda*) has only long leaves, flowers and capsules that are urn-shaped and nod downwards, and no spicy scent; and it barely crosses into Washington from Canada. Both *Kalmia* and *Andromeda* are toxic plants, grow in similar bogs, and are sometimes mistaken for *Ledum*. Crush the leaves to make sure. If you find one of its toxic relatives, look around in the same area, for Labrador Tea is usually far more abundant than the others in their mutual habitats.

HABITAT The *Ledums*, like most Ericaceae, need acidic, poorly drained, or boggy soil. Look for *Vacciniums*, Bog Orchids, Bayberry stands, and

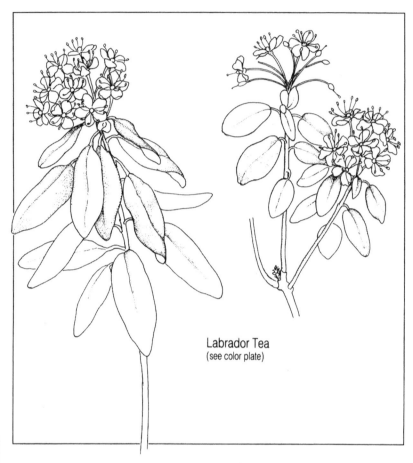

Labrador Tea
(see color plate)

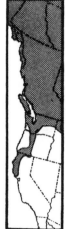

open wet meadows, in the mountains of the coastal ranges, the Cascades, the Rockies south to Wyoming, along the coastal bogs north to Alaska, and as far south as Sonoma County in California (or perhaps as far south as Santa Cruz). In coastal bogs, look for Skunk Cabbage first, then check around the swamp for Labrador Tea.

CONSTITUENTS Ericolin, arbutoside, ursolic acid, about 3% tannins, and a volatile oil that includes ledol (Ledum camphor).

COLLECTING Gather the leaves in the summer and fall (after seeding), break off the leaf tips, and dry loosely in a paper bag (for tea). If you can, gather the spring or early summer leaves for fresh tincturing. If you can't, don't worry. The aromatics are higher in the late spring and therefore stronger externally; the leaves are better collected after midsummer. With somewhat less aromatic oil content, this makes for a better tea.

STABILITY Usually at least two years, if the leaves are kept whole until using. The tincture is good for three or four years, but eventually the active constituents precipitate out (unlike with most tinctures).

PREPARATION Fresh Leaf Tincture, 1:2 (for external use). Dried leaves separated from stems for interleaving between layers of stored clothes. Dried leaves for tea, up to a handful for a pot.

MEDICINAL USES The tea tastes great: a little bitter, aromatic, salty, and tart, all at once. You will find that several pots can be made from the same leaves. It is slightly laxative, yet helps soothe diarrhea. It is both slightly expectorant and drying to the bronchi and sinuses if you have a head cold or allergies. Most of all, if you have an upset stomach, have been vomiting, or have a yellow-green hangover, drink at least a cup or two of the strong tea. Labrador Tea has that ability, like Yerba Mate, to taste good fresh and steaming, lukewarm, or left-in-the-pot cold. Ledol, one of the aromatics found in the spicy oils, is somewhat toxic in excess, but it is not water soluble. It is a sedative and slightly narcotic substance and, like camphor, can cause palpitations and cerebral irritability in large amounts. Scandinavians used to (and may still) crush a handful of leaves into their booze, leave them there, and use that liquor for a nighttime sedative nip.

The fresh tincture can be applied to kill scabies, lice, and chiggers, and works very nicely as an antifungal for various skin tineas.

OTHER USES Schofield recommends using the leaves in stored grain to discourage mice and rats. The leaves may be added (in moderation) to herbal smoking mixtures to improve the taste.

Lemon Balm

Melissa officinalis   (Labiatae)
OTHER NAMES Balm, Melissa

APPEARANCE Lemon Balm is a medium-sized plant, Mintlike, hairy, and with frequently branched, sharply four-sided, brittle stems. The leaves are light to medium green, 1 to 3 inches long (much smaller towards the top), with a distinct petiole, round to somewhat triangular, and scalloped to bluntly toothed. The flowers are borne on thin axillary stems, themselves axillary to small leaves, and new flowers bloom higher up the plant in response to moisture, sometimes long after the older blossoms have matured to seed. The flowers themselves are light yellow to white and somewhat inconspicuous. The scent of the foliage is sweetly lemony.

HABITAT Lemon Balm is an escaped garden plant and can be found in

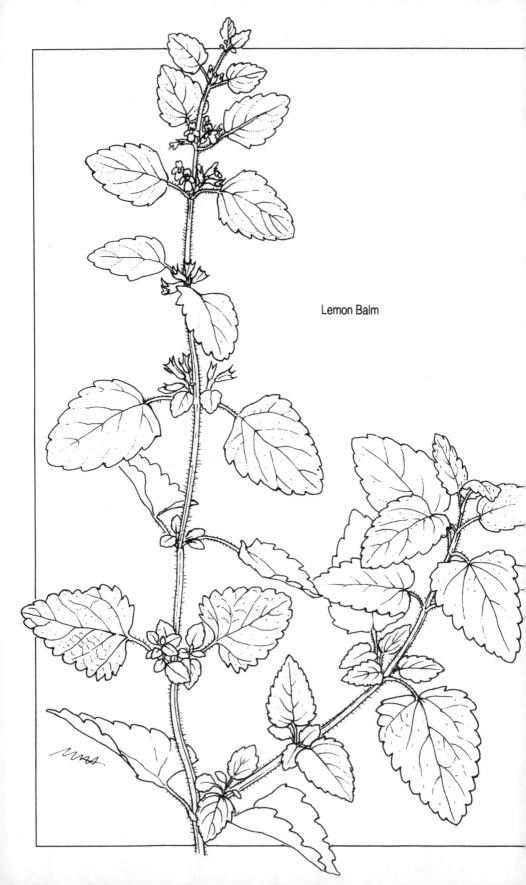

Lemon Balm

a variety of moist, shady circumstances. It is most frequent in the coastal lowlands and foothills, from Santa Cruz northwards through what is left of the Redwood belt to Tillamook Bay in Oregon. I have seen it inland west of the Cascades in Oregon and Washington, but it occurs in greatest abundance along the coast.

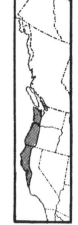

CONSTITUENTS A volatile oil including citral, citronellal, eugenol acetate, geraniol, polyphenols, tannins, flavonoids, rosmarinic acid, and triterpenoids.

COLLECTING Gather whole aerial parts from early summer to mid-fall and dry Method A. Its hairiness and the fact that it can be found by roadsides make it important to gather it from clean areas.

STABILITY Lemon Balm is not stable for very long. Its leaves are thin and fragile, and the overall content of volatile oils is, at best, only a small fraction of what it is in other members of the Mint family. I haven't found that it survives much past a year; if you discover that the plant works well for you, I would suggest either making a tincture of recently dried herbs or storing the dried tea in airtight bags in the freezer.

PREPARATION Standard Infusion, 3 to 4 fluid ounces; Dry Herb Tincture, 1:5, 50% alcohol, ½ to 1 teaspoon in hot water, or several cups of the tea if needed. Lemon Balm smells great, tastes pleasant though a bit bland, and combines well with other herbs.

MEDICINAL USES Lemon Balm is not a potent medicine, works predictably, has no side effects, and can be combined with other herbs in a beneficial way. It is a simple sedative and a surprisingly effective mood elevator and antidepressant. If you are tired, burned out, nervous, or under extended emotional stress, the tea will relax you nicely. The tea is a useful antispasmodic for a variety of conditions, from menstrual cramps to stomachache to diarrhea and gas pain. It is mildly antiviral and can be drunk every several hours for flu, bad head colds, and fevers, as well as to induce sweating, promote relaxation, decrease aches and pains, and perhaps help with the virus. It has been shown to be moderately effective against herpes viruses, especially cold sores. Good stuff.

Licorice Fern

Polypodium glycyrrhiza (Polypodiaceae)
OTHER NAMES Common Polypody, Rock Brake, Sweet Fern; *P. vulgare*, var. *occidentale, P. occidentale*

APPEARANCE This is a small fern, often with only one or two fronds growing from a rhizome. The fronds are usually around a foot long, of

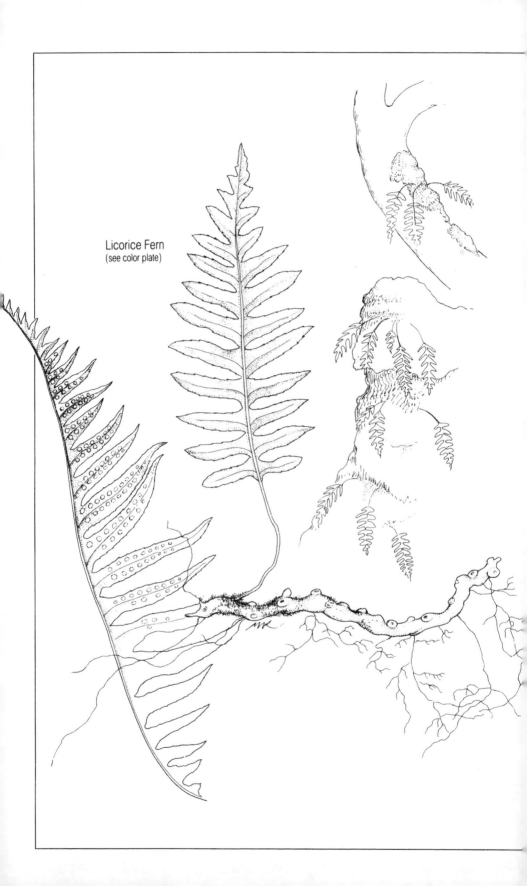

Licorice Fern
(see color plate)

which a third of the length is the naked stalk that extends from the root to the lowest leaflets (pinnae). The pinnae are smaller at the bottom, flare out to their greatest length (2 to 3 inches) a quarter of the way up the frond, and decrease in length to the tip, forming an extended pyramid in shape. The pinnae are lanceolate, somewhat alternate along the stem, and pinnatifid, with the clefts almost through to the midrib. The whole appearance is of a delicate little fog-forest fern, growing mostly as an epiphyte, from mossy rocks, trees, nurse logs, even old cabins and Civilian Conservation Corps rock work. The main things to remember about Licorice Fern are that the entire width of the leaflet or pinnule is attached to the stem, splaying out to web with the pinnae above and below, and that the dark brown, horizontal, scaly rhizome is translucent-fleshed and has an overripe licorice-sweet taste.

HABITAT Licorice Fern is an epiphyte, and is completely a plant of the moist temperate rain forests of the Pacific Coast, from the region of the coastal Redwoods in northern California (as far south as Marin County), all the way up to coastal Alaska; west to the Aleutians; and inland in the wettest localities of the Columbia Gorge; the western edges of the Cascades of Oregon and Washington; the inland valleys of British Columbia; and so forth. It is rarely found outside of the ranges of coastal and river fogs. Find moss-covered logs, trees, rocks, and slopes, avoid stepping on the slugs, and you will probably find Licorice Fern. Other species of *Polypodium* fern are sometimes encountered, and one, *P. vulgare*, a common fern of temperate northern circumboreal wet places, resembles Licorice Fern; but although it has a similar sweet root taste, it has an unpleasant, gagging aftertaste and is much less elegant than our plant.

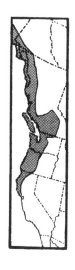

CONSTITUENTS Two steroidal glycosides, polypodine B, polypodoside A, (+)-catechin, (+)-afzelechin, and the steroid saponin, osladin. There have been periodic reports of the presence of glycyrrhizic acid, the sweet substance and predominant bioactive compound found in Licorice Root (*Glycyrrhiza glabra*), but this is not the case. Licorice Root mimics some adrenocortical functions and can aggravate sodium retention in some individuals. Licorice Fern does not appear to share these effects/side effects. Its close relative, Common Polypody (*P. vulgare*), contains methyl salicylate, a fairly common plant substance with Wintergreen scent and some aspirinlike effects. Licorice Fern probably has some salicylate constituents, perhaps accounting for some of its anti-inflammatory effects, but I have found no reference to that fact in the literature. Still, I would probably not use the plant if I had an allergy to aspirin, was taking anticoagulants, or had any clotting disorder.

COLLECTING Gather the rhizomes in late summer to mid-fall, scrub them clean of chuff, and dry. The fresh root is not the best form to use internally, as it can cause mild nausea. The dry root is the preferable form. The dried rhizomes are tough and brittle, and it may be preferable to cut them into small sections when fresh, drying them in that form. You should avoid gathering roots in the spring, both because it prevents the fern from reproducing by spore and the high sugar content of the rapidly growing spring plant can cause the drying rhizomes to easily mold.

STABILITY The roots are stable for several years.

PREPARATION The Strong Decoction, 2 to 4 fluid ounces, up to three times a day.

MEDICINAL USES The main value of Licorice Fern is in helping to decrease inflammatory and hypersensitivity states. Let's say you have been stung by a bee and your skin is sensitive and itchy for days afterwards, or you ate some marginal shrimp, got a mild case of hives, and you find that your stomach hurts, your lungs are sore, or your hemorrhoids are flaring up. Maybe you took some ampicillin, got a mild reaction, and your skin and mucosa have been oversensitive for months now. These are variously mast-cell excitability, allergy-induced IgE (Immunoglobulin E; see Glossary) reactivity, atopic allergies, and slow-histamine responses. All that means is that something caused a specific allergic reaction (bee venom, shrimp, or ampicillin), the specific antibody (acquired or learned immunity) acted, you got the hives, diarrhea, or swollen lips, and the response went away. You are left with a lingering wheal or inflammatory excitability, not specific to anything, just pissed-off and irritable. In such a state, irritations to the bronchial membranes, throat, stomach, bowels, skin, and joints can result in frequent, short-lived but aggravating inflammatory responses that are hard to figure out. Things that don't normally bother you act up, food that you often eat causes indigestion or rapid heartbeat, normally innocuous pets make you itch, and so forth. Try this: lightly scratch the inside of your forearm or the skin below your navel with your fingernail. If the scratch raises a red wheal that goes away within an hour, you are reactive. It won't help to keep treating the specific inflammation; it will crop up somewhere else since *you* are inflamed. You can take antihistamines (very efficient but with lots of side effects) or use Licorice Fern (less efficient but with no side effects) and decrease your environmental and food irritants as the inflammatory response gradually subsides.

Generally, this plant works best for lung irritations, stomach and colon irritability, and for inflamed throat, mouth, and gums. I have seen it help cervix and prostate irritability as well, although I would usually start with the more usual approaches (Trillium, Peony, Yerba Mansa, and the like), using Licorice Fern if the inflammatory response still continues.

CONTRAINDICATIONS As mentioned, Licorice Fern may contain salicylates. Therefore, it probably shouldn't be used with aspirin allergies, anticoagulant drugs, or blood dyscrasias; and, lacking thorough knowledge as to its constituents, it is best to not use it during pregnancy.

Lomatium

Lomatium dissectum   (Umbelliferae)

OTHER NAMES   Desert Parsley, Fern-leafed Lomatium, Indian (Desert) Parsnip, Wild Carrot; *Tohza, Leptotaenia dissecta*. The species has a number of name variations, both as *Leptotaenia* (*dissecta, multifida, purpurea, eatonii,* and *foliosa*) and *Lomatium dissectum,* vars. *dissectum, multifidum, eatonii,* and *occidentalis.*

APPEARANCE Lomatium is a large, substantial plant, sending up fernlike, bright green leaves in the spring, the whole basal leaf sometimes a foot long, divided into three or four sections, which in turn multiply into threadlike leaflets. Larger plants may have a dozen basal leaves. The flowering stalks are 2 to 5 feet tall, stout, and nearly leafless, extending well above the foliage. When growing on rocky outcroppings, as they often do, the stems arc out and upwards, a distinctive pattern that aids in their identification. The flowering stems may branch on occasion, but there is usually a single umbel of yellow or purple flowers at the end of the stem. By summer they have matured into large, flat, oval seeds, with shallow wings and barely visible oil tubes. Each seed splits from the base to form two separate carpels, splaying out from the top. By early fall these occasional single seed halves clinging to tall stems may be all that is distinctive about the died-back aerial parts. Many botanical texts describe the large, woody, thickened root. Actually, the root is fleshy, thick at the top, lumpy, and irregular, like a mutant cross between a carrot and rutabaga, with odd parts left over. The skin is pearly grey, with many oil glands spread throughout the variously cream- and yellow-colored flesh.

In the spring the roots ooze milky aromatic sap; by fall the sap is more resinous and balsamic; but in any case, the sticky, bitter aromatic sap and the soft, fibrous flesh (not at all woody) differentiate this big Lomatium from the others of the genus. The Lomatium clan is huge, with eighty closely related species in the western states. For many years, the large size of a few of these plants (most Lomatiums are quite small) caused botanists to class them apart in the genus *Leptotaenia*. The larger Lomatiums, by whatever name, are an amorphous group, and I have found several strikingly varied stands whose *roots* are typical of *L. dissectum* in their morphology and constituents, which *act* like *L. dissectum* when tinctured, have identical contents as measured by TLC (thin-layer chromatography), but don't particularly *look* like *L. dissectum*. I have found these plants in such varied locations as Modoc County, California, northwestern Wyoming, and the front range of northern Colorado. I have a hunch that other of the larger plants in the old *Leptotaenia*

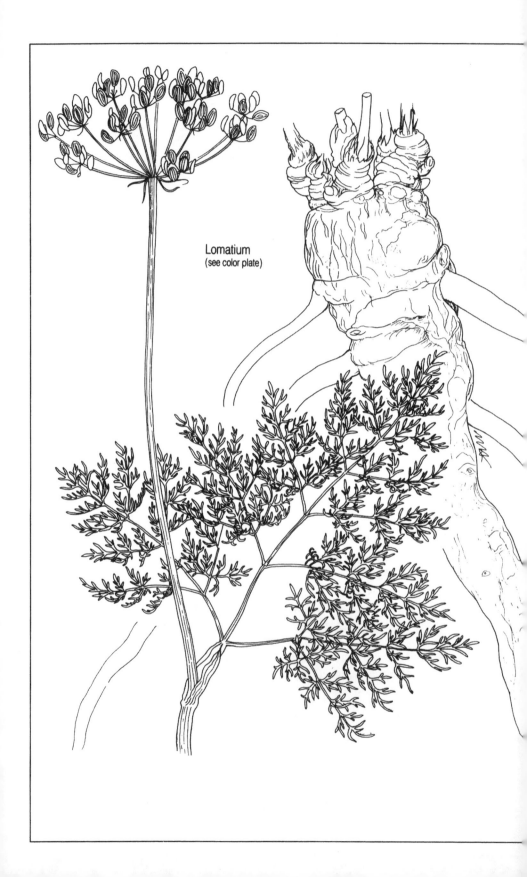

Lomatium
(see color plate)

genus can be used in the same way, but in any case, *L. dissectum* and its varieties are the most widespread and successful of the group and what I am familiar with. Most of the other large Lomatiums that grow in the range of *L. dissectum* have sweet, starchy parsniplike roots and could not be confused with this bitter, aromatic, oily- and waxy-rooted giant.

HABITAT Lomatium is found sporadically in rocky localities on Vancouver Island, across to southern British Columbia and Alberta; but its main turf is the Great Basin, from eastern Washington, south through Oregon and the dry slopes of the Sierra Nevada; most of Idaho, east to western Montana; south through Wyoming, Utah, and Nevada; the northwest corner of Colorado; and with a few large but disjunct pockets in central Arizona. Look for a creek or river valley cut through a mesa, with steep slopes, some trees, boulders, rocks, and (usually) stands of Balsam Root. You will probably find some Lomatium in such localities—if you look long enough, that is. If not, try further downcreek towards the beginning of the canyon, where the alluvial fan widens out, and check along the slopes overlooking the water. Finding your first *Lomatium dissectum* can be maddening, since large stands, growing in the right circumstances, may be 100 miles apart, only to grow in every nook and cranny once you have found them. Check with an herbalist, botanist, or your local university herbarium if you get too frustrated.

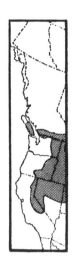

CONSTITUENTS A mixed bag of essential oils, gums, resins, and resinoids, with antimicrobial tetronic acids, luteolin, coumarin glycosides, including columbianin, luvangetin, and at least one furanocoumarin.

COLLECTING I have dug the roots in late spring, summer, and early fall, and find that I like using the earlier roots for fresh root tincture and the fall roots for dry root tincture. Conversely, unless you have a lot of time on your hands to look for dried, overhanging flower stalks with a few large, flat seeds still adhering, and you like hanging out over narrow canyons in eastern Washington in late August (I do, but I do it for a living), stick to the spring growth (bright green and in flower) or the early summer growth (yellow-green basal foliage and nearly mature, large seed umbels). Be practical; it is far easier to find, identify, and dig Lomatium earlier in the year.

I have no qualms about high-grading an area. You will often see large numbers of plants up the gorge, difficult to access without rock climbing equipment, and a few plants towards the bottom of the hill that you can get to. Just dig those that have roots embedded in dirt, leave those anchored between rocks (and all those up the slope you can't get to), and you will have anywhere from 1 to 5 pounds of huge, dark, oozy roots, a creek a few steps away to wash them in, and nearly all of the plants remaining to reseed. If you plan to dry some roots, let them wilt whole for a few days in the open or in a paper bag, then slice them crosswise about ½ inch thick, and finish drying them in cardboard flats. If you were to slice them right away, the milky sap would be absorbed into the flats; letting them wilt allows the sap to harden a bit, and little absorption occurs.

STABILITY The dried root is strong for at least eighteen months; both dry and fresh root tinctures are stable for years.

PREPARATION Fresh Root Tincture, 1:2, Dry Root Tincture, 1:5, 70% alcohol, both 10 to 30 drops, up to five times a day. Cold Infusion, 2 to 3 fluid ounces, up to five times a day.

MEDICINAL USES Lomatium has been used for centuries as a medicine by Native Americans who live in the Great Basin; it was used by many Mormon settlers in Utah and Nevada, and it was well known by some Oregon pioneers. They all used it for lung problems, bad fevers, and pneumonia, and there are many references to its value for persistent winter fevers; *Leptonaenia* preparations were used by regular school, eclectic, and homeopathic doctors in the Pacific region as late as the turn of the century. Except for a brief reference to it in the *Journal of the American Pharmaceutical Society* (1925), outside of the region it was pretty much ignored until Percy Train, operating on a shoestring in Nevada, put together a group of remarkably intelligent screening protocols; he published a government evaluation of the potentials of Nevada medicinal plants, at the beginning of the Second World War (naturally nobody noticed), and found that Lomatium soared above them all. It killed just about every microbe his research group tested it against, and you could douse rats in it without hurting them. He also reiterated the information that had excited Nevada physicians earlier: morbidity among Nevada Indians and whites who had used Lomatium against the influenza epidemic of 1920–1922 was far lower than among the general population. In the last decade it has been used with great success by naturopathic physicians, all of whom are trained in the Northwest.

Although Lomatium effectively inhibits most gram-positive bacteria, and I have seen it work quickly (combined with Echinacea) against shigella infections (including my own), its main value is for respiratory virus infections. Its aromatic resins act as an expectorant, some of the fractions (as with Eucalyptus) are exhaled as gases by the lungs, and some of the resins are excreted in the bronchial mucus, all aiding lung cleansing and reducing bronchial microbes. Further, several of the aromatics have been shown to limit replication or shedding in many viruses, and they also seem to shorten the duration of the viral infection and limit the surface area of mucus membranes that become infected. Lomatium definitely helps simple head colds and shortens the duration of overt influenza viral infections.

Several of the coumarin glycocides and the furan-based acids have, in other plants, been shown to stimulate the rate of phagocytosis (eating bad stuff) in white blood cells, and Lomatium can be expected to be a mild immune stimulant. I would recommend combining it with a diaphoretic, such as Wild Ginger, European Pennyroyal, or Elder; a stimulant to liver function and bile secretion, such as Dandelion; and something to stimulate mucus secretion in the respiratory tract, such as Balsam Root, Grindelia, or Osha. One of the side effects that some people get from Lomatium is a rash of hives. It seems to occur more frequently with the stronger fresh root preparation, but, a month later, in the same person, it produces no skin eruption, so it would not appear to be an allergic reaction. While using other herbs in combination with Lomatium, as mentioned above, I have seen no such reactions occur. The rashes seem to be a short-term nitrogenous waste-product overload from immunologic stimulation, cytokine excess, or the waste products of viral die-off. If you use other herbs to stimulate waste-product metabolism and excretion, you get no rashes. If you use Lomatium as a "little-drug" antiviral, trying to kill the bugs as if it were some plant antibiotic without supporting the whole person, side effects can occur.

Lomatium seems to also be very helpful in limiting the severity and number of respiratory infections in those with slow viruses, such as Epstein-Barr virus and cytomegalovirus, the kind of stuff they now call chronic fatigue syndrome. It should also be tried with HIV infections, since all these immunosuppressive viruses decrease the general resistance to respiratory infections.

Otherwise, the tincture is an excellent first aid for skin infections, a gargle for sore throats, and a topical aid for gum and mouth inflammations; and the cold infusion, warmed to body temperature, can be used as a douche for candida and other vaginal infections. For gardnerella infections, the vaginal pH (normally acidic) needs to be normalized afterwards with lactobacillus from a yogurt douche.

OTHER USES The milky sap that oozes from spring roots is an excellent skin-moisturizing agent.

Madrone

Arbutus Menziesii (Ericaceae)
OTHER NAMES Madrono; *A. procera*

APPEARANCE Madrone is a widely branching, red-barked tree with large, leathery leaves that are bright matte green, elliptical in shape, and from

3 to 6 inches long; there are always a few, usually lower down on the branches, that are turning reddish brown and falling. The bark is at first yellow-green, then reddish brown like Manzanita bark, then darker and shedding in long, shaggy sections. The trunk and limbs are spreading, erratic, and have foliage equally spreading and quite visible. The spring brings clusters of small, urn-shaped, white to flesh-colored flowers that mature into berries of a butterscotch or buff-red color, and are sweet to blah tasting, rough-skinned, and full of hard little seeds. A 30-to 40-foot tree may be one hundred years old.

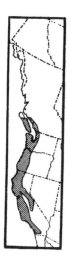

HABITAT In southern California, there are some stands in the San Gabriel and San Bernardino mountains and the Cleveland National Forest. They don't take to basin smog, so look for them between 3,000 and 5,000 feet. They are fairly common from the Ventura County southern edge of the coastal range, up through the Redwoods (both sides), north to British Columbia. Madrone also grows on the west side of the Sierra Nevada, up through the western side of the Cascades. It is most abundant in northern California and southern Oregon. Arizona Madrone (the closely related *A. arizonica*) is found in the mountains of southern Arizona. *A. Menziesii* can be found from northern Baja California, northwards to Prince George, British Columbia.

CONSTITUENTS Arbutin and several other related phenol glycosides; at least two alkanes; ursolic, arbutic, and ursolic acids; and gallotannic acid.

COLLECTING Collect the whole green leaves, dry Method B or just loose in a paper bag (they may be stored in this fashion as well). If you plan to use them regularly, crush the dried leaves into small fragments, fill a quart jar, pour 1 tablespoon of grain alcohol or 2 tablespoons of brandy on top of them, and close the jar tightly. This slight amount of alcohol, dispersed through the leaves by evaporation, makes the glycosides far more soluble in water when you make the tea.

STABILITY Loose or pickled leaves are stable for several years.

PREPARATION Make the tea as a Standard Infusion, and take doses of 3 to 4 fluid ounces three times a day. For a sitz bath, boil ½ cup of the pickled leaves in 2 quarts water for at least thirty minutes, pour into a bathtub, and *then* add tap water to the desired temperature and deep enough to cover the hips. Sit in the water for at least four chapters of a standard-formula murder mystery or two feature articles in *National Geographic*.

MEDICINAL USES Madrone serves the same function as the Manzanita–Uva Ursi group, although it is a little less astringent and may be taken for a day or two longer without having to worry about gastric irritability. Take the tea for acute bladder infections instigated by food binging and unusual consumption of veggies and fruit (or Ding Dongs and Oreo cook-

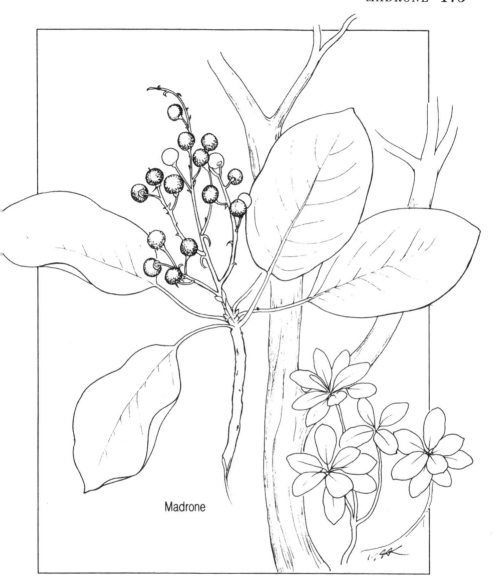

Madrone

ies, for that matter)—the things that are likely to make the urine alkaline. I wouldn't suggest using the tea for more than a week because of the high tannin content in the leaves. Conversely, in acidic urine bladder infections (premenstrual; meat or coffee excess) try half as much tea combined with Thuja, Grindelia, Yerba Santa, or Juniper.

The sitz bath works wonders for postpartum mothers as well as for vaginitis, bacterial vaginosis, and (at least superficially) for yeast infections. You might want to add some Yerba Mansa, Sweet Root, or Usnea tea or tincture to the sitz bath, as they are all rather effective antifungals.

OTHER USES The berries can be boiled and strained, the puree added to apple juice and pectin (and lots of sweetening) to make a jelly. To be perfectly frank, leave out the berries and it is just as good a jelly, although it will lack the panache of food gathering.

Maidenhair Fern

Adiantum pedatum   (Polypodiaceae)
OTHER NAMES Five-Finger Fern; *Culantrillo*

APPEARANCE To describe this lovely is almost redundant. The fronds form colonies that arise from creeping, scaly rootstalks, and the individual fronds splay out palmately and fanlike from 1- to 2-foot shiny black or brown wire-stems. The colonies and the places they grow evoke images of salamanders, deva-magic, and the cool shade of the world before Man. The fronds are kind of groovy too: water won't wet them. There are two other species you may encounter. In warm, clean canyons of coastal California you may find California Maidenhair (*A. Jordanii*); it is irregular-leaved, dark brown, shiny-stemmed, and with the leaflets (pinnules) shaped like little fans that are more broad than long. The European Venus-Hair Fern (*A. capillus-veneris*) is to be found occasionally, with greater ferny side stems and leaflets more long than broad. I don't like gathering it, as a rule, only because of its relative scarcity.

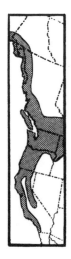

HABITAT Our primary Maidenhair Fern can be found throughout the Pacific Coast, from central California (the San Francisco Bay Area and the Sierra Nevada) north to Alaska and east through cool forests, from nearly the beaches to the middle mountains. Cool, damp, shady, and clean is the ticket. The California Maidenhair is found mostly in the coastal mountains, from Santa Cruz to San Diego, rarely east of the Central Valley, up warm, wet canyons, near seeps and Monkey Flowers.

CONSTITUENTS Filicine, filicinal, fernene, adiantone, adipedifol (hopane-type triterpenes); b-sitosterol, stigmasterol, campesterol (phytosterols); mucilage, and tannin.

COLLECTING Gather the fronds and stems, removed at ground level, bundle, and dry Method A. The bundles look so nice hanging around the house on hooks that sometimes it's tempting to leave them up as decorations until they are needed. Sadly, they fade rather quickly, so store them in the dark, away from the appreciative glances of friends.

STABILITY If stored in the dark, Maidenhair Fern is stable for at least two years.

PREPARATION Standard Infusion, 1 to 4 fluid ounces, or just any old way you want.

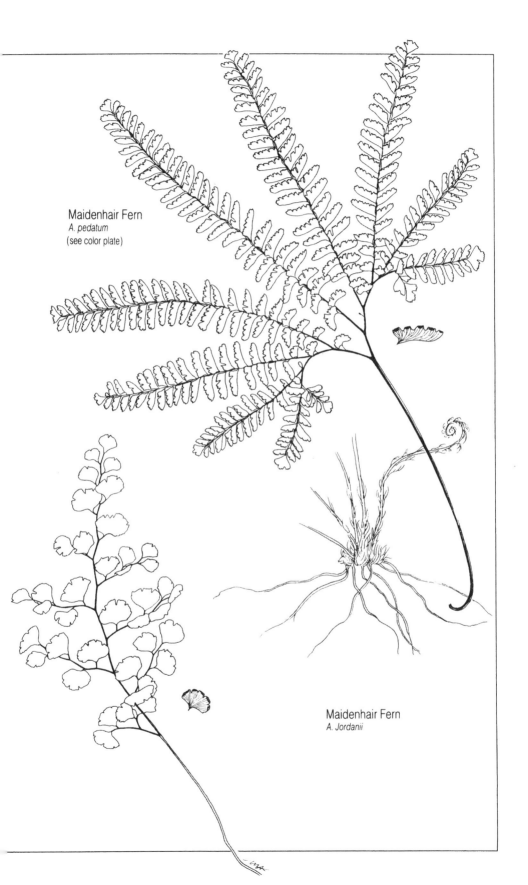

Maidenhair Fern
A. pedatum
(see color plate)

Maidenhair Fern
A. Jordanii

MEDICINAL USES Maidenhair Fern is a gentle remedy and is not for the heroic of inclination. It does work quite nicely, however, for a variety of common imbalances. It is astringent, hemostatic, and slightly stimulant to mucus membrane functions. The widest use is for coughing and heaviness in the lungs, either from an actual bronchial infection or from tiredness and weakness in those who seem to show every little problem by wheezing, gurgling, and throat clearing. I have found it helps to drink a cup of the tea in the morning if you are particularly susceptible to smog and air pollution. In Europe and Latin America it has a long history of stimulating slow and crampy menses to organize. It seems most effective for young women and those having trouble getting back on cycle after birthing, nursing, or coming off birth control pills.

In a far subtler fashion, Maidenhair Fern combines well with Horsetail, another botanical source of silica, for strengthening, over a period of time, chronic stress on connective tissues, particularly in filtering organs. This makes it helpful for liver weakness, especially from alcohol, early borderline emphysema, and kidney weaknesses that might, in time, become overt renal failure. It has mild vasopressor and diuretic effects in rats.

OTHER USES The tea, either infusion or decoction, is an excellent hair rinse, adding some body (particularly in sun-dried or over-processed conditions) and, with Chamomile or Yarrow added to the tea, some sheen and, dare I say it, luster.

Manzanita

Arctostaphylos spp.   (Ericaceae)
OTHER NAMES *Madroño Borracho, Pinguica*

APPEARANCE We have dozens of species of Manzanita in the Pacific West. They are so alike in appearance and have such similar constituents that I lump them all together. They are variable in size, ranging from prostrate bushes a couple of feet tall to shrub-trees 10 feet high or taller. They all have thick, leathery leaves, smooth or a bit raspy, pointed-oval, on short petioles, blue-green to grey-green and universally 1 to 1½ inches long. They like somewhat acid soil, but don't need much moisture. The bark is the most distinctive part of the plants, with its famous Manzanita red-brown. Trunks and large stems twist and turn, flashing red through the thick foliage, and only in the oldest trunks does it shed a bit in strips. The flowers show in spring as masses of mostly terminal white to pink urns, maturing into orange, reddish, or red-brown berries, mealy-bland to the taste, but with a little tartness. *Manzanita* means

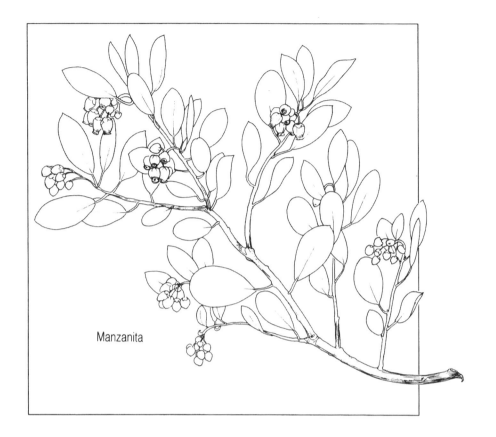

Manzanita

"little apple" in English. The leaves are astringent but otherwise bitter-bland to the taste. If it is intensely bitter and found growing in the western ranges from southern Washington southwards, and the leaves are opposite (not alternate as in Manzanita), you have found some Silk Tassel (*Garrya* sp.). If the bark is right, but the leaves are much larger, you have a small Madrone.

HABITAT The Manzanitas are most common in California, found in almost all the counties, in foothills and moderately dry mountains that usually have enough moisture to support some Live Oak, Juniper, or Pine. It ranges east into Nevada, Arizona, and New Mexico; north through Oregon (mostly west of the Cascades); and into southern Washington.

CONSTITUENTS Arbutin, methylarbutin, ericolin, ursone, and a high level of tannins.

COLLECTING Gather from late spring to mid-fall, picking branches high in foliage; dry in paper bags, and, after dry, sort through to remove branches and stems, retaining the leaves.

STABILITY Left whole and protected from light, the leaves are good for two or three years.

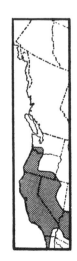

PREPARATION Dry Herb Tincture, 1:5, 50% alcohol, 30 to 60 drops in 8 ounces of warm water, up to four times a day; Standard Infusion 3 to 4 fluid ounces, up to four times a day. For a sitz bath, the Standard Infusion, 8 to 12 fluid ounces in warm water, up to twice a day.

MEDICINAL USES The tea or tincture has one distinct and appropriate use: it is used for cystitis and urethritis that occur after food or alcohol binging, with resultant alkaline urine. With a relatively stable diet and lifestyle, the number of hydrogen ions consumed (acids), minus the amount needed to digest proteins and butterfats in the stomach (the normal alkaline-acid metabolism of the body being stable), leave enough hydrogen ions remaining to keep the urine slightly acid (6 to 6.5 pH) and antimicrobial against the normally present intestinal flora. With carbohydrate binging, and a short-term decrease in dietary proteins and therefore a decrease in the main food source of acids, the stomach will secrete its normal acids, causing a short-term deficit of hydrogen ions in the urine. Alkaline urine (above 7 pH) is more likely to allow coliform bacterial growth in the urethra and irritated mucosa, resulting in pain on urination. The glycosides in Manzanita, especially arbutin, are metabolized and excreted in the urine as hydroquinone, an antimicrobial waste product that is most active in an alkaline pH. So, you drink several cups of the tea or take the tincture in water, do it for a couple of days, take a little cranberry juice (acidifying to the urine and also antimicrobial), and it should back off the infection and get things back to normal. If it doesn't help enough, change your approach. Shift to Yerba Mansa and Mallow tea or some Bidens and Redwood; even Yerba Santa will sometimes help the bladder infection that doesn't respond to Manzanita or its therapeutic and botanical relatives, Madrone and Uva Ursi.

Manzanita is so high in tannins that more than a couple or three days of regular use of the herb will start to irritate the stomach lining and even the kidneys. If the painful urination is getting better but the tannins are a problem, you can change to Blueberry or Pipsissewa, two relatives with similar but weaker effects and little astringency.

The sitz bath is remarkably effective for birth recuperation, but I have been told by midwives that it is best to wait twenty-four hours after birthing to start the bath. It also helps hot, irritative inflammation in bacterial vaginosis and yeast infections, vulvitis, and the acute pain in the initial outbreaks of genital herpes and venereal warts (either sex will be helped). The boiled tea is excellent as a wash for abrasions, infections, contusions, and burns. The astringency is high, shrinking, and cooling, and the other constituents are rather antiseptic for the broken skin. After a few washings or applications, the skin will be dry and tight and probably need a little salve, skin dressing, or oiling.

CONTRAINDICATIONS You shouldn't use the herb internally for more than about four days. It is astringent to the mucosa, and, especially in the last trimester of pregnancy, it can decrease placenta-uterine membrane permeability; consequently, it is probably not a good idea to use Manzanita during pregnancy.

OTHER USES Like Uva Ursi, the dried, crushed leaves can be added to herbal smoking mixtures. They taste best if you brown them lightly in a frying pan before adding them to the blend.

Matilija Poppy

Romneya Coulteri   (Papaveraceae)

OTHER NAMES   *R. trichocalyx, R. Coulteri*, var. *trichocalyx*

APPEARANCE Matilija Poppy is a tall, attractive bush, with many stems and branches arising from thickened, softly woody lower trunks. The foliage and most of the stems are grey-green in color, sometimes tending, in shaded areas, to blue-green; the leaves are alternate and variously cleft into irregular lobes, three to nine in number, and clammy-glaucous. The whole plant exudes a clear to slightly yellow sap when broken, the kind of weeping you would expect from a Milkweed, but without the opacity. The flowers are sheer delight, up to 5 or 6 inches across, with six snow-white, papery-silk petals and a busy yellow center, resembling in color a large Prickly Poppy without the spines. The showy flowers are terminal and upright, maturing into 1½-inch-long terminal pods, slightly bristly, filled with small, rough, grey-brown seeds. With its immense, fragrant, showy flowers and large, blue-green leaves, Matilija Poppy, and its varietals and hybrids, are widely cultivated in gardens of the West.

HABITAT Matilija Poppy grows in the washes, canyons, and leeward ridges of the coastal ranges of southern California and northern Baja California, below the hard-frost levels (2,500 feet), from Santa Barbara County southwards, inland to the San Bernardino Mountains and the western edge of the Imperial Valley. It may be confused with Bush Poppy (*Dendromecon rigida*), a tall, straggly shrub with smaller flowers (2 inches across on the average), simple leaves that tend more to yellowish green, and with long, skinny, pointed seedpods. Although not as potent a medicine, Bush Poppy may be used similarly.

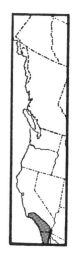

CONSTITUENTS Coulteropine (1-methoxy-protopine), protopine, 1-reticuline, romneine, d-romneine, and sanguinarine and its derivatives.

COLLECTING Gather the leafy stems in May through late July, dry Method A; retain leaves, whatever floral parts you collected, and the smaller green stems, discarding the larger stems.

STABILITY A couple of years.

PREPARATION Dry Herb Tincture, 1:5, 40% to 50% alcohol, 20 to 30 drops, up to five times a day; 1 teaspoon with 2 teaspoons of water and a pinch of salt for a mouthwash; Standard Infusion, 1 to 2 fluid ounces, up to five times a day, or use topically as a cleansing wash; the powdered herb mixed with an equal part of Alum Root, California Bayberry bark, or Yerba Reuma (powdered), makes a disinfectant astringent first aid powder. Since Matilija Poppy grows in the same places as White Sage, I like adding another part of the latter herb, powdered, to mix with the other two.

MEDICINAL USES This lovely plant does a number of low-tech but useful things. Like Prickly Poppy, it is a good external wash for skin pain and inflammation due to an allergic reaction, chemical irritation, heat rash, or mild but painful burns and sunburns on soft, tender flesh. The tea is best, but the diluted tincture is also usable. The powdered herb or above-mentioned mixture is a good first aid, since the plant, with its many alkaloids, is a quality antimicrobial. Add the astringent and the White Sage, and you will inhibit bacteria (aerobic and anaerobic) and the more common skin fungi; and lessen the inflammation and pain with the drug analgesia of the Poppy, the tissue shrinking of the astringent, and the aromatic anesthesia of the Sage.

The diluted tincture, although nasty tasting, inhibits microbes in the mouth, lessens gum sensitivity, and, with its sanguinarine alkaloids, helps to lessen plaque buildup. If you really want to do a whole mouth thing, try this approach in the morning. Brush your teeth with a little baking soda, thereby alkalizing the mouth (and cleaning the teeth). Use the mouthwash, holding it in the mouth for a minute then spitting it out. Wait a couple of minutes, then add a teaspoon of Cinnamon tincture to half a cup of water, and rinse your mouth out. For Cinnamon tincture, grind up a couple of ounces of Cinnamon quills (don't use the powder; it is often of only marginal strength), and steep in 10 ounces of vodka for a week, after mixing them both in a blender for several minutes. The Cinnamon tastes good, thereby removing the taste of the Matilija Poppy; it is also antimicrobial and has a nice astringent effect on the mouth and gums. In addition, it also eventually stops gum bleeding that is from poor mouth health and not from dietary deficiency.

Finally, the tea or tincture is a pretty good remedy for bacterial gastroenteritis from bad food that is not serious enough to warrant medical intervention, but is bad enough to give you the runs at both ends and make you feel hungover in the way that, otherwise, could only result from gorging on lamb and ouzo at a three-day Armenian wedding in Fresno. The herb helps inhibit the bug, lessen the cramps and pain, and is mildly sedative at the same time.

CONTRAINDICATIONS Matilija Poppy is probably not appropriate for internal use during pregnancy and is not appropriate internally in conjunction with prescription medication. It may produce a false positive in urine testing for opiates (if used internally).

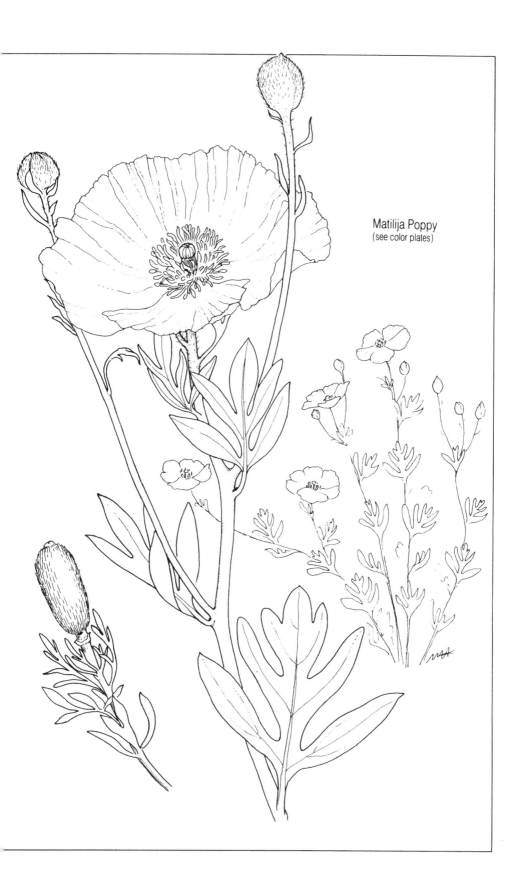

Matilija Poppy
(see color plates)

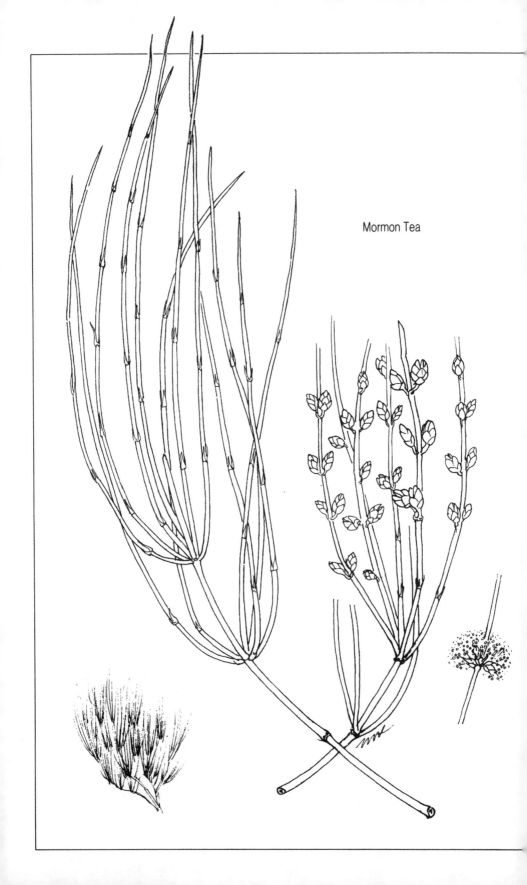

Mormon Tea

Mormon Tea

Ephedra viridis, Ephedra nevadensis   (Ephedraceae/Gnetaceae)

OTHER NAMES   Mexican Tea, Joint Fir, Brigham Tea; *Canutillo, Popotillo, Tepopote*

APPEARANCE   Mormon Tea is often loosely lumped botanically with the conifers, but in reality it is a relic of a far older class of plants, and has no close living relative. There are around fifty species of *Ephedra*, with the Mediterranean and Asian species differing from the North American varieties in that they contain the drug alkaloid ephedrine, but otherwise look alike. Years ago I remember seeing Mormon Tea in the background of several of Sergio Leone's spaghetti westerns and was astonished to find out that the movies were filmed in North Africa and eastern Spain. They looked like they were filmed in Arizona or Nevada (even if everyone but Clint Eastwood needed to be dubbed into English for American release), what with all that *Ephedra* all over the place. Well, same genus, different continent, different species . . . and different constituents.

Mormon Tea is a woody shrub, covered in long, reedlike, jointed stems. It lacks any apparent leaves, with only a reduced little band of scalelike leaves around each joint, either two (in our two species) or three in some inland *Ephedras*. *E. viridis* is bright green and densely stemmed, often resembling a bunch of green plastic brooms, with the woody branches concealed by the "foliage." The new growth in the spring has red bark, which becomes reddish brown by the second year and grey later on. The inner pith of the green stems is reddish and mealy, the joints often covered in a reddish brown resin, particularly in dry seasons; and in drought, with the color a bit faded to yellow-green, the resined joints are quite visible. The plants are usually 2 or 3 feet high, although I have encountered old plants around Frazier Park in California that are 5 feet high. The surface of the stems is crepey and finely ridged, the leaf scales are two in number, and the plants are either male or female, putting out little chunky catkins or conelets from their nodes in the early spring. I don't usually gather Mormon Tea in "flower," waiting till later, but there seems to be little variation in constituents during the year.

Ephedra nevadensis is a lower growing plant, with long, olive green stems that often seem to arise directly from the ground, with the woody branches nearly buried in grass or dirt. The stem surface is less ridged, and the diameter is a little larger than *E. viridis*. The scales are two in number also, but the flowers/cones are more numerous and busier. The pith has little red, and there is very little resin at the joints. Another species, *Ephedra californica,* with a blue-green or yellow-green color, is found in our range, but the taste is bitter and the stems are much thicker and waxy, making it the least desirable of our coastal plants, although the constituents are the same and it can be used if necessary. The scales and stem branches are in threes, easily setting it apart from the other two. *Ephedra trifurca* is a big, spiny-tipped Mormon Tea that can be found as far as southeastern California, but it is so tough I would ignore it if I were you.

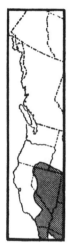

HABITAT *Ephedra viridis* is a mountain species, usually growing between 4,000 and 7,000 feet, liking slopes and Juniper flats, often covering lower mountain valleys and mesa tops. It is found along the slopes of the San Bernardino Mountains and into the eastern edge of the coastal range in Ventura County; back along the desert side of the Sierra Nevada in California; all the way up the Great Basin into southeastern Oregon; in all of Nevada; and all around the Four Corners Area of Utah, Arizona, Colorado, and New Mexico. *Ephedra nevadensis* is found in the same areas, only at lower altitudes, usually from 1,500 to 4,000 feet, and also eastwards to the Big Bend area of Texas. *Ephedra californica* grows at low altitudes from Kern County south through San Diego County, into Baja California, and east to the Mojave Desert and Las Vegas. *Ephedra trifurca* can be found as far west as the Mojave River near Barstow, and likes it *low* and *hot*; it even grows near Yuma, Arizona.

CONSTITUENTS Traces of pseudo-ephedrine, together with related ephedrates; tannin, silica, and the astringent compound catechin.

COLLECTING *Ephedra viridis* has long, green sprays of stems, and they can be pulled off intact and dried in bags or bundled with rubber bands. The stems have joints that are closer together towards the tips, and because of their thin diameter, they can be broken apart at the joints quite easily after they dry. *Ephedra nevadensis,* when growing under ideal circumstances—that is, with long, extended, broomlike stems from the ground up—can be snipped, bundled, and dried in bags. Although the stems may break at the joints, you might have to snip them down into small pieces. With both species, gather the long plumes, not the short, stubby older growth. Processing such chunky stuff is maddening; it is preferable to look around for plants with broomlike newer growth. The other two species have to be cut, not broken, since they are so thick and wiry: last resort Mormon Tea.

If you have gathered *Ephedra viridis* in any quantity, you also can collect the little reddish brown resin that falls off the joints; separate it, and use it for a nearly pure astringent-hemostatic powder. It is easily powdered and stays potent for years; just dust it on scratches, abrasions, and chafed skin.

STABILITY The broken stems are stable for up to two years, although they should be stored away from light, as they fade easily.

PREPARATION The herb can be taken as a Simple Infusion, Decoction, or even a Cold Infusion. Too much at one time may irritate the stomach (all those astringents), so use the tea intermittently during the day.

MEDICINAL USES The main uses of Mormon Tea are for helping to decrease lung and sinus congestion before and during allergic reactions, and as a simple diuretic for water retention and to dilute the urine during mild cystitis and urethritis. Generally, although the tea contains no ephedrine alkaloid, the potent adrenalin-mimic used for asthma, it contains discrete relatives of the drug. They have just enough potency so the tea can be remarkably effective when drunk *before* a seasonal allergy occurs. A couple of cups a day for an adult will usually abort most of the allergy, and you can add a Mint or Lemon Balm for flavor. The tea is astringent enough that it helps diarrhea as well as mucus membrane ulcers in the stomach, duodenum, or colon. It isn't really strong, but it tastes pretty good and is safe. Mormon Tea is not a therapeutic giant, but it is something that most households should have around. And don't forget the powdered resin.

Nettle

Urtica dioica, U. urens   (Urticaceae)

OTHER NAMES   Stinging Nettle, and the taxa *U. gracilis, U. holosericea, U. californica, U. Lyallii,* etc. Hitchcock and Cronquist list these as varieties of *U. dioica* (sounds reasonable to me), but many texts list them as a wide range of separate species, so don't get upset. If it's tall, like a large Mint, and perennial, call it *U. dioica;* if it's a short, stubby annual, with startlingly efficient stingers, it's *U. urens.*

APPEARANCE *Urtica dioica* (along with its varieties) is a tall, handsome plant, with opposite leaves and a square stem. I am embarrassed to admit how many times I have seen a Nettle leaf in the late spring, mistaken it for a Mint, crushed it to check the scent (Peppermint, perhaps?) . . . and stung my nose. Nettle leaves are brilliant dark green, variously round or lanceolate, and have neat, regular serrations along the edges. Some varieties have round-shaped leaves, and some have narrow and long leaves; but they all form a sharp tip and have stinging hairs on the light green underside; and most have a few on the dark green upper surface. The stems, of course, are covered with stingers.

The plants sometimes form extensive stands, connected by underground roots, and may range from 2 or 3 feet in height to as tall as 10 feet. Plants in moist, open areas and along the coast tend to be shorter, with larger leaves; mountain plants or stands growing from out of deep shade into the light are taller, often with leaf pairs widely separated and shade-stunted. The plant blooms in spring (coastal) and early summer (mountains), producing flowers that grow from small stems which arise from below the leaf axils and sprout from the main stem, with male flowers usually on separate and shorter stems above the female flowers. The clusters of green seeds are mature by mid- to late summer.

Dwarf Nettle (*Urtica urens*) is an annual European weed, usually around a foot or so in height; with a square stem, opposite leaves that are rounded, coarsely toothed, and crowded towards the top; and many short, stubby seed clusters of mixed sex. The plant is well armored with particularly potent stinging hairs. All of the Nettles form single stalks and seldom branch—and they all sting.

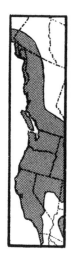

HABITAT Nettle is found everywhere in the Pacific West. Along the coast it will grow in meadows, in water, or in any moist place. In the mountains it is found along waterways, and in drier inland mountains it only grows along year-round creeks. Dwarf Nettle is a sporadic weed in rural areas of the inland agricultural valleys of California, Oregon, and Washington; and although common locally, it is maddeningly unpredictable. It is important to be aware that Nettle is a plant high in nitrogen and minerals. Both types of Nettle can thrive obscenely well below agribusiness runoff that is high in inorganic nitrates and heavy metals. This is probably not particularly important in the short-lived annual Dwarf Nettle, but with the rest, which have perennial growth and long root life, soil metals will form substitute compounds that, more poorly metabolized, begin to concentrate in the plant's heavier parts and, in spring and summer, the leaves. Since the same substitute heavy metal compounds are formed in our tissues if taken from the leaves, carefully avoid agribusiness and industrial areas. Besides, which gives more pleasure: gathering plants in an irrigation ditch southeast of Portland or picking plants below a waterfall with a view of Mount Hood? (Rhetorical question.)

CONSTITUENTS Formic acid (fresh plant only), galacturonic acid, ascorbic acid, histamine, 5-hydroxytryptamine, choline and acetylcholine, vitamins A and D, iron, sodium, potassium, phosphorus, calcium, silica, and albuminoids.

COLLECTING The plant should be juiced in the spring and early summer, up to the time it begins flowering. For the dried herb, gather anytime from mid-spring to full seed (late summer). Gather carefully with gloves, bundling by the stems, dry Method A, and strip the leaves when dry. The stinging hairs are inactive when dry, but large plants with thick

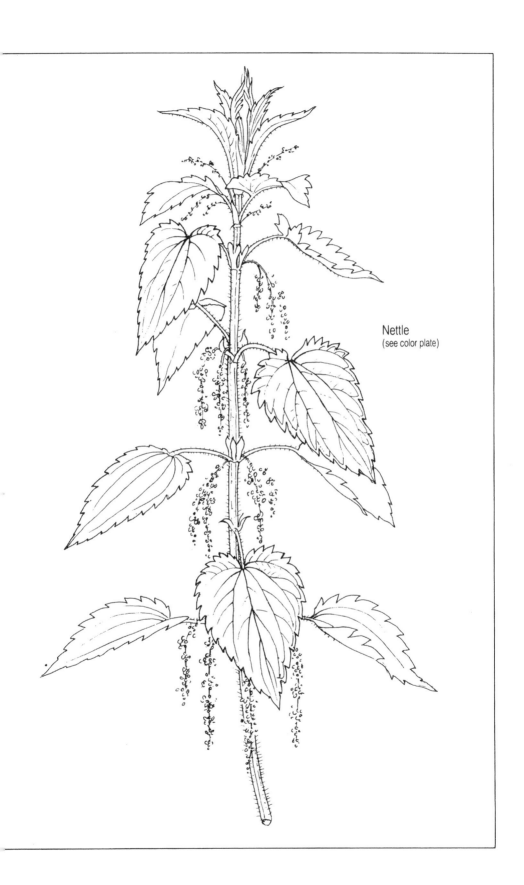

Nettle
(see color plate)

stems may have hairs that are coarse enough to irritate the skin mechanically, so it may be necessary to still use gloves.

STABILITY The dried leaves are stable for at least eighteen months; the preserved juice should be used within six months.

PREPARATION The fresh juice can be preserved for a month with the addition of 25% alcohol, and, if refrigerated, will last for up to six months. The juice can be frozen in those little cocktail cublet ice trays, removed after a couple of days, and stored loose in freezer bags, a cube melted for a dose. Use the herb for tea as a Cold or Standard Infusion, 2 to 4 ounces as often as needed. The Mineral Tea is made with equal parts by weight of Nettle, Red Clover tops, and wild or organic Alfalfa; put a rounded tablespoon in a cup of tea, three or four times a day. When using Nettle in tea, it needs to be brewed fresh each time, as the constituents start to precipitate and become less active after an hour or so in solution. As a food supplement, powder the dried leaves and store them in a closed container in the refrigerator. If the idea really appeals to you, large quantities of the powdered leaves can be frozen in individual bags and pulled out for use one bag at a time. This gives you the chance to fondle the dark green powder of summer past, as the snow piles up outside.

MEDICINAL USES The fresh juice, preserved or defrosted, should be used in tablespoon doses, added to 4 to 6 ounces of water, and taken up to three times a day for a strong diuretic. Weiss recommends its use for mild cardiac edema and venous insufficiency as well as for stimulating uric acid excretion by the kidneys. Be that as it may, the fresh juice is a strong and efficient diuretic, increasing both the volume of urine and to a lesser degree, the wastes. It works well for major premenstrual water retention, particularly since it also has astringent effects that keep it from overstimulating the uterine lining. Some volume diuretics such as Juniper, Parsley, and Celery can stimulate the uterus and create the potential for a disorganized menses. Others, such as Uva Ursi or Manzanita, can be so astringent as to impede the flow.

Nettle, as juice or tea, is an especially useful diuretic for those in a relatively "acid" state, with an increase in nitrogen metabolism, increased hydrogen ion excretion in the urine, and a lower, more acidic pH. This occurs together with an increased stress on the blood-buffering system. Since the blood must maintain its slightly alkaline pH, and since nearly all the waste products the body produces are acid, something like Nettle tea or the mineral tea described above helps to add electrolytes and alkali to assist the buffering system when under stress, and Nettle specifically helps increase the transport and excretion of blood nitrogen waste products. This makes it very useful in arthritis, eczema, and psoriasis— particularly when the problem is aggravated by anxieties, freak outs, or *really* bad food (and combinations thereof).

The tea, in general, is a useful agent for decreasing bleeding, either from acute irritation (like nosebleeds and constipation-induced rectal spotting) or from congestion with ulceration. It is second only to Shepherd's Purse for uterine bleeding and has the advantage of being a tonic or strengthening herb that can be taken for a long time or as a preventative, whereas the other is for bad stuff, right now!

Dwarf Nettle tea is also a very effective urinary tract astringent, shrinking inflamed urethral and bladder membranes and lessening the pain of urination. Some painful urination occurs because of an infection, and in this case it is necessary to deal with the organism; but some urethritis and cystitis is just the result of irritation, friction, or overacidic urine, and responds well to Dwarf Nettle and, to a lesser degree, *Urtica dioica.*

Nettle has a spotty record as a remedy for sinus allergies. Some claims made for it seem a bit excessive, but I have found it is a good adjunct to Ma Huang (Chinese *Ephedra*) or ephedrine or pseudoephedrine preparations. These can have hypertensive and CNS-stimulation effects that can be lessened by taking half the amount of herb or alkaloid and drinking some Nettle tea. Nettle is a synergistic decongestant, and besides increasing the effect of smaller amounts of *Ephedra* alkaloids, it will combine well with Eyebright, Goldenseal, California Bayberry, Yerba Mansa, Yerba Santa, and other such allergy-head cold-coughy-wheezy-red eye-type herbs.

The tea, made of isotonic water, can be used as a douche, enema, eyewash, and gargle (at separate times, of course), and will shrink, tighten, and generally act as an anti-inflammatory astringent for simple redness and irritation of the mucosa.

The dried, green seeds, gathered in late summer, can be moistened with a little alcohol and steeped in three times their volume of olive oil for a week. Blend the mix briefly, let it resettle, and squeeze it through a cloth. Add a little oil of Rosemary or oil of Lavender, and the green oil can be used to rub in the scalp before shampooing or swimming, to lessen dryness, stimulate the scalp, and (so this bald herbalist has been *told*) increase hair growth.

OTHER USES The powdered leaves are high in chlorophyll (*very* high) and in useful minerals, including iron; they are also high in protein, at least for plant leaves. All over the country people are taking arcane, obscure food supplements, often with little information to go on, and with the side effects and other problems seldom mentioned; and they cost a *lot* of money. Spirulina and chlorella are algae—dried pond scum that is excellent food for pollywogs, but so high in nucleoproteins (DNA, RNA) that it can cause nitrogen overload, purine buildup, and uric acid excess. Bee pollen is high in sugar and protein, well digested, and gives one a nice lift; but it is also expensive, especially considering what it is: the genetic information of plants mixed with worker-bee spit and enzymes—

high in uric acid potential, with the possibility of giving one an allergic reaction to the bee source *and* whatever pollen they collected. Every year we see some new harebrained food supplement derived from weird sources, containing new stuff that we didn't know we needed (or even existed), and which we can *now* obtain . . . usually at great expense. Most of these hustles are elaborations of valid concepts or discoveries that, with flights of marketing fancy, packaging, and product development, are presented as *stuff you need* (but didn't know until now). This is simply the health food industry's version of the corruption of much of American retailing: marketing and image strategies to create the impression that there is a necessary product inside. It is seldom done with such cynicism; I am sure most folks believe most or all of what they try to sell.

Nettle powder is something that you can gather yourself in places that you trust, and you can add it to smoothies and salad dressings; put it in bread; add it to your tea, home beer, and so forth. It is green food your body recognizes and can help build blood, tissue, and self-empowerment.

Oregon Grape

Mahonia (Berberis) aquifolia, M. nervosa, M. repens, M. pinnata (Berberidaceae)

OTHER NAMES Barberry, Mahonia, *Odostemon*, Creeping Barberry, Mountain Holly; *Yerba de Sangre*

APPEARANCE I guess, when push comes to shove, *Mahonia aquifolia* is *the* Oregon Grape, since it is the state flower of Oregon and the former official drug plant up until its last listing in the 1935 *National Formulary*. It is a leafy bush, from 2 to 5 or 6 feet in height, covered in wavy, prickly, hollylike pinnate leaves. The leaflets are oblong-oval, and 1½ to 3 inches long; shiny dark green above, dull below; and are opposite, with a single terminal leaflet, so the number of them that make up the compound leaf is five, seven, or nine. The compound leaves are alternate, and on long, wiry petioles branching out from tough, brown-barked stems. The bark is yellow or yellow-green, the lower stems have yellowish wood as well, and the roots have the greatest pigment, sometimes bordering on orange. The flowers are bright yellow clusters, upright or hanging downwards, and bloom in March and April. They mature into juicy clusters of blue-purple pseudo-grapes. These are usually intensely sour and sweet, although some have a bitter aftertaste. The bush, like all of our Oregon Grapes, is an evergreen, but after two or three

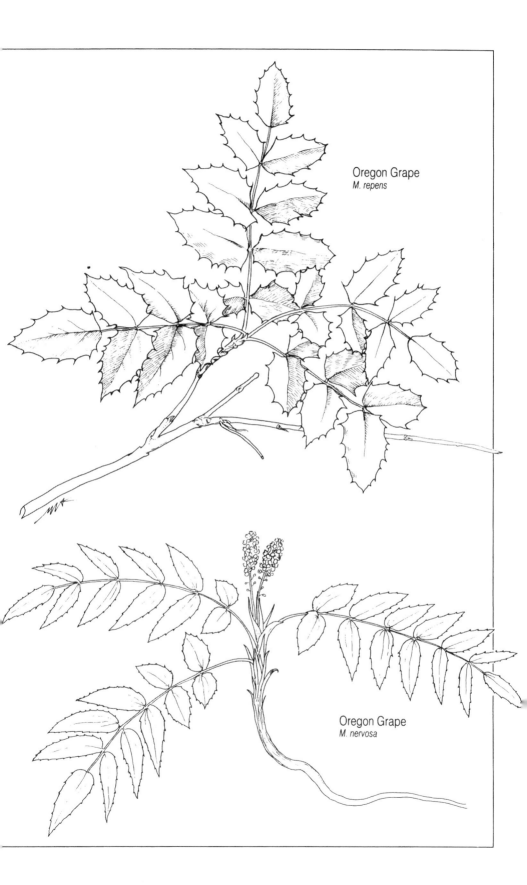

Oregon Grape
M. repens

Oregon Grape
M. nervosa

years, an individual leaflet or a whole compound leaf will get senescent and turn orange or even flaming red.

Mahonia nervosa is a broad plant, but with short stems that seldom exceed a foot in height sending out tufts of long compound leaves that may extend out well over a foot. The central leaf stem is often reddish brown, and the leaflets are leathery, 2 or 3 inches long, and so neat and regular as to appear artificial. They may number up to nineteen or more, but thirteen or fifteen is more common. The flowers are borne in an elongated yellow bunch arising from the end of the stem along with the compound leaves, and mature also into bunches of grapelets. Although folks use these fruits extensively as well as *aquifolia*, I have found their taste to be like sucking on a vitamin C tablet and an aspirin simultaneously. I suppose they can make a serviceable jelly, much as Manzanita fruit can; just add sufficient apple juice and pectin.

Mahonia repens is a little munchkin version of the previous two. It has a short stem like the second, with wavy, ivylike leaves that resemble *M. aquifolia*. Since a dozen plants may branch off the same underground root system, the buried bush can be fairly bulky when the dust settles. The flowers are the typical yellow clusters, with juicy grapelets that taste sour and unripe even when long shriveled on the stem.

Mahonia pinnata is a stout-stemmed, low shrublet, with densely crowded compound leaves that resemble *M. aquifolia* in leaflet shape, but with more twisted and undulating, even backward-pointed, leaflets. The leaves are the spiniest of the four, and the lowest pair of leaflets are close to the base of the petiole, almost clasping the main stem. They number between five and fifteen but when crowded around the flowering stalks may be three- or single-leaved. For flowers and fruit, round up the usual suspects; although nobody claims the viciously sour fruits are anything like edible, with some sugar, they make a nice lemonade . . . barbade. (Mahonade, maybe pinnade?)

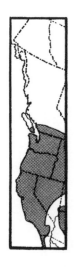

HABITAT *M. aquifolia* grows in shade in the north coastal range of California, from Mendocino County northwards; or the western slopes of the Sierra Nevada from east of Sacramento northwards; and in shady lower forests all the way through Oregon and Washington, southern British Columbia, into northern Idaho, and sporadically down the east side of the Cascades.

Mahonia nervosa grows on higher shady forested slopes of the coastal ranges from Monterey County, California, north to the Oregon border; east across the Siskiyou Mountains to the base of the Cascades; and in higher old-growth (or second-generation) forests on the coast and the west side of the Cascades, north to British Columbia.

Mahonia repens grows on the east slopes of the Sierra Nevada, from Inyo County, California; northwards across the Siskiyou Mountains (sporadic), and up the east side of the Cascades; north to British Columbia and Alberta; south along the Rocky Mountain Cordillera to New Mexico; and east to the Dakotas. It likes open, forested canyons, and is drought-tolerant, as long as it has shade and a good slope.

Mahonia pinnata is a plant of California, liking rocky, exposed places within the forest and along open rocky ridges, from Del Norte County southwards along the coastal ranges all the way to Baja California, and the inner ranges of southern California. It is most common south of the San Francisco Bay and may come down the mountains to lower altitudes tucked along the edges of streamside thickets.

CONSTITUENTS The primary bioactive agents in Oregon Grape are the many isoquinoline alkaloids. Besides the main yellow alkaloid berberine, the roots and foliage contain berbamine, oxyacanthine, and oxyberberine; the roots have others, including canadine, mahonine, magnoflorine, and jatrorrhizine, depending on the species and other esoteric factors.

COLLECTING Gather the roots and lower yellow stems from midsummer to winter, the leaves from May through mid-fall. *M. aquifolia* and *M. pinnata* often have upper stem bark and wood with little or no color, and these should not be used. The stems of the other two are so short and stubby that it doesn't matter. The washed roots and stems should be chopped while still fresh, especially if you have some larger diameter taproots. They are tougher than they look—take my word for it. The leaves can just be stuffed into a paper bag and dried. *M. pinnata* can grow in some pretty gnarly places and will have very high levels of berberine if growing upside down in dislodged boulders or experiencing other botanical ordeals (similar to the desert *Mahonias* of the Southwest). The other three have genial and predictably lower alkaloid content.

STABILITY The dried leaves, stored out of any light, will last for up to a year; the dried roots and stems will last for several years.

PREPARATION The Fresh Root Tincture, 1:2, or the Dry Root Tincture, 1:5, 50% alcohol, 15 to 30 drops, up to four times a day (before meals and upon retiring) as a hepatic bitter; or 30 to 45 drops, up to three times a day (midmorning, midafternoon, and before retiring) as a liver stimulant. Use the tinctures or Chopped Root or Leaf Tea as needed topically or as a mouthwash; the leaves as a Salve or Oil, Method A. The oil preparation should be made of olive oil, or an antioxidant added, such as *Larrea,* vitamin E, or gum benzoin, as the constituents of the leaf are inadequate alone to prevent rancidity. The recently dried leaf may be powdered and sifted, kept in a lightproof container, and dusted on skin abrasions as an antibacterial.

MEDICINAL USES Oregon Grape has three main functions: as a bitter tonic for impaired salivary and gastric secretions, as a stimulant to liver and skin protein metabolism, and as an antimicrobial for the skin and intestinal tract.

As a bitter tonic, it has the simple, predictable effect of stimulating salivary secretions (both lubricating and digestive) and, by reflex, gastric secretions. These include hydrochloric acid, pepsinogen, hormones to stimulate the pancreas and gallbladder, and the protein carriers for vitamin B_{12} transport. Take 15 to 20 drops in a little water ten or fifteen minutes before eating. An easy rule of thumb is the following: if you have indigestion regularly, have teeth or gum problems, and a white or yellowish coat on your tongue in the morning, use the herb as a bitter tonic. If, on the other hand, your indigestion is accompanied by excessive salivation and the tip of your tongue is red, then your stomach lining is probably irritated and inflamed, and you should try Yerba Reuma, Bidens, Hedge Nettle, or Oxeye Daisy instead—even Hypericum oil; in this case you don't need a stimulus to secretion, but something to cool and soothe. The bitter tonic use (as well as the liver-stimulating doses) are useful for stomach problems of the chronic drinker (subacute, congested membranes) but not for the gastritis of the occasional binge drinker (inflamed, hot membranes)—unless you want to use it for a hangover treatment.

Oregon Grape is a stimulant to liver and skin metabolism of dietary and blood proteins and is helpful for those people who show signs of moderately or constitutionally impaired hepatic function. This shows as dry skin, poorly healing skin, delicate mucus membranes, constant bad breath, coated tongue in the A.M., and difficulty in digesting fats and proteins or even an aversion to them. Other symptoms are rapid shifts in blood sugar levels, a lifelong preference for sweets, salads, fruit, and cola drinks, and a history of food or environmental allergies—adrenalin junkies with chronic constipation. Try the tincture (30 to 45 drops) three times a day for at least two weeks, and gradually add a bit more quality proteins, lipids, legumes, and the like to your diet. Remember the constipation part, as much of that chronic problem derives from poor upper digestive reflex and deficient bile release from the gallbladder.

The oil, salve, dusting powder, tincture, or tea is a first-rate skin disinfectant and antimicrobial, since just about any kind of abrasion has been shown to be aided by the alkaloids in Oregon Grape. Further, the tea or tincture can be taken every several hours for manageable intestinal infections, from mild salmonella infections to shigellosis; it even helps amebic dysentery a bit. Best of all, it helps to become regulated after you have recovered. You know what I mean; you have segments and functions you never even *dreamed* of, and every one of them hurts . . . for days.

Oxeye Daisy

Chrysanthemum leucanthemum (Compositae)
OTHER NAMES Field Daisy, Leucanthemum; *Leucanthemum vulgare*

APPEARANCE This is a well-known plant, found sporadically throughout North America. When mature, the flowering stems are 2 to 3 feet tall. This perennial has from one to ten stems, each one with at least one white and yellow daisy flower; it sometimes bears secondary flowering stems, but on these there is only one flower per stem. The stems are irregularly ridged, with alternate, widely spaced, strap-shaped leaves, erratically toothed. The lower, sometimes basal leaves are petioled, the upper ones stem-clasping. The foliage has a Yarrow-Chamomile scent when crushed, and the flowers are bitter.

HABITAT Oxeye Daisy is found in abundance along roadsides, in vacant lots, fields, meadows, and in the mountains throughout our area. It is much less common in the southern half of California and the dry inland valleys.

CONSTITUENTS An essential oil containing chrysanthenone, verbenone, pyrethrins, and over twenty known polyacetylenes.

COLLECTING Gather flowering stems and dry them, Method A. The plant is strongest when first flowering (usually mid-June), but it is serviceable up until early September. Discard dead flowers and leaves before drying. Include the stems with the herb.

STABILITY Oxeye Daisy will stay effective for about a year as the dried herb.

PREPARATION Standard Infusion, 2 to 4 fluid ounces, up to three times a day. Dry Herb Tincture (recent herb only), 1:5, 50% alcohol, ½ to 1 teaspoon, up to three times a day. As an insecticide, Fresh Flower Tincture, 1:2, add 1 tablespoon dish detergent per cup of finished tincture for spraying; as a powder, the recently dried flowers, ground in a blender, then stored in a closed container in the freezer.

MEDICINAL USES Oxeye Daisy decreases secretions when taken internally, and dries up and disinfects when applied externally. It is usually best when taken warm (not hot) or simply at room temperature. Use it for bronchitis or asthma characterized by moist, hypersecreting mucosa, with copious watery secretions, and red, inflamed membranes. It has some of the anti-inflammatory effects found in its relative Feverfew, although not enough to induce possible side effects. Oxeye is safe and effective for excess sweating, excess secretions, vaginal discharges, runny eyes, and, oddly enough, overconcentrated, acidic urine (where it acts

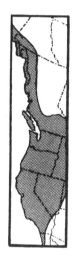

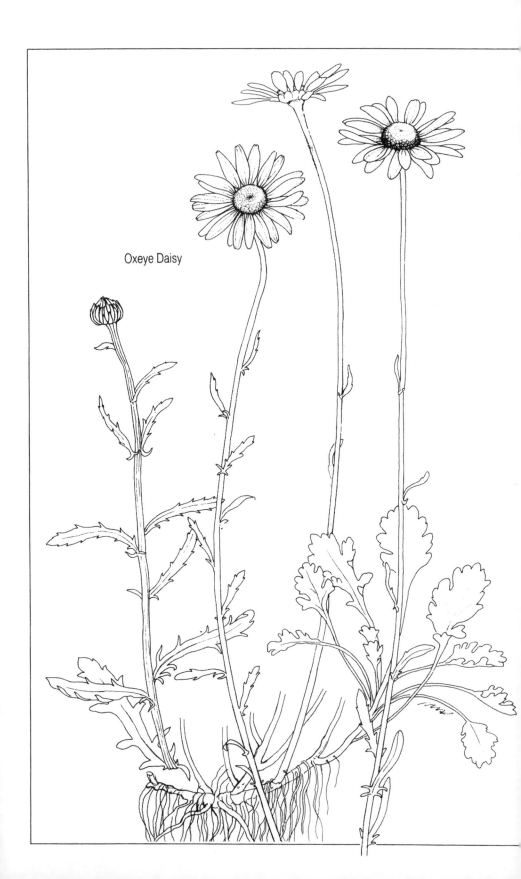

Oxeye Daisy

as a simple diuretic). Although not as strong as Canadian Fleabane or Shepherd's Purse, it is a serviceable hemostatic, especially for mucus membrane bleeding, and is one of our better herbs for gastritis with hypersecretions of the stomach and mouth, as well as for a gastric ulcer that lingers, irritates, and won't quite heal. The tea is a good douche, mixed with Yerba Reuma, Yerba Mansa, California Bayberry, or Hedge Nettle for an astringent. It is antifungal and antibacterial, and besides being a useful douche, it may be used as a cleansing, disinfecting wash. It can be used as a hair and beard rinse for scalp and skin fungal infections.

OTHER USES The preparations of the flowers are fairly useful insecticides, as the flowers contain pyrethrins. It isn't as useful as commercial preparations, but it's *your* preparation. The powder can be fluffed into the fur of pets for repelling fleas.

Pearly Everlasting

Anaphalis margaritacea   (Compositae)

OTHER NAMES   Everlasting, Life Everlasting, *Gnaphalium margaritacea, Antennaria margaritacea*

APPEARANCE Pearly Everlasting is another of those typical composite colony plants, like Yarrow and California Mugwort, with upright aerial stems arising off of parallel woody underground root systems. Just imagine a buried shrub, with the ends of the branches sticking up from the ground, and the lower branches, stems, and trunks below ground with the roots. The unbranching stems bear long, linear leaves, dark green above, furry below, and alternating closely, one upon the other. The leaves are thin and gracefully extended, and don't appear to be as crowded as a broad-leaf plant, with similar numbers, would be. The whole plant is downy, and the dark green upper leaf surface may be nearly grey in hue when growing in the full sun, darker (with fewer hairs) in the shade. The flowers are distinctive: large white pearly puffs arranged in loose pseudo-umbels at the top, each the size of a pea. When newly blooming, the individual flowers are opalescent beads, each with a bright yellow center. After a while, the white bracts start to spread out, and the yellow center—the actual flower—starts to turn towards brown in color. The bracted flowers retain their shape and color long after drying, and have been used for floral decorations and winter bouquets for centuries; hence the name Everlasting.

If you run across a similar plant, but less fuzzy, with yellowish white blossoms, and with crushed foliage that smells balsamic or piney, it is a closely related *Gnaphalium* (Field Balsam or Cudweed), with the same uses and greater expectoration effects. If you run across a similar plant that has short flowering stems rising out of dense mats of silvery basal leaves (usually in the mountains), it is another relative, *Antennaria* (Cat's Foot or Pussy Toes). These three genera are closely related, some of the taxonomic differences are moot, and to some degree they are interchangeable as remedies. Pearly Everlasting is the most common of the group, and this single species is found widely in temperate North America and Asia. The flowers are usually single-sexed, with pistillate yellow centers on one plant and stamenate flowers on another—a difference important to the plants and botanists, not to us. Isolated stands may have flowers with both stamens and pistils. The mature plants (August) will normally be 2 or 3 feet in height.

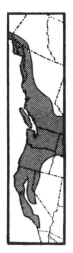

HABITAT Pearly Everlasting is usually a mountain or forest plant, growing from the San Bernardino Mountains; north from central California, in both the coastal ranges and the Sierra Nevada; northwards to Alaska along the coast of the Panhandle; southeast to Alberta and western Montana; and in logging areas, road cuts, and burns everywhere there is (or was) forests. In California and southern Oregon, if you find the plant growing at low altitudes by the coast, it is a Cudweed *(Gnaphalium)*. Use it anyway.

CONSTITUENTS Anaphalin and gnaphalin (monoterpenes) and the flavones luteolin and quercitin, together with volatile oils, varying from very little in *Anaphalis* and *Antennaria* to a fair amount (and therapeutically important) in *Gnaphalium*.

COLLECTING Gather the herb in flower, preferably in late summer when the blossoms are still compacted; dry Method A.

STABILITY Pearly Everlasting should be usable for a couple of years, the aromatic *Gnaphalium* (Cudweed) perhaps for eighteen months.

PREPARATION Standard Infusion or a strong simple infused tea of the whole dried herb, as needed; the dried leaves, rubbed into fuzzy wads, used with water as a poultice; the dried leaves, partially rubbed, as a smoking herb; the dried flowers, briefly simmered in a little water, cooled to warm, applied to burns, and covered with a moist cloth.

MEDICINAL USES The tea is soothing, anti-inflammatory, and astringent, acting as a feeble antihistamine and decreasing edema in swollen membranes. It is a safe and palatable tea for diarrhea, gastroenteritis (stomach flu), and an irritable stomach and esophagus, with moist mouth and red-tipped tongue. The tea and, at least for tobacco smokers, the smoked herb, acts similarly in helping cool the membranes, decreasing their inflammation and edema, and acting as a mild expectorant. Although a smoker myself, I would hesitate to recommend smoking herbs

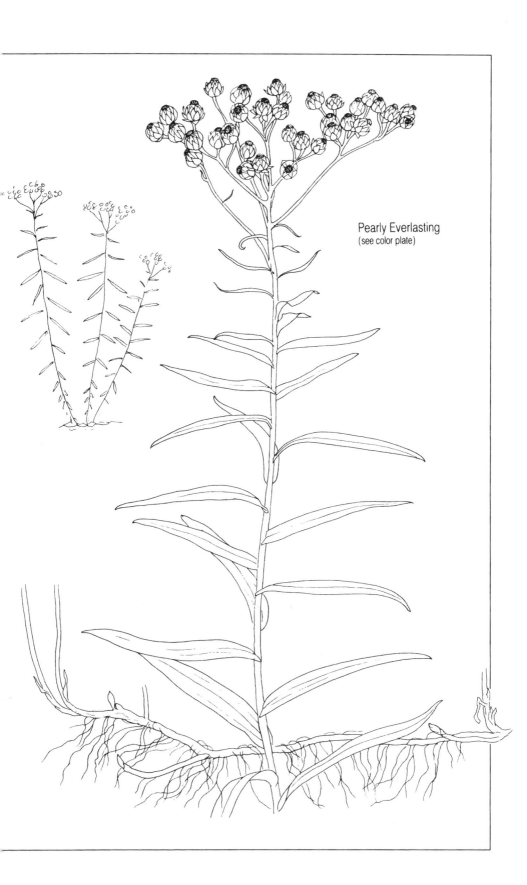

Pearly Everlasting
(see color plate)

as a therapy for anyone other than a smoker. The leaves, however, have long been used as an herb for smoking mixes by Native Americans, both as a flavoring agent and as the base for other herbs, including Tobacco. Dried leaves, uncured for smoking, are harsh and unpleasant. The best uncured leaves for smoking mixtures, for pleasure or ritual, have always been those that have a lot of fuzz and not much mass. These include Coltsfoot, Mullein, Raspberry leaves, and Pearly Everlasting.

As a poultice the leaf is helpful for bruises and contusions, soothing and decreasing redness and swelling. It does not seem too useful for joint pain, or inflammation that is multitissued or deep, although it has a long history of folk use for that purpose. The leaf poultice and especially the flower poultice are stimulating and healing to sunburns and other moderate burns from heat and friction. The aromatic *Gnaphaliums* are a little better, but *Anaphalis margaritacea* works quite nicely as well. This is another one of our gentle, almost forgotten, and frequently usable homely medicines.

Peppermint

Mentha piperita   (Labiatae)

OTHER NAMES   *Menta* (Spanish); the most common plant to be called "Mint"

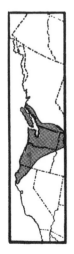

APPEARANCE Peppermint forms stands connected by underground roots, and sends up, at maturity in summer, 1 ½- to 3-foot-tall stems. They are erect, unbranching below the flowers, and dark green. The leaves are rounded to pointed, with small, sharp teeth, petioled and opposite. The stems are square, dark green, and sometimes purple tinged. Occasionally, plants in a more open, atypical habitat will form secondary branches from the lower stems, but the volatile oils of these marginal plants are often unpleasant and less predictable. Look for the herds. Flowers are terminal on one or more upper stems, from separate balls to a nearly united spike, and pink to lavender-blue or even purple in color. Peppermint closely resembles Bergamot Mint and even Spearmint, so crush the foliage. Bergamot Mint is perfumy-lemony; Spearmint smells sweet and edible; Peppermint is sharp, pungent, and with little subtlety. Just remember the taste of Peppermint Life Savers.

HABITAT A European plant, Peppermint has escaped from gardens and can be encountered in almost any cool, damp stream in the lower altitudes. It is seldom found in southern California; and in California in general, most of the stands are on the north coast. In the rest of our

Peppermint

area, any cool, moist place is a possible locality. Most secondary streams have a "heart" where alluvial deposits are broadest, trees are densest, and species diversity is greatest. Such a place, which may be where a stream drains into a larger waterway, or up a mile in a shady bowl, is where you will usually find Peppermint (or other Mints).

CONSTITUENTS The volatile oil, containing menthol, methone, menthofuran, methyl acetate, and other terpenes, is the active part. Other constituents, such as resins and gums, have little therapeutic importance.

COLLECTING Gather in late summer, when the larger stems are in early bloom. Since the foliage arises from common roots, all the stems will have the same chemistry, so you may gather both the flowering and unflowering stems. The menthols are derived from simpler terpenes, including pulegone and menthofuran. Menthofuran gives the leaves a sweet, somewhat unpleasant aroma, with less medicinal value; and the pulegone, the main constituent of immature Peppermint (and Peppermint that matures too early in the year in cultivation), is the active compound in Pennyroyal, with pronounced effects on the sweat glands and the uterine lining. In a cool, moist locality, the stands mature in late summer (August through mid-September), and almost everything has been synthesized into menthol and menthone; this is the desirable stuff. Collect it in bundles, and dry Method A. The most practical processing is to strip off the leaves and flowers carefully, so as to keep them unbroken, and chop up the aromatic stems into short segments, combining with the rest. If you need the leaves only, such as for cooking, keep the chopped stems separate and use them for tea.

STABILITY As long as the leaves have their pepperminty scent, usually rather subdued after two years.

PREPARATION The tea, as needed. The Dry Tincture, 1:5, 50% alcohol, ½ teaspoon in ½ cup warm water. As powdering up the leaves, even briefly, allows too much loss of aromatics in the air, try this method of tincturing: put 25 ounces of the menstruum (or even 80 proof vodka) in a blender, add a third of the 5 ounces of whole dried herb, cover, blend until a slurry, add another third of the leaves, reblend until thoroughly pureed, then add the final third. There should be enough liquid to mix and grind up the herb (although with a little blender-panting). Scrape the mash into a quart jar and let set for a week, then squeeze or press out the tincture. If you have picked some truly exquisite Peppermint, just dried it and made the tincture, the finished product will knock your socks off (or stockings or whatever). The whole plant, tinctured this way, has a breadth of taste and aroma far greater than any other Peppermint extract. For internal use of Peppermint Oil (purchased from a pharmacy), take a tablespoon (½ ounce) of the oil, add to 4 tablespoons of Marshmallow Root powder or Kudzu (Kuzu) root powder, mix thoroughly with a fork, and put into #00 capsules. Dose, for acute pain, 3 to 4 capsules, three times a day; for irritable bowel syndrome or chronic colitis, 2 capsules, three times a day. Freeze unneeded capsules to prevent evaporation of the oil.

MEDICINAL USES There is nothing as effective as Peppermint for simple dyspepsia, stomach cramps, and nausea. Drink it, drink it, drink it. Angelica and Catnip have a low-level drug antispasmodic effect, whereas Peppermint anesthetizes the nerves in the intestinal tract by local action. Its effect is simple, straightforward, and limited to the mucosa, but it is familiar, safe, and without the complexities and occasional side effects of the other two. Because it does not stimulate the uterus, it is safe for morning sickness; the other two are not. The only disadvantage of Peppermint tea or tincture is that most of its anesthesia is exhausted by the middle small intestine, so taking enough to affect the cramps and pain of diarrhea and colon spasms is to risk feeling like a two-legged mint candy; you radiate "Eau de Life Saver" on top, and have fewer cramps on the bottom. Your breath makes your eyes water.

This is the reason for taking the pharmaceutically distilled Oil of Peppermint and powdered root mucilage in capsules. The Marshmallow or Kudzu binds the volatile oil, slows down the absorption in the stomach, and disperses it further down the intestinal tract. If you have irritable bowel syndrome (IBS), alternating constipation and diarrhea brought on by emotional stress, with cramps during the loose phase (a bit like asthma of the bowels), nothing, including prescription medication, works better than Peppermint oil. In Europe you can get enteric-coated capsules that only begin to dissolve in the small intestine, but this is a reasonable facsimile. If you still find that the oil is too rapidly absorbed in the stomach, add a tablespoon of coconut oil to the mix, and only use 3 tablespoons of root powder. I have seen the capsules *with* several cups of the tea work wonders on occasion for the pain of ulcerative colitis and Crohn's disease. It isn't curative, but it removes much of the pain. These are often serious disorders (unlike IBS), with much danger, much iatrogenesis from medications, so anything safe to help the pain will lessen the overall side effect from anti-inflammatory drugs.

Both the tea and the capsules are helpful for gas pains, palpitations, and the heaviness associated with a hiatus hernia; and they tend to lessen the frequency of heartburn and esophageal acidity from gastroesophageal reflux if it is associated with such a hernia. Often times it will work as well as cimetidine, and without the low-level side effects of that drug.

OTHER USES The tincture makes a great schnapps.

Pitcher Sage

Lepechinia calycina   (Labiatae)
OTHER NAMES   *Betonica (Bretonica); Sphacele calycina*

APPEARANCE Pitcher Sage is (in good years) a large, handsome, fuzzy, lime green shrub, growing from 2 to 6 feet tall, and resembling a cross between California Sage and Lemon Balm. The shrub forms many heavily leaved, brittle branches, with the lower leaves 2 to 4 inches long, borne

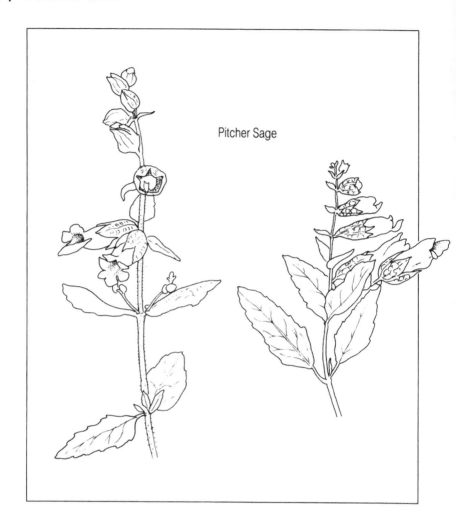

Pitcher Sage

on ½-inch-long petioles, the upper leaves stem-clasping and strongly veined. The showy flowers crowd the terminal leaf axils, usually predominately on one side of the stem. The calyx is large, inflated, and strongly veined, becoming an inflated inch-long fruit filled with little fuzzy black seeds. The flowers are light pink to white, with lavender blotches, and are showy, inflated tubes with an extended lower lip. The shrubs are really rather striking when encountered in a stand in the foothills. The lower parts of the plants have a distinctive dark green matte texture, while the upper parts are two tones lighter green, with the large calices forming an even lighter, nearly chartreuse accent to the tips of the branches. The color coordination alone, even without the big ballooned flowers, makes the bushes distinguishable from rather long distances. Of course, the scent of the crushed foliage gives it away in a second. It has a strong, almost unpleasant odor, reminiscent of Sage, Catnip, and Lemon Balm. Pitcher Sage is a surprisingly little-known plant, even though it is found in the foothills of the most populated parts of California. It would be an ideal cultivated native: it is drought-resistant, with large, showy flowers and striking foliage; it reproduces well from seed and simply needs a slope, some plants to provide it with partial shade, and water.

HABITAT Pitcher Sage is found in the foothills and canyons of the California coastal ranges. This primary species (the others are really varieties) is found from Ojai and Mount Pinos north to Sonoma, Napa, and Lake counties. There are some substantial but more sporadic stands in the Sierra Nevada foothills, from Mariposa to Butte counties. Other varieties grow in the foothills of the Santa Monica, San Gabriel, Santa Ana, and Laguna mountains of southern California. It seldom grows much above 3,000 feet, and plants in higher, colder canyons have smaller, sand-papery leaves. Their scent is often unpleasant.

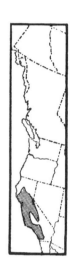

CONSTITUENTS Carnosic acid, carnosol, salvidin, ursolic acid, salvia-tannins, and several unspecified mono- and diterpenoids.

COLLECTING Gather the clean flowering or fruiting tops (discard brown or discolored leaves) and dry Method A.

STABILITY Usually a year, or as long as the complex aroma is intact and not reduced, by age, to a sage-skunk scent.

PREPARATION As a therapeutic agent, the Standard Infusion, 3 to 4 fluid ounces, up to four times a day. As a tea, to taste.

MEDICINAL USES The standard infusion, although at that strength rather unpleasant tasting, is a very useful uterine tonic, especially for chronic low-level pelvic irritability that may occur for several days following menses. Severe pain is symptomatic of such problems as salpingitis or pelvic inflammatory disease (PID), so I am talking here about a benign but uncomfortable condition that some women have, not an overt pathology. Try it three or four times a day starting the third day of menses. Although not a primary approach, it will help heal uterine infections more quickly if taken along with primary therapy. Further, I have seen it help acute pain in the occasional inflammatory episodes that benign prostatic hypertrophy induces in men. Otherwise, this herb, like many of its relatives—Sage, Desert Lavender, and Rosemary—acts as a general astringent for the intestinal tract and lungs when there are irritative hypersecretions and overt inflammations, such as gastritis, diverticulitis, and hemorrhoids. It contains several active antioxidants, which may explain the folk use of a Brazilian relative for a crude sunscreen. Steep a cup of the crushed leaves and ½ cup of Chaparral (*Larrea tridentata*) leaves in enough olive oil to cover, set for a month, strain out, and use. I have no idea about its protectant rating, but the oil seems, subjectively, to do the job nicely. The combination of these two aromatic herbs makes for a somewhat funky scent, but you get used to it. Besides, it will decrease the free radical damage from those old UVs.

As a simple tea, it combines well with Lemon Balm, Lemon Mint, Crimson Sage, or Spearmint. If you add several leaves to a pot of Mormon Tea, it seems to cut the bitterness, and the slight therapeutic value is complementary.

Prickly Poppy

Argemone corymbosa, A. munita　　(Papaveraceae)

OTHER NAMES　Thistle Poppy; *Chicalote, Cardo Santo; A. intermedia, A. platyceras, A. hispida*

APPEARANCE All the Prickly Poppies have the same general appearance; they are 2- to 5-foot-tall branching thistles that somebody has stapled big white and yellow Poppy flowers onto (aliens, perhaps? tiring from doing the Dracula with cattle and making circles in wheat fields . . . on the next Geraldo). The stout stems are covered in spiny leaves and, in our area, are olive-blue-green in color. *Argemone munita* has dense foliage—variously shaped, stem-clasping, rumpled leaves. *A. corymbosa* has longer leaves that arc out from the stem rather attractively, and it secretes orange sap when broken *A. munita* has a watery yellow sap. Both have horned and prickly flower buds, large crepe paper white petals (usually six), and a thicket of bright yellow stamens. The many fruits are armored little resin-tipped footballs, containing many small, dark poppy seeds. As the sides of the capsule gradually open, the seeds are slowly dispersed, some by simply falling out, the lower ones remaining until blown out by strong winds weeks or months later. Both plants are perennials, but *A. munita* can often propagate as an annual.

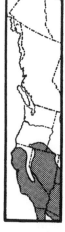

HABITAT *Argemone corymbosa* is a plant of the southern Great Basin, ranging from Nevada south to the Mojave Desert of California and the Mogollon Plateau of Arizona. *A. munita* is found all along the California coastal and inland ranges, south to Baja California; on both sides of the Sierra Nevada; into Nevada; north into southeastern Oregon; and it should be expected in southern Idaho. Both species are most common in middle and lower mountains and hills, from 1,000 to 5,000 feet, especially in rain shadows. They are a classic indicator of overgrazing by cattle, and with the general drought of the second half of the 1980s, their range and frequency can be expected to permanently increase. Although na-

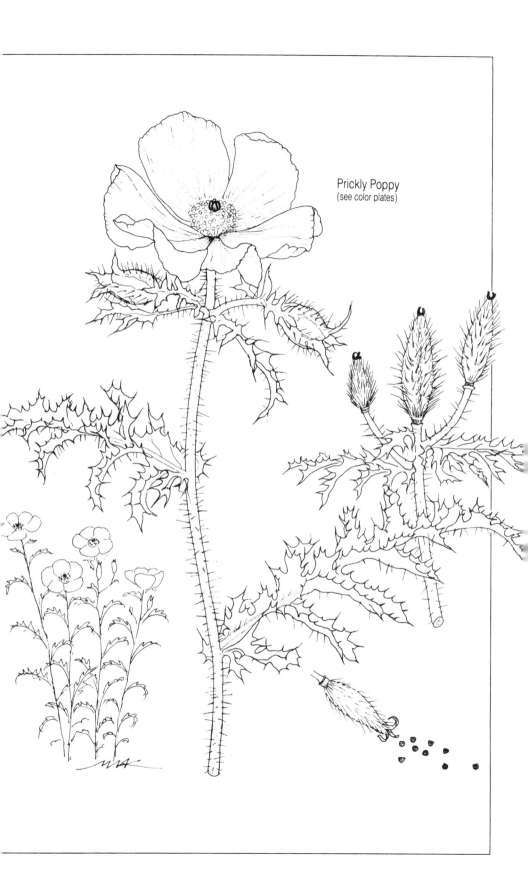

Prickly Poppy
(see color plates)

tive, they are becoming troublesome weeds in many parts of California, just as they are in Arizona, New Mexico, and Texas.

CONSTITUENTS Protopine, berberine, sanguinarine, cryptopine, allocryptopine, and other isoquinoline alkaloids; the seeds are high in a drying, fixed oil containing linolenic, acetic, valerianic, butyric, cinnamic, and benzoic acids, along with the alkaloids berberine and sanguinarine.

COLLECTING Although the whole plant has potency, the strongest part is the flowering upper third of the stems; gather with gloves and dry loose in paper bags. The strength can be increased by pulling the whole plant, root and all, hanging it upside down until somewhat wilted, *then* removing the flowering third and the roots, and discarding the rest. It is best to do this in the late spring and early summer in wet years. Gathering the seeds a few weeks later when the spiny pods cover the plants, with the older and larger pods starting to turn tan, is a laborious, painstaking (pain *giving*) process. Snip them individually or in bunches directly into paper bags. Allow them to dry, gradually shaking the ejected seeds out of the bag as they are shed from the pods. Some pods may not open, even when dry, and may need to be mashed, crushed, or stomped open, and the seeds winnowed or sieved.

STABILITY The dried herb will stay strong for at least a year; the seeds are good for a couple of years, the root even longer.

PREPARATION The herb as a Cold Infusion, 2 to 3 fluid ounces, up to four times a day; topically as needed; the root as a Decoction for topical application, or powdered and moistened for a poultice. The seeds may be added to foods as a mild laxative, ground and encapsulated (3 to 4 #00 with warm water in the evening), or 1 part freshly ground seeds steeped in 3 parts olive oil in a warm (not hot) place for a week, and the oil decanted from the seeds. The best of all methods for a skin dressing is to mix 1 part freshly ground seeds with 1 part ghee (rectified sweet butter), melting them together over a low heat, removing to harden overnight, remelting and hardening the same batch for several days, and finally melting and pouring off the resultant impregnated ghee into a container. Scrape the remaining seed-ghee glurch into a square of clean cloth after it hardens, tie it up in the cloth with a string or rubber band, and simmer the tied bundle in a pot of water. The remaining fat and oil will rise to the top, harden after the water cools, and can be lifted off and added to the first batch, both parts remelted to mix evenly, and then returned to the final container. You now have a proper, top-of-the-line burn and irritated skin ointment (and a rather messy kitchen).

MEDICINAL USES The seeds, taken internally, either with food or in capsules, are an excellent laxative for those with poor digestion and sluggish colon function that causes a dull frontal headache. The laxative effect is not for the person who has the dry constipation of adrenalin stress but for the person with sluggish lower-GI with achy legs, rectal pain, dull ache on urination, and soft bowels.

The cold infusion taken internally is a strong sedative and pain reliever for intestinal cramps and painful urination that lingers around after an infection has been dealt with but the membranes still hurt. Difficulty in urinating after childbirth or catheterization can be helped by the tea, which relaxes the trigone muscle and urethral sphincter, and decreases sacral nerve irritation and local pain in the process. The tea should only be used for several days at a time; because it contains small amounts of a number of somewhat toxic alkaloids that are fine for short-term use but not so cool for long-term use, and also has a truly disgusting taste; the tea can start to get nauseating after the third day.

The tea and the root poultice will relieve local pain from muscle trauma, hyperextensions, contusions, and painful swellings. For moderate burns from the sun, heat, or friction, bathe the parts with tea, dry, and apply the oil or salve made from the seeds. The seed preparations, particularly the ghee salve, will lessen skin pain, decrease distension pain, and protect the skin. Hand injuries from sports or martial arts benefit from the salve, and sore feet can be buttered up as well.

Red Cedar

Thuja plicata   (Cupressaceae)

OTHER NAMES   Western Red Cedar, Giant Cedar, Arborvitae, Western Flat Cedar, Thuja

APPEARANCE Red Cedar is Juniperlike, with large, fanlike branches, and with cinnamon red bark, which becomes grey-brown with age. The leaves are reduced to scales, growing laterally, flat, and drooping, with a yellow-green to bright green color, and a strong lemon-pine scent. Large trees are sometimes rare these days, being a preferred timber, but may grow to 150 feet or more; they are conical and almost Redwoodlike in shape, buttressed, with fluted, fibrous trunks. Smaller trees are more common, with trunks hidden by large fan-branches—rich, aromatic, reptilian. The occasional stand of old-growth giants is so striking, it's little wonder that some of the Native Americans of the Northwest hold them in religious regard.

HABITAT Red Cedar grows in moist lowlands and middle mountains, from western Montana through Idaho, Alberta, and British Columbia; to the southern edge of the Alaska Panhandle; and south to northwestern California, where there are occasional stands.

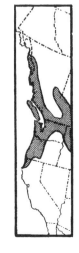

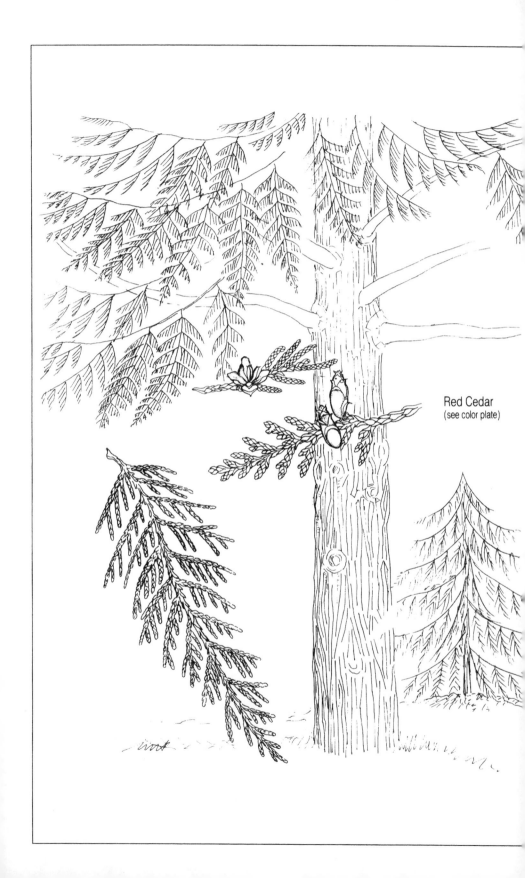

Red Cedar
(see color plate)

CONSTITUENTS Plicatic acid, mearnsitrin (a flavonolglycoside), procyanidins, prodelphinidin, umbelliferon, p-coumaric acid, myricetin, quercetin, kaempferol-3-0-a-rhamnoside, catechin, gallocatechin, and volatile oils containing thujone, fenchone, and umbelliferone.

COLLECTING Gather the fanlike branches of younger trees in summer or fall (highest oil content), and process for fresh plant tincture or dry, Method A, and garble to remove the red stems. For incense, you may use whole branches for smudging, or run the leaves loosely through a hand grinder and use the pieces on coals.

STABILITY The dried fans, stored well, will usually retain their aromatics and potency for a couple of years.

PREPARATION Fresh Herb Tincture, 1:2; Glycerin Tincture (fresh herb), 1:2; menstruum, 50% glycerin, 40% water, 10% alcohol; Cold Infusion, 2 to 3 fluid ounces.

MEDICINAL USES Red Cedar is strongly antifungal and antibacterial, and stimulates innate immunity scavenging. The fresh tinctures work best, with the glycerin tincture being better for application to tender tissue. For various tineas, such as tinea versicolor, athlete's foot, ringworm, jock itch ("crotch rot"), and nail fungi, apply the tincture two or three times a day, with consistency. It may take a week, but Red Cedar works. For chronic vaginitis, with long, sluggish menses, use the infusion for a douche (alternating days) and take some of the tea (also on alternate days).

The tincture or tea acts as a stimulus to many smooth muscles, and this can be used to advantage in respiratory, urinary tract, and reproductive problems. For chronic, mucus-heavy bronchial conditions, some tea is useful, but the best remedy is to put a teaspoon of the tincture into some simmering water and inhale the steam. Simmering some herb or inhaling the scent from a cotton ball impregnated with the tincture (alcoholic) may be adequate alternatives. The cold infusion, internally, is effective for a heavy, boggy uterus with dull aches, long cycles, and frequent low-level vaginal irritation, or for the male equivalent, a boggy, enlarged prostate, with ache on urination or ejaculation, and periodic mucus in the urine; for women, the douche is effective as well. Red Cedar stimulates the vascular capillary beds (and the subtle musculature that responds to local environmental changes) to expand and contract, heat and cool, and it is this effect that makes the *Thujas* so useful for chronic bladder and urethral irritability. For these conditions use the cold infusion twice a day.

Red Cedar is an immunostimulant, increasing phagocytosis (scavenging) by granulocytes (scavenging white blood cells); and small, daily doses (in the absence of kidney disorders or pregnancy) can increase resistance to chronic respiratory and intestinal infections. It can be combined with small amounts of California Snakeroot and *Astragalus* to broaden the type of responses, and Devil's Club and Oregon Grape to increase the catabolism or cleansing of metabolites produced by the immunologic stimulus.

CONTRAINDICATIONS Red Cedar is not for extended use by those with kidney weakness, and is not an appropriate herb for internal use during pregnancy.

OTHER USES The leaves are a lovely incense.

Red Root

Ceanothus velutinus, C. cuneatus, C. integerrimus, etc. (Rhamnaceae)

OTHER NAMES Buckbrush, Tobacco Brush, Deerbrush, Mahala Mat, Lilac Bush, Oregon Tea Tree, Sweet Birch, etc.

APPEARANCE This is tough. There are more than thirty species of *Ceanothus* in the Pacific West, all are at least locally abundant, and, as with Sages and Manzanitas, California is the center of great species diversity and rampant (perhaps even immoral) hybridization. Several of the genus grow to become small trees, such as *C. thyrsiflorus* and *C. spinosus*. With their size and lovely blue and lavender flowers, they are some of the most decorative native trees to be found in coastal California. For our purposes, the ideal Red Root is a short, chunky subshrub, usually spiny, with white aromatic and soapy flowers, dark green foliage, and tough, obstinate roots spreading out from a tough taproot. The root bark should be red or wine-colored, the inner wood at least Caucasian flesh-colored. The three species listed above are the most widespread of this type, found up and down the coast, so I will talk about them. Other Red Roots match this description and can be used, but finding them (and identifying them) is up to you.

Ceanothus velutinus, called Tobacco Brush, Sticky Laurel, Mountain Balm, and Snowbrush (as well as other names) is a rounded, dark green bush, sometimes 3 feet tall in the center, often only a foot in height, and formed of many short, thick stems covered with large, generally sticky leaves. Plants may be spread out to 10 feet in width, but most plants in a stand will be from 2 to 4 feet in diameter. Like most *Ceanothus* species, the oval leaves have three or five primary veins running from tip to tip, and well-delineated secondary veins branching out from them; but the upper surface may be so covered with shiny resin that this is not always apparent. The underside is lighter, the stems are sticky, and the big, leathery leaves often tend to stand upright, somewhat vertical to the ground. The flowers are large oval clusters of small, snow-white blossoms, shockingly white against the dark green, varnished leaves; they bloom from late spring to fall, depending on the rain and heat. The flowers are aromatic, and the leaves have a strong, pleasant, spicy taste. The plant is not spined.

Ceanothus cuneatus is most commonly called Buckbrush; it is all stems, branches, and spines, is stubby, and has grey bark; the branches spread out in complete disarray from larger ones, stems from branches, sometimes opposite, sometimes not, and usually at a predictable angle halfway between 45 degrees and 90 degrees, with one opposite stem 2 inches long and its twin maybe a foot long with its own stems. The leaves are small, oval to oblong, and have almost no stem, bursting from the branch in bunches, pairs, or singly, light green on top, lighter still below, with a strong central vein. The spines barely qualify as such (unless they stick you), being little more than short stems, with or without leaves. The flowers also are tiny, white to cream-colored, forming oval balls, crowded erratically at the ends of stems or along their length. They are sweet-spicy scented and foam up with a little water.

Ceanothus integerrimus is usually called Deerbrush. It is a tall, somewhat lyrical bush, with many long, yellow-green branches, from 4 to 10 feet tall, nodding, flexible, and covered in three-veined, pointed-oval leaves. They are blue-green above, lighter below, and usually from 1 to 2 inches long. The flowers form graceful pyramidal terminal clusters of a snow-white to light blue color. All three of these species (and most *Ceanothus*) have flowers that mature into little three-horned, acornlike seed capsules.

HABITAT *Ceanothus velutinus,* var. *laevigatus* is a somewhat taller coastal variety, found from Marin County, California, northwards into Oregon, Washington, and British Columbia, along the west side of the Cascades. It is really more a difference of size, since it may resemble the main, smaller variety in less favorable locations. The more widespread, small type is found from Tulare County northwards in the Sierra Nevada range of California, and may be quite sparse in the southern edges of its range. It grows northwards into Alberta; all along the east side of the Cascades; and eastwards into Idaho, Montana, Nevada, Utah, and Wyoming. It is a mountain and foothill plant, abundant in clearings, on open slopes, and where there has been burning and clear-cutting of the main conifer forests in the West. In old-growth or uncut forest, it is limited to occasional stands filling in places too rocky, steep, or dry for the conifers to grow.

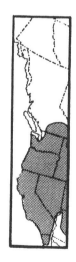

Ceanothus cuneatus is a plant of dry slopes, hillsides, and ridges, from Baja California del Norte northwards to central Oregon; and in California in the drier lower slopes of the Sierra Nevada all the way to the coast, and points in between. Look for it on the dry side of any mountain and foothill in most of California; it will usually be there. Sometimes it may be all that is there.

Ceanothus integerrimus grows in the area between the previous two,

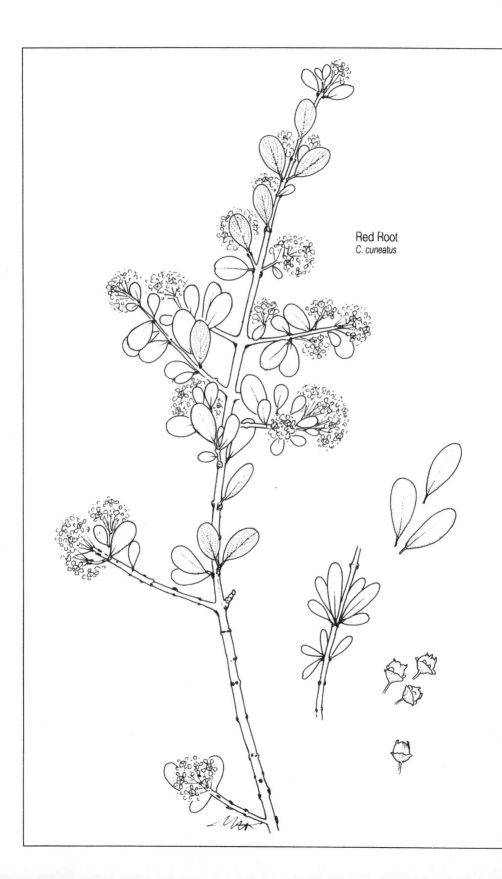

Red Root
C. cuneatus

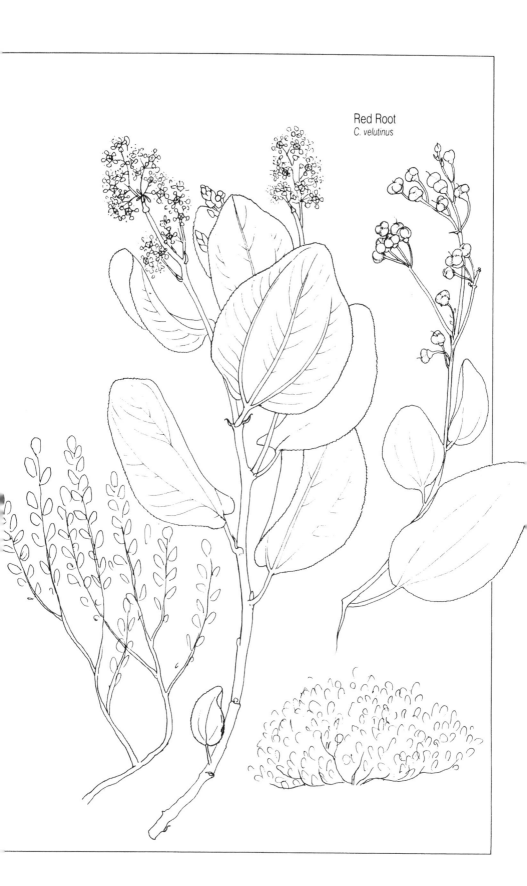

Red Root
C. velutinus

usually below the forest; it needs more water and shade than Buckbrush. In the coastal ranges of California it grows at 1,000 feet or lower; in the inner southern California mountains, it is seldom encountered below 4,000 feet, but along the Sierra Nevada it may descend down to 2,500 feet. It extends up the coast to southwestern Oregon; along the east side of the Cascades up to Washington; and east and south as far as New Mexico.

CONSTITUENTS *Leaves:* Nonacosane, 1-hexacosanol, velutin, and traces of caffeine reported in several species. *Root and bark:* betulinic acid, ceanothic acid, ceanothenic acid, methyl salicylate, and the alkaloids ceanothine, ceanothamine, integerressine, integerrenine, integerrine, and americine. Other constituents are tannins, phlobaphenes, resins, and oils, with succinic, oxalic, malonic, malic, orthophosphoric, and pyrophosphoric acids.

COLLECTING The roots are usually best gathered from midsummer to mid-winter. The most desirable roots have a reddish or wine-colored bark. The inner wood varies from cream-colored to reddish purple. If the wood has at least some reddish color, use it with the bark; if it is pale cream-colored and lacking in tint, use just the bark. If the main taproots have some color in the wood, I go ahead and use all the side roots as well, discarding the stems at the level that tan root bark changes to green stem bark.

Plants growing in difficult or marginal places usually have stronger root color, and greater therapeutic value. *Ceanothus* is a nitrogen-fixing plant, somewhat unique because it has a soil fungus as a symbiote, rather than the nitrogen-fixing bacteria found in legumes. It seems that the more difficult the environment, the more the reliance on nitrogen-fixing, the stronger the root color, and the stronger the medicine. The roots are tough and intractable, so you will need limb shears, good pruning shears, sometimes a sharp hatchet, and good gloves or good calluses. No matter what you are doing, you will need to work the roots while they are fresh; dry roots need a band saw to process.

STABILITY The dried root and bark are stable for at least two years, even longer. The leaves are good for up to a year.

PREPARATION Fresh Root Tincture, 1:2, 30 to 60 drops, up to four times a day. If you are able, by some miracle, to grind up the roots, the Dry Tincture, 1:5, 50% alcohol, is quite nice as well. The Cold Infusion can be taken in doses of 2 to 4 fluid ounces.

MEDICINAL USES Red Root is one of the best examples of and recommendations for using herbs in the subclinical grey area that precedes overt disease. It is an astringent to membranes, and is a good gargle and mouthwash for a sore throat or sores in the mouth. Beyond this, much of its value comes from its effect on the integrity of blood proteins. It helps increase the quality of blood charge, thereby increasing the repelling charge of the capillary cells. With improved charges, there is improved transport of blood fluid out into the interstitial colloids and more efficient uptake of lymph, as well as return of fluid back into the blood exiting the capillaries into the veins. Remember, the lymph is simply part of the blood, temporarily shunted through back alleys, cleaning up garbage too large to be absorbed directly into the venous capillaries, and with its trash gradually broken down and nosed through by white blood cells, it is returned back into the subclavian veins.

One of the best uses of Red Root is for liver headaches and inflammation from blood fats. Picture this: late evening, a meal of green chile chicken enchiladas with sour cream and cheese, a couple of glasses of wine, and greasy sopaipillas with honey. The green chile and alcohol dilate the intestinal membranes; the sour cream and cheese contain butterfat, the fat that doesn't need bile to digest, and it is absorbed rapidly into the portal blood that drains from the GI tract to the liver. The fats, rapidly absorbed, flood through the liver into general circulation. Blood fats have little or no electrical charge, unlike the blood proteins, and they can exit the capillaries easily, particularly when you are tired and greased out. Fats stimulate the mast cells that are found around the capillaries, those cells that are responsible for histamine release during tissue stress. Histamines dilate the capillaries, making them more permeable, and your eyes get red, your head starts to ache, you itch, your joints get painful—whatever you are prone to, you get. Take some Red Root, get that blood charge back a bit, decrease the effects of the blood fats, feel better. You see, Red Root isn't for headaches, just certain kinds; it isn't for arthritis, just certain kinds; this differentiation is too subtle for use in medicine, but just right for herbology. I use a dark-field microscope to observe live blood, and after such a meal, my blood is full of blood fats (chylomicrons), and my red blood cells (RBC), normally repelling each other by a like membrane charge, stick together in long rolls, or *rouleau*. You can imagine how hard it is to squeeze these adhering RBC rolls through the fine capillary beds in the brain—or the fingers or lungs. If I take some Red Root (a couple of squirts of the tincture will do it), an hour later the blood fats may still be there, but the red blood cells are no longer clumped in rolls; instead, they are dispersed across the slide.

In general, with its positive effects on the blood charges and its improvement of interstitial fluid and lymph passage, Red Root is helpful in a variety of conditions. It won't *cure* you—just make you better able to cure yourself. The tea is very effective when used during tonsillitis; make up a quart of the cold infusion and sip the whole thing during the day. For inflammation or swelling of the lymph nodes, the tincture or tea helps immensely. It won't get rid of the cause of the inflammation (usually an infection or allergy), but it strengthens the node tissues while immunologic responses continue. In portal congestion, with aching hemorrhoids, varicose veins, and cervical or prostate congestion, use Red Root. Because it stimulates fluid drainage from congested tissues, it is always helpful with breast cysts, ovarian cysts, or other hydroceles, if taken with something that stimulates the blood supply to those tissues. For ovarian and testicular cysts, it can be combined with Don Quai, Blue Cohosh, or *Helonias*. For breast cysts (Chamaelirium) that enlarge and shrink with your hormone cycle, combine the Red Root with Milkweed, Cotton Rootbark, or 3 to 5 drop doses of *Phytolacca* tincture (fresh Poke Root tincture available from an N.D. or, as a mother tincture, from an M.D. homeopath).

Because it acts to tonify the structure of lymph tissue, Red Root is often helpful for hepatitis or mononucleosis, when the spleen is enlarged and painful but the actual infection is on the way out. I am not claiming cure in such cases, only a strengthening of certain tissues during a disease process. In the alphabet viruses, CFS, EBV, or CMV (even HIV), the chronic congestion of lymph pulp can be helped with regular use of Red Root. In the lymph "system," you have cells that do stuff, such as lymphocytes like T-Cells (parenchymal cells), and cells that act to hold things together in a tight, controlled package (mesenchymal or structural cells). Red Root doesn't stimulate the active cells of immunity; it stimulates the structural or connective cells that form the organ within which the lymph cells work.

Red Root is an excellent home remedy for menstrual hemorrhage, nosebleeds, bleeding piles, hemorrhoids and old ulcers, and capillary ruptures from vomiting or coughing; it should also be used by heavy drinkers with gastritis, whiskey nose, and other symptoms of capillary fragility. The tincture of California Lilac was used by the homeopath Boericke for sore throat, inflamed tonsils, sinus inflammations, and diphtheria, both internally and as a gargle. The leaves can be used for tea, especially *C. velutinus,* and the fresh flowers can be used for a feeble but elegant soap.

CONTRAINDICATIONS Red Root has been used experimentally to improve blood coagulation (in people) and as an anticoagulant (in veterinary medicine). Both uses have been discarded, since the effects are *tonic* to the blood proteins and have no predictable drug effect in medical practice. Still, you may wish to avoid it if you have overt blood disorders or if you are taking medication that is meant to affect blood clotting. If you have a specific allergy to aspirin products, you might find that some species of Red Root may trigger a mild response. Just out of normal conservatism, I would recommend only moderate use during pregnancy.

In general, there is little information regarding drug reactions with Red Root. It is a rather benign but complex herbal medicine, and, except to aid lymph structure in slow viruses and tonify the spleen during liver and lymph viruses, I would suggest not using Red Root if you are under medical care for an overt disease. Red Root is for healthy people under stress, not for sick folks under treatment—the best kind of herb.

Redwood

Sequoia sempervirens   (Taxodiaceae)

OTHER NAMES   *Keilth* (Yurok) and several other California Indian names

APPEARANCE The Redwood almost needs no description, being one of the most famous trees in the world. Redwoods may reach over 300 feet in height, and they have a majestic, almost conical shape. The trunks are covered in furrowed reddish brown, spongy bark and have many slender branches that are totally out of reach on mature trees. The leaves are ½ to 1 inch long, flat, and dark green on top, forming typical sprays. The foliage is lightly, gently aromatic when crushed, more so in the younger saplings. This is advantageous because these are the branches we *can* reach.

HABITAT The Redwoods, in their present, depleted biomass, are found from south of Santa Cruz in California north to just inside the Oregon border, as high as 2,000 feet, but only within the range of coastal fog. Ninety percent of all the Redwood forests have been clear-cut, and half of what's left will be gone by the end of the century, but there is still more than enough to maintain huge stands of the trees in protected public and private lands. What is gone are the huge tracts of *forest,* the ecology that is a thousand or ten thousand life-forms that have now been reduced to the small protected enclaves of "Redwood Forest." The trees, of course, are just the big, erect, macho parts of the *forest,* and because the trees are great lumber—cheap, large, easily harvested, straight-grained, and rot-resistant—they have been clear-cut for a century. Without the big trees, the thousands of other organisms that make up the *forest* die. The Redwoods are not Southern Pine, which forms Pine farms in huge tracts of boring monoculture in the southeastern U.S. The Redwoods only grow in irreversible, irreplaceable *forests.* You can't farm them in neat rows; you can only cut down the ones that are already growing, thereby permanently destroying the ecology that they are a necessary part of. So you have to go where there are Redwoods, find some young ones you can reach, and clip a branch or two. Go to the edges of a state park or national park or to the little insipid riverside belts of old forest that the lumber companies maintain for the sake of appearance on the

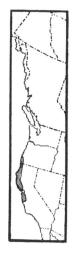

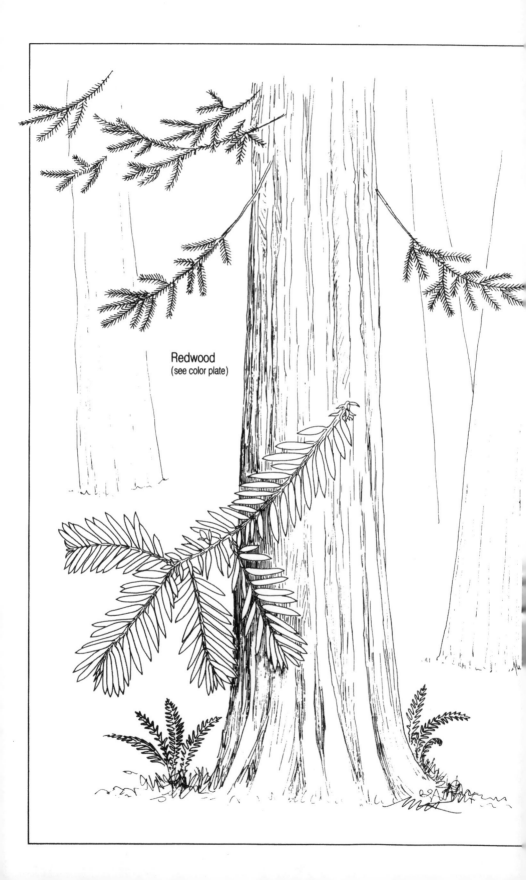

Redwood
(see color plate)

northern coast of California. Good luck trying to fish there; the erosion from clear-cutting upstream has seriously depleted the game fish, but you can gather a little Redwood foliage and maybe some Wild Ginger and Yarrow while you're at it.

CONSTITUENTS Monoterpenes, procyanidin, prodelphinidin, and (+)-catechin and (+)-gallocatechin in the stems.

COLLECTING Gather a couple of branches, dry Method A, and process the whole branch, leaves and stems together. Spring foliage seems the strongest for medicinal use, but it is alright later in the year as well.

STABILITY Stored properly, the tea should be strong for at least eighteen months.

PREPARATION Standard Infusion, 2 to 3 fluid ounces, up to three times a day.

MEDICINAL USES The tea is an elegant-tasting remedy for the recuperative stage of a lung infection, when the mucus is slow to loosen and you cough your brains out in the morning trying to expectorate the stuff that accumulated during sleep. Coming down from breaking the fever can be a trying time when a simple bronchial virus can linger and, with impaired resistance, a secondary infection or viral reinfection can occur. The tea will introduce aromatics into the bloodstream, which are excreted as waste gases by the lungs. This helps to disinfect the mucus membranes and the passive air in the lungs themselves and to stimulate secretions by the membranes that help soften the mucus. If you wish, you can add some Balsam Root, Grindelia, or Osha to the tea to increase the expectoration. But for a simple chest cold, most of the time Redwood should be enough.

Further, the tea, with its aromatics and astringents, acts as a simple, soothing disinfectant to the urinary tract; it is helpful for mild bladder infections without causing complications.

OTHER USES The leaves make a lovely incense when placed on charcoal or embers.

Salal

Gaultheria shallon   (Ericaceae)
OTHER NAMES   Oregon Wintergreen

APPEARANCE Salal is a handsome plant, with large 2- to 4-inch-long oval leaves that are shiny dark green on top, rough and lighter underneath, with a pronounced central vein. The foliage is thick and leathery.

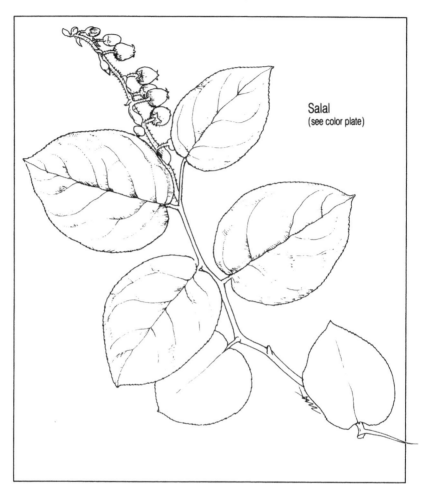

Salal
(see color plate)

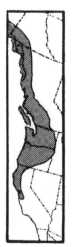

The leaves are alternate, with varying lengths of petioles, and, at least on the newer terminal branches, they zigzag off the red-mealy barked stems. Older central stems, thicker and browner, usually straighten out, so the zigzag pattern of leaves is primarily exhibited by new growth. The flowers are the typical little pink urns of the Heath family, clustering off the sides of small, forking auxiliary or terminal racemes, usually with little pink oval bracts on the opposite side of the stem. By late summer or early fall these have matured into purple-black berries—succulent, bland, sweet, tart, and a little spicy to the taste. The plants may form low-growing semivines a foot tall along roadsides and in open areas, and form 6- or 7-foot-tall thicket plants in shady, moist places.

HABITAT Salal can be found growing along the coast and the coastal mountains from Santa Cruz to the Alaska Panhandle; south through western British Columbia; as far east as the eastern slopes of the Cascades in Washington; and in Oregon, m̄   y on the west side of the Cascades. I have found it in the Sweetwater River drainage in Idaho, but it isn't supposed to grow there, so never mind. Its range does not extend from the Oregon Cascades into the California Sierra Nevada, and it stops somewhere near where Ed Smith lives in south-central Oregon.

CONSTITUENTS Flavonoid aglycones, sideroxylin, latifolin, tannic acid, and gallic acids (leaves); an abundance of flavonoids in the berries.

COLLECTING Although Salal is an evergreen, it is best to gather the young, reddish, zigzag branches from late spring to mid-fall. Bundle them and dry them, Method A. The berries should be collected in early to mid-fall, when fully mature.

STABILITY The leaves are good for several years; the dried berries, whole or made into cakes, last until the next season.

PREPARATION A Simple Infusion of five or six crushed leaves is the easiest media for the medicine. The powdered leaves can be applied topically as needed or mixed with water for a short-term poultice.

MEDICINAL USES The tea is astringent and anti-inflammatory, both locally to the throat and upper intestinal mucosa, and, through the bloodstream, to the urinary tract, sinuses, and lungs. It is a safe, frequently repeatable tea for diarrhea, accompanied by heat, cramps, and moderate fever. It can combine well with Silk Tassel for use in the acute stage, and, after usually a day, you can use it with Mallow and Yerba Mansa for the colon inflammation, maybe adding Angelica, Peony, or Skunk Cabbage for the cramps.

Although there are stronger therapies, the tea helps scratchy, irritated coughs from allergies or dusty, dry air that provokes a low-level raspy throat and lungs, which is phlegmy on waking, dry by afternoon, and becomes a pathetic little toad-croak cough before retiring. You know what I mean: Chinook winds, the Santa Anas, dry air from the Palouse into Portland—that sort of stuff—giving some folks a dry wheeze for a week or two.

For young children the tea is helpful for colic and gas pains resulting from subtle food hypersensitivities to such items as soya milk, pea soup, whole grains, or garlic. Similarly, for adults with gastritis or a pre-ulcer stomach condition that causes distress two or three hours after meals, the tea is safe and helpful. For bladder irritation, particularly in those types of cystitis that don't necessarily cause the urge to urinate but cause pain *after* urination, the tea is almost a specific.

The tea and the powdered herb are an effective astringent, hemostatic, and pain reliever when applied to scrapes, abrasions, burns, and insect bites. This herb isn't a major medicine, but it is common, comely, and effective against common problems in a commonsense fashion, has almost disappeared in use as a healing plant, and needs reintroduction.

OTHER USES The berries were and are a major food for lots of birds and mammals, including us. Salal and Shallon are derived from the Nootka name for the fruit, which translates as "bland berry that tastes a bit better than tree bark during February blizzards" (just kidding). The traditional way of storing them is to lay a covering of the leaves in a flat box, pour the fresh berries on top, mash them semiflat, and dry. If you want, use them in this form like raisins (with crunchy little seeds inside), or crush some fresh berries, enough to hold the dried ones together in a cake, and dry again. This mixture will store easily all winter and can be used in a variety of ways. I like to defrost some whole Blueberries and use them to moisten and form the cake; they add some needed flavor as well. Whether you use fresh Salal berries or Blueberries, you end up with ridiculously purple hands. Salal berries are incredibly high in flavonoids, and can be used as a free, nutritional therapy for strengthening capillaries in chronic skin and mucus membrane fragility; use a chunk twice a day.

Sarsaparilla

Smilax californica   (Liliaceae)

OTHER NAMES   California Smilax, Western Greenbrier; *Smilax Jamesii, Smilax rotundifolia,* var. *californica*

APPEARANCE When I first found this *Smilax,* I couldn't believe my eyes, since I usually traveled to Arkansas and Oklahoma to gather Sarsaparilla. I don't think I have ever run across a western herbalist who even knows this anomaly exists. *Smilax californica* is a stout, woody vine, moderately prickly, sometimes smooth and glaucous, and sometimes fiercely barbed. The lower stems are glandular and swollen around the former leaf nodes, greenish brown, and vaguely ridged or quadrangular. Like other plants that can climb high with their tendrils, Sarsaparilla has leaves beginning several feet off the ground; they are alternate, short-stemmed, rounded, 2 to 4 inches in diameter, with five or seven parallel veins, and crosshatched with secondary veins. (Plants without trees or shrubs to climb on often have smaller leaves that start close to the ground, as well as long, straight tendrils.) In good Willow thickets the stems may grow to 10 or 15 feet high. The plants are dioecious (separate sexed), and the females bear short, stubby umbels of black, juicy berries which are hard to find and apparently not present every year.

HABITAT Our Sarsaparilla grows along the banks of slow-moving streams and in the thickets next to them. It is common in the basin of the Illinois and Rogue rivers of southwest Oregon and the northern lower tributaries of the Sacramento River, growing as far south as Sacramento

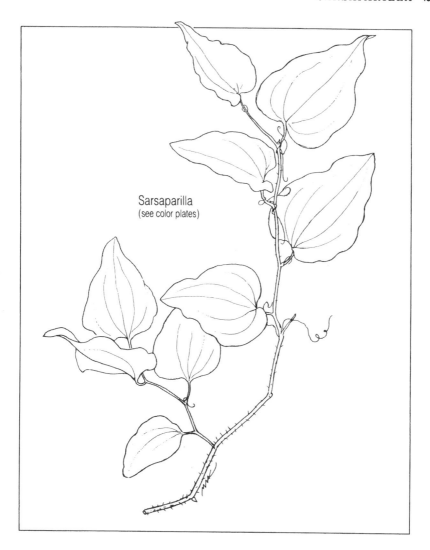

Sarsaparilla
(see color plates)

itself. Considering recent toxic chemical spillage in northern California, stick to the tributaries. If you find minnows along the river's edge, it's clean enough to dig the plant.

CONSTITUENTS Although I have found no direct study of this species, the closely related S. *rotundifolia* of the southeastern U.S. contains moderate amounts of the *Smilax* group of saponins and steroid glycosides. Natural products chemists may cover their eyes and groan, but I have gathered four species of eastern *Smilax* and this California one. Sarsaparilla from the Caribbean has always been the most sought after, and is the formerly official drug plant. Its light red color has been the hallmark of its strength. The California *Smilax* and S. *glauca* of the south-central states, with its outrageous, warty root nodes, dry to a good red color. The fresh root tincture of S. *californica* forms the most foam of any of the American Sarsaparillas I have tinctured fresh and, since the saponins (soaps) are generally indicative of the strength, and this species has lots of soap in its root, I hereby declare it groovy stuff.

COLLECTING Sarsaparillas, growing high and gnarly in thickets, competing with many other plants, have long, skinny, and intractable roots. They seldom have underground tubers, or at least none I have been able to locate without a backhoe. Individuals out in the semiopen are more likely to have more root mass and shorter, more intertwined stems. These roots are grey to reddish brown, with many nodes, side runners, and tuberous masses (if you are lucky). Always leave some runners and foliage for regeneration, fill in the sandy holes, and cover well. They will regrow rapidly with root culling; and a fresh section with nodes at both ends, if planted beside some other moist, sandy place, will usually take by the following year. It is a robust plant, growing in a somewhat limited area, and needs some spreading around. You will only have a male or a female, but in a couple of years you might bring it a "friend," or at least do some root dividing to increase the unisexual colony. If you are going to use it dry, chop the roots while they are fresh; they dry very tough. I usually include a foot of the stem.

STABILITY At least two years.

PREPARATION Fresh Root Tincture, 1:2, 60 to 90 drops, up to three times a day. Dry Root Tincture, 1:5, 50% alcohol, 30 to 90 drops, up to three times a day. Cold Infusion 1 to 4 fluid ounces, up to three times a day, made from finely chopped or ground root.

MEDICINAL USES A subtle plant, so many claims have been made for Sarsaparilla that it has been discarded long ago as a useful medicine. For one thing, it doesn't cure a specific disorder. It is a gentle and accumulative anabolic and adrenocortical stimulus, useful for those with what I call a liver-deficient constitution—that is, with dry skin, chronic constipation, allergies, labile blood sugar, poor fat and protein absorption, dry mouth, poor gums, and a tendency to an adrenalin-stress habit. It helps modify innate immunity hyperactivity, with allergies and chronic inflammations, while strengthening acquired immunity and specific response to a particular confrontation. I have seen it help benign prostatic hypertrophy and the tendency to cervical erosion, but only with long-term use.

Sarsaparilla needs helpers, such as Devil's Club, Licorice Fern, California Spikenard, and Oregon Grape root. If you have predictable nighttime urination, moderate or low blood pressure, cold extremities, and the dry skin/dry gut syndrome, combine it with Devil's Club, American Ginseng, or Dong Quai (cured Chinese Angelica). For prostate problems, combine it with White Sage, Saw Palmetto, Shepherd's Purse, or

Yerba Mansa. It is distinctly beneficial by itself, over a period of time, with appropriate changes in lifestyle and diet. Just don't expect it to cure a pathology. Weightlifters and bodybuilders have turned to Sarsaparilla with the same ferocity with which they work out. Rumor has it that it's "as good as steroids, and good for you, too!" Rumor has always implied that it contains testosterone and "makes you a man!" (What if you're a woman?). Twaddle.

Silk Tassel

Garrya spp.   (Garryaceae)
OTHER NAMES   Quinine Bush; *Cuauchichic*

APPEARANCE The several *Garryas* are Oak and Manzanitalike shrubs, with generally smooth bark, and stout, leathery, evergreen leaves. The leaves are opposite, and most of the twigs and branches are paired as well. The short leaf petioles often form a connecting sheath around the stem, giving the younger growth a segmented appearance. Both Oaks and Manzanitas have alternate leaves, and either corky or red bark; Silk Tassel bark, especially in younger branches, is mostly greenish. *Garrya flavescens* is the most common species of the genus; it is typical of the several others, with the exception of *G. elliptica,* a larger, dark-barked semitree of the northern California and southern Oregon coasts that I have not seen, picked, or used—so I won't talk about it. As for the usual floppy, unkempt, and many branched *Garryas,* the flowers are separate sexes (mostly) and form short or long catkins of a yellow or cream color. In wet years the catkins may form spectacular drooping displays; hence the name Silk Tassel. The seeds are dry little blackish berries around ¼ inch in diameter, borne at the ends of the branches. The bushes range up to 10 feet in height and are substantial in demeanor, although sometimes sparsely branched.

HABITAT *Garrya flavescens,* the most common of the genus in California, grows in dry mountains and foothills, between 4,500 and 7,000 feet, and from San Benito County and Fresno County south into the inland ranges as far as San Diego County and the inland ranges of Baja California. It is found as well in the mountains around the Mojave and Colorado deserts of California; from the Providence and Granite mountains of San Bernardino County of that state; into the Charleston Mountains near Las Vegas; and east across the Mogollon Rim. It hybridizes with *G. buxifolia* and *G. fremontii* (and in Arizona with *G. Wrightii*); there is such difficulty telling these species apart where they meet (and they share many localities) that it is hard to be specific. *Garrya buxifolia* (or

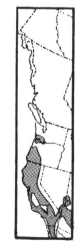

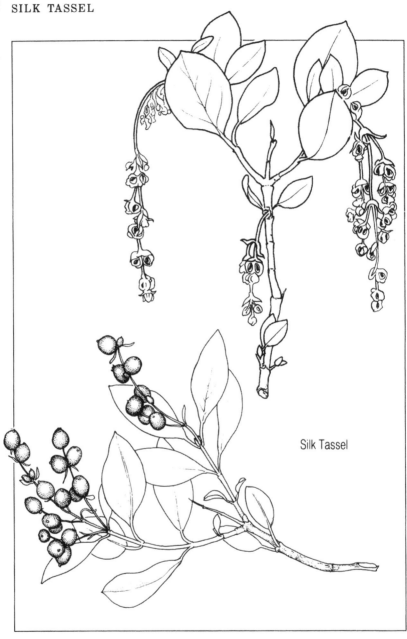

Silk Tassel

G. flavescens, var. *buxifolia*), with smaller leaves and a bushier growth, occurs in similar dry mountains from Curry and Josephine counties in Oregon, south to Mendocino County in California. *Garrya fremontii* grows up past the Columbia River into southwestern Washington; from Eugene, Oregon, south through the north coastal range to Monterey County in California; from Modoc County, California, south along the Sierra Nevada and disjunct into Orange, Riverside, and San Diego counties; and to Baja California along the inner coastal mountains—in all areas on dry hillsides and mountains above 2,500 feet. *Garrya veatchii* is another species, found along the central coastal range from Santa Cruz south to Ventura County; and east to the central Sierra Nevada. Frankly, I can't tell most of these plants apart a lot of the time, and I suggest that you not worry as well, since they all have similar chemistry, appearance, and use. Silk Tassel is Silk Tassel.

CONSTITUENTS Garryine, garryfoline, veatchine, delphinine, cuauchichicine, and two unnamed diterpene alkaloids.

COLLECTING Although the bark and root can be used (they are more potent, and perhaps riskier), I find the leaves of summer (poetic?) to be the best. Gather the leaves after they bloom and before the berries are ripe, or by late August. They may be pickable at other times, but the evergreen leaves can be distinctly weaker after they have aged, and I like the newer, fresher leaves on younger branches; these are strongest from mid-spring through late summer. The leaves can be dried loosely in a paper bag or Method B.

STABILITY The dried leaves will stay strong for at least two years, if kept whole.

PREPARATION Fresh Leaf Tincture, 1:2, Dry Leaf Tincture, 1:5, 50% alcohol, 60 to 90 drops of either, up to five times a day. Sometimes you will need to take a couple of doses an hour apart to initiate the antispasmodic effect, and then take a smaller dose every four hours afterwards. A Cold Infusion, 2 to 3 fluid ounces at a time, can be taken similarly, although the intensely bitter taste of the tea may be repulsive; the tincture, although every bit as disgusting, can be swallowed quickly, followed by some pleasant mineral water as a chaser. If you don't mind the bitter taste, all constituents are relatively water soluble, the leaves are quite stable, and the tea works fine. Just be aware that Silk Tassel is an overt crude drug, not a tonic or strengthener like so many of our herbs; it should be taken as you would aspirin, with awareness of frequency and dose.

MEDICINAL USES Our Silk Tassels are strong and reliable smooth-muscle relaxers, of the type generally classed as parasympathetic inhibitors or anticholinergics. In proper amounts they will have little sedative effect on the central nervous system, but they slow down and moderately suppress the vagus nerve, the myenteric plexus, and the sacral ganglia of the parasympathetic nerves. What this means is that they are useful pain relievers and antispasmodic for the cramps or tenesmus from diarrhea, dysentery, gallbladder pain, urethral or bladder cramps, and menstrual cramps. The Mohave and Kawaiisu Indians use it for stomach cramps and diarrhea, and it can work near miracles for bad cramps from gas or flatus, of both the upwards and downwards type. I have also seen it be effective for the disquieting distress from hiatus hernia gas pain. Although gallbladder spasms from stones are symptoms of a potentially dangerous condition, for many people they come and go for years; Silk Tassel can aid gallbladder flare-ups. Consider this scenario: it's 3:00 A.M. after Thanksgiving dinner, which consisted of lots of dressing, gravy with lipid bubbles not quite congealed, candied and buttered yams with marshmallows, cornbread with butter, plum pudding with hard sauce, and several glasses of somebody's pet wine from Napa Valley, then some pumpkin pie with a delicious Crisco crust; three hours later, at 11:00 P.M., you eat some mincemeat pie and later after you've gone to bed you have dull, sulphur-green pains in your belly that just awoke you. Stand up, walk around, try to burp, and take some Silk Tassel for your gallbladder that cries out in distress, in mortal need of some more bile acids. A more prosaic scenario: you gobble up a can of cashews in munchies frenzy and get similar gallbladder and common duct cramps.

I have known a number of women who have found Silk Tassel to be excellent for *bad* cramps, especially with accompanying colon pain. I can vouch for its usefulness in passing kidney stones, along with Hydrangea, Gravel Root *(Eupatorium purpureum)*, and hot baths. Silk Tassel lessened the cramps with a sure hand.

Silk Tassel has several advantages over the classic anticholinergic medicines of the atropine or Belladonna type because it has little secretory suppression, won't cause the dry mouth and constipation syndrome, and won't make you feel weird and disjunct.

CONTRAINDICATIONS Prescription and over-the-counter drugs should be avoided when using Silk Tassel, and it is not appropriate for younger children or use during pregnancy. If you start to get cold-clammy and a little short of breath, you have taken *far* too much. Take a break, watch CNN for a couple hours, and get restimulated.

Spearmint

Mentha spicata   (Labiatae)
OTHER NAMES   *Yerba Buena; Mentha viridis*

APPEARANCE Spearmint propagates by rootstalk, forming extended colonies of upright, 2- to 4-foot-high, bright green aerial parts. Like other Mints, it has a square stem, opposite leaves, and strong scent, but the foliage is a bit lighter green, and the plants tend to be a little hairy. The flowers bloom in late summer, forming long, pyramidal spikes from several to many branches; they are terminal and lavender-pink in color. The

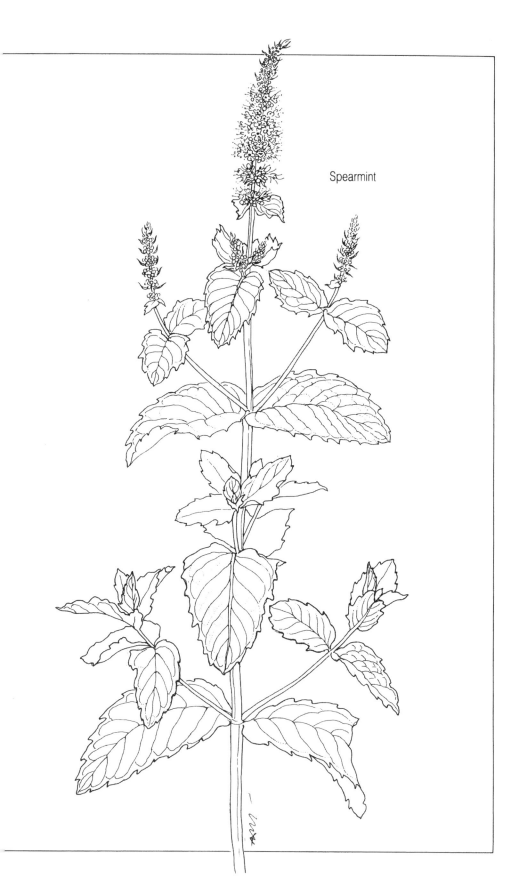

Spearmint

leaves have almost no petiole and in open areas may be 3 or 4 inches long towards the base of the stem, although 1 to 2 inches is normal. Spearmint branches more than Peppermint and less than Bergamot Mint; and the side branches, emerging at 45-degree angles in pairs from the main stem, have subtending leaves.

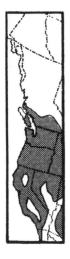

HABITAT Spearmint grows in streams, ditches, and along riversides throughout the West and can be found from San Diego County to British Columbia. The scent of different stands varies greatly; some, growing in warm, sunny localities, smell like cat piss. The choicest plants grow in cool, shady areas and have to be plucked out from between thickets. The best places to look are where streams make turns; if the stream turns to the right, check the banks on the left, and vice versa.

CONSTITUENTS Volatile oils, composed primarily of carvone, with l-limonene and pinene, are the active components.

COLLECTING Gather aboveground parts when the plant is beginning to bloom or is in full bloom. Plants around the edges of stands with insect holes and discolorations often have inferior oils, so go for the main section of the stand. Bundle and dry, Method A. Strip the leaves, flowering tops, and small stems, discard the main stems. Unlike other Mints, the taste of Spearmint stems is inferior. Store whole in an airtight container; crush the leaves when making tea.

STABILITY If stored properly, the herb can remain pleasantly aromatic for up to two years, although with diminished strength.

PREPARATION A simple tea can be used as much or as often as needed. A tincture can be made from the recently dried, best-you-can-pick herb for flavoring, using the method outlined under Peppermint.

MEDICINAL USES Although not as strong as Peppermint, Spearmint, with its lovely, pleasant taste, can be used for almost any stomach or digestive problem. It does not have the anesthetic strength of Peppermint, but it also does not have the stimulation of the latter. Its lack of circulatory stimulation makes it preferable for nausea and indigestion from a sick headache or migraine, and also for acid indigestion from a nervous stomach.

A pot or two of the tea is very helpful for irritative urination with acidity and high specific-gravity urine; after overindulgence in meat, fats, spices, and alcohol; for adrenalin stress; or following the use of anabolic steroids, cocaine, or amphetamines. Drink the tea cool or cold.

OTHER USES Try adding a shot of the tincture to lemonade, fruit punch, carrot juice, or apple cider. Add a little to applesauce served with lamb dishes; cranberry or raspberry preserves; stout or too yeasty homemade beer; or mix with a little yogurt for fruit salads.

Stream Orchid

Epipactis gigantea   (Orchidaceae)

OTHER NAMES   Helleborine, Giant Helleborine; *Helleborine gigantea*

APPEARANCE Stream Orchid grows in stands, generally 2 or 3 feet high, although around the edges of a preferred habitat there may be plants only a foot high. In shady, warm creeks they may reach 4 or 5 feet, but this is unusual. The orchid flowers bloom in mid-spring, in leafy terminal and lateral clusters, usually six to eight in number. They have three right-angled sepals, two upper petals (all five similarly marked), and an extended, heart-shaped lower lip. The whole flower is yellowish green, with orange and red stripes on the lip and similarly colored (or drab) sepals and upper petals. In some areas the flowers are rather bright and colorful, but they are often more a light green with just a little lip pigment. They may be an inch long but are usually smaller. They form ½- to 1-inch-long seed capsules that hang down like little footballs from the stems and are usually gone by late summer. The leaves are furled and stem-clasping, from 3 to 5 inches long, and marked by strong parallel veins, broad at the base and lanceolate towards the top. The stems are singular, unbranching, and rubbery-succulent; they may have from three to seven leaves by maturity in summer, and they rise from creeping, often connected root stalks that are fleshy and light grey-brown, with a peculiar yeasty scent.

HABITAT Stream Orchid is found sporadically but abundantly from Baja California to British Columbia, and eastwards to the Rocky Mountains in the north, and New Mexico and Texas in the south. It likes low springs in desert areas and slow-moving rivers and shaded tributaries along middle and upper mountains. Unlike other Orchids, it doesn't need special root environments, fungi symbiosis, or the obscure pollination strategies that make the family so delicate in the world we are creating with logging, pollution, and insecticides. It is found with some difficulty, but is widespread, especially along the coast and the dwindling riparian areas of southern California and Arizona. The roots can be transplanted in the fall, and the seeds have a fairly high germination rate (for an Orchid) if you want to spread it in moist banks nearer to where you live. I have gathered it in such diverse localities as a city park in Seattle, the Rogue River Wilderness Area in Oregon, the eastern slopes of the Sierra Nevada, near a spring in the Santa Monica Mountains, and east of Death Valley in Nevada. Good luck.

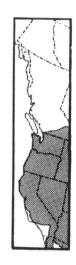

CONSTITUENTS A volatile oil and resins that are known to contain alpha spinasterol, stigmasterol, campesterol, b-sitosterol, as well as some bitter glycosides.

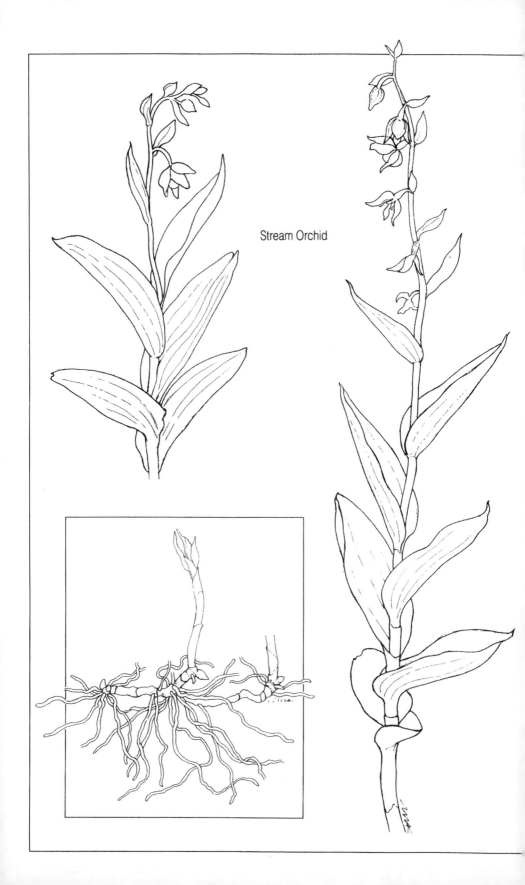

Stream Orchid

COLLECTING Gather the roots in the fall after the seed capsules have emptied and dropped and the clasping leaves are starting to get a yellowish tinge. I have found that (at least in extended stands along streams) pulling up small root masses intermittently, upstream to downstream, leaves most of the plants intact and able to fill in the spaces the next year. Snip off the stems, wash, and either tincture fresh or dry whole, Method B.

STABILITY Whole roots will stay strong for up to two years or as long as the characteristic smell is present.

PREPARATION Fresh Root Tincture, 1:2, Dry Root Tincture, 1:5, 60% alcohol, 30 to 60 drops, up to four times a day. The dried root is not water soluble, so grind up as needed, and take 2 to 4 #00 capsules, up to four times a day. If you plan to encapsulate a large amount, refrigerate or freeze them for storage.

MEDICINAL USES Stream Orchid has the same effects, although feebler, as the scarce and protected Lady Slipper Orchid (*Cypripedium* spp.). Although Lady Slipper Orchid is still relatively abundant in a few areas of the north country, it is disappearing permanently from vast areas where it used to grow. Our plant is abundant, successful, and nonspecialized; and judicious harvesting, coupled with some seeding or transplanting, will keep it that way.

Stream Orchid is a mood-elevating antispasmodic and sedative for those with a cold nature and generally deficient constitution. It is especially useful for menstrual cramps and hypersensitivity to pain that prevents sleep. If you have a lot of PMS distress, with cold hands and feet, a clammy, sweaty brow, and nameless unspeakable dreads suitable only for one of Poe's lesser poems (" . . . lest I be buried alive amongst the miasma of the spirit . . . ," etc.) or a Sylvia Plath dread-alike contest, try a few doses of this friendly plant. I have seen it help depression resulting from cocaine burnout; it can also aid people with a lot of emotional stress, in whom every little ache and pain is magnified and whose tolerance for noises, smells, and bright light is virtually nonexistent. If you have sprained your knee (or whatever), and you can't get to sleep, try Stream Orchid. It is mild but eventually useful for depression or hysteria, with respiratory and vascular guarding, yawning, and ghost pains in the belly, pelvis, or limbs.

CONTRAINDICATIONS It is not particularly recommended for those with strong, emphatic, and neck-bulgy states; and it is not advisable to combine it with depressant drugs or alcohol. It also probably should not be used during pregnancy.

Sweet Root

Osmorhiza occidentalis   (Umbelliferae)

OTHER NAMES   Western Sweet Cicely, Mountain Sweet Cicely; *O. ambigua, Washingtonia occidentalis*

APPEARANCE   Sweet Root is a mountain plant, usually forming dispersed stands of mixed young and older plants. Older plants may have dozens of stems reaching 3 or 4 feet in height; younger plants may only have two or three stems, 2 or 3 feet in height, and more basal leaf growth. The stems are sparsely leaved, at least compared to some other large umbels, and have small trifoliates emerging from stem sheaths in the spring blooming stages, spreading out by late summer to extended, long-petioled bipinnate or ternate-pinnate leaves, finely serrated, strongly licorice-scented, and spicy-tasting. The spring umbels are pale yellow or yellowish green. By summer they have matured into long, angular, thin, dark seeds that taste like anise candy. Of all the *Osmorhizas* or Sweet Cicelys that grow in North America, this is the only one I know of that does not have barbed or clinging seeds. If the plant you have in front of you has very little scent and clinging seeds, it is probably *O. chilensis* or Western Sweet Cicely. This is a nice, widespread plant that leaves your clothes covered in little skinny, hairy seeds, but it ain't Sweet Root. Besides, the stems of Sweet Root are thick and fairly upright, whereas Western Sweet Cicely has thin and spreading stems. Close, but no cigar . . . and no taste.

The root reflects the foliage: older plants with many stems have larger (and more aromatic) roots. The roots are dark brown-grey externally and cream-colored internally, sometimes forming one single mass of tapering roots, other times forming extended lateral rhizome growth, with many descending roots that tightly bind dirt and gravel into a big, happy mess. As soon as you uncover the roots, whatever their size, there is no doubt that you have the right plant. They have a strong scent of Sassafras or root beer, with a sweet, spicy flavor that leaves a tingling aftertaste.

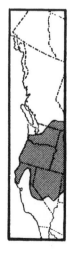

HABITAT   Sweet Root is found in nearly all the mountains of the Pacific West. In California it is found on wooded slopes above 3,000 feet in the Sierra Nevada and sporadically along the upper edges of the north coastal range as far south as Mendocino County. In Oregon, Washington, and British Columbia, it favors the higher, cleaner forest areas, and it is most common in the older forests of Alberta, Idaho, Montana, Utah, Wyoming, Nevada, and Colorado. In the northern and eastern parts of its range, it is often found with *Lomatium dissectum* and Balsam Root. Look for Sweet Root along the lower slopes of mountain creeks and along switchbacks and shady higher slopes close to logging roads.

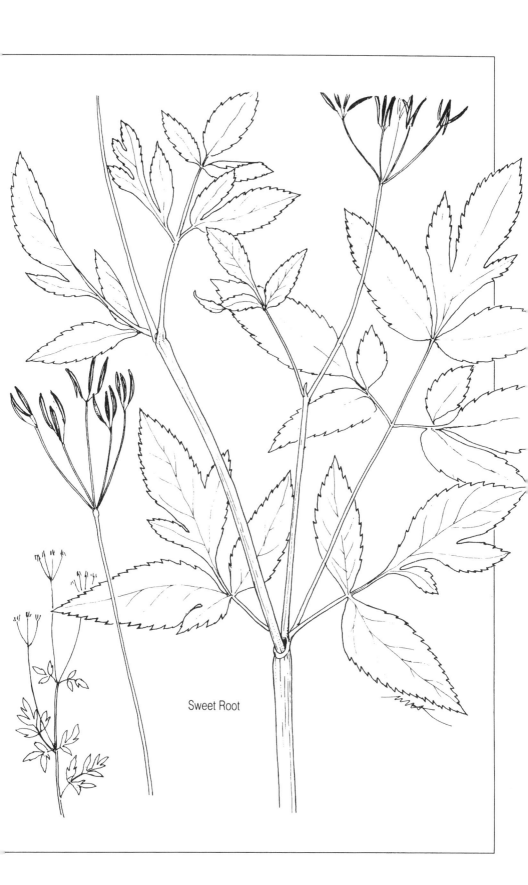

Sweet Root

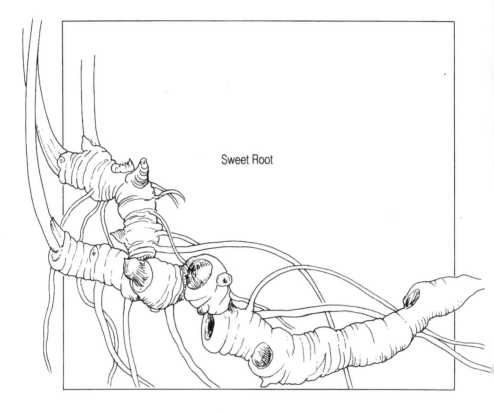

Sweet Root

CONSTITUENTS Although little is known about this species, its volatile oils contain anethole and other phenylalanine-derived phenolic ethers, as well as the important antifungal falcarindiol and (probably) 3-O-methyl-falcarindiol.

COLLECTING The root should be gathered from late summer to mid-fall. The root seems to be stable and strong all year long, but gathering from late summer on allows for the plant to set seed first. The leaves are best collected from late spring to late summer. To clean large root masses, snip them into smaller sections, shake out the dirt and gravel, and wash well in running water, which can usually be found nearby.

STABILITY Whole dried roots are stable for at least a couple of years, although the scent softens with age. The leaves are strong for six months but still have a pleasant flavor for at least a year if kept whole.

PREPARATION Fresh Root Tincture, 1:2; Dry Root Tincture, 1:5, 65% alcohol. The root tinctures may be used topically as needed, or used internally, 45 to 60 drops in warm water, up to three times a day. For tea, prepare the dried root as a Strong Decoction and use 2 to 3 fluid ounces, up to three times a day. The roots can be added to other roots or barks for tea; the leaves can be added to other herbs also for tea; both improve the flavor, apart from any intended therapeutic effects. The crushed leaves can be added to salad dressings and marinades to contribute their fennel-tarragon flavor. Those of you out there who brew your own goodies should seriously consider using the roots, leaves, or seeds in making beer, mead, or root beer; and Sweet Root would certainly improve the taste of such potentially insipid wines as Dandelion, Mountain Ash, and Service Berry. The antifungal effects of the root may limit the alcohol content a bit, but the taste should make up for the lack of giggle-juice.

MEDICINAL USES The tincture can be diluted with 2 or 3 parts of water and applied freely to tineas and other fungal conditions; and the tincture or root tea is definitely helpful for upper-intestinal candidiasis or lingering sulphurous burps from bad food or a low-level stomach infection. The warm decoction has been useful as a douche for vaginal yeast infections and as an enema for candidiasis suprainfections of the descending colon. This seems especially effective when the infections have followed antibiotic or immunosuppressant anti-inflammatory therapy; it is less helpful in chronic immunodepression or when the infection is well established and regularly aggravated by sugar binging.

A tea made up of 2 parts Sarsaparilla (*Aralia nudicaulis* or *Smilax* species), 1 part Licorice Root, and 1 part Sweet Root can be very useful in modifying blood sugar imbalances, even when they border on adult onset, insulin-resistant diabetes. Further, in the adrenalin-dominant, stress-addicted ectomorph, with gum problems, dry skin, and chronic dry feces, a couple of cups a day of the tea will act as a surprisingly effective laxative and stool softener. Clarissa Smith, the Wyoming herbalist, recommends chewing a few seeds as a stimulus to the defecation reflex. This would probably be very useful for those who have stopped smoking or drinking coffee and have gotten *very* cranky and constipated.

Trillium

Trillium ovatum   (Liliaceae)
OTHER NAMES   Wake Robin

APPEARANCE Trillium is an easy plant to identify, with its single, succulent stalk and its three oval leaves. In spring it bears a large three-petaled flower, white at first, then turning pink as it matures. This is not important to us as herbalists, since we just look, don't pick, until late summer and fall. The flower forms a fleshy, yellow, three-sided capsule in early summer, filled with tiny seeds. The root/bulb is several inches to a foot below the ground and is tan to white, with many descending rootlets.

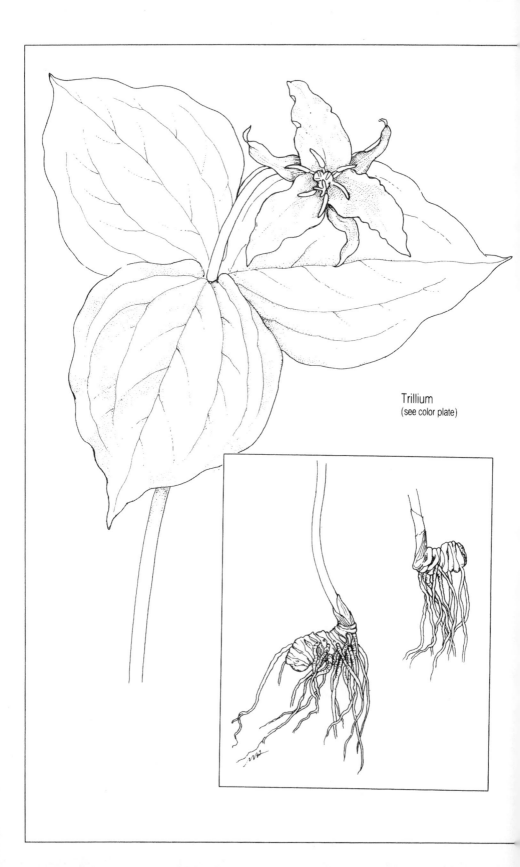

Trillium
(see color plate)

HABITAT Trillium is widely distributed in moist old-growth forests, from the coastal Redwoods in California; north along the coast to British Columbia; on both sides of the Cascades in Oregon and Washington; across the northern half of Idaho; into mountainous Alberta and Montana; and down into Wyoming. Find a creek starting in the forest, follow it down through the trees to where it begins to broaden out, and you will usually find some Trillium. Logging, people, and pollution have decreased the number of plants, especially in California. I used to find them in abundance in the Santa Cruz Mountains . . . no more. I would recommend the Northwest for gathering your Trillium.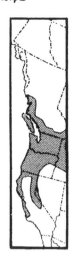

CONSTITUENTS Saponins, especially trillarin and diosgenin; fixed and volatile oils; tannins; trilline.

COLLECTING Gather the green leaves, stems, and roots in August and September, after blooming, seeding, and just before the leaves begin to change color. Frankly, I have moderate distress gathering too many of these plants, even in areas where they are abundant, so I compromise by collecting a few dozen whole plants and top off the tincture with just foliage and stems of some more plants, leaving the roots of these for the next year. If you gather leaves when they are in bloom or in early summer, you will deprive the plants of their annual reproduction and deny the bulbs adequate photosynthesis, which may kill them. If you time it right and wait until they are just about to turn yellow, the roots will have plumped up for the winter, the foliage will still have full potency as a medicine, and everyone will be happy. The roots are stronger, and doses are based on at least half of the volume of tincture containing the whole plant, but if you only wish to gather the leaves and stems for moral reasons, then double the recommended dosage. The dry roots are the form normally encountered in commerce, but they are much feebler than fresh ones and are little more than an astringent agent, similar to Geranium Root. Fresh roots dry to a fifth of their fresh weight and lose most of their specific effects; and gathering them is wasteful of the plant.

STABILITY Trillium lasts for years in the form of the tincture.

PREPARATION Fresh Whole Plant Tincture, 1:2, 15 to 30 drops, up to four times a day.

MEDICINAL USES First and foremost, Trillium is for uterine bleeding. But large doses (over 30 drops) may, in fact, aggravate the problem; I have found that 20 drops is the best average dose within this therapeutic window. It works remarkably well for fibroid (myomas and fibromyomas) bleeding, combined with 30 drops of Shepherd's Purse. In some cases, by decreasing the endometrial bleeding, the fibroids may even stabilize and become quiescent. For mid-cycle spotting, especially during ovulation, use the same approach, taking the Trillium and Shepherd's Purse doses for at least a couple of days. For heavy, sustained periods and following a D & C, the Trillium alone may be adequate; and for home birthing, with a history of heavy menses or previous birthing hemorrhage, use the Trillium with some Cotton Root bark tincture during the placental stage. In the postpartum period, if the lochia has started to turn red after being relatively clear, use Trillium.

For males with benign prostatic hypertrophy who are going through an acute episode, with inflammation and pain on urination, Trillium is effective along with Bidens or White Sage tea. For hematuria from urethral or bladder irritation (and not from kidney cause), even from kidney stones or gravel, use Trillium and Bidens for several days, followed by several days of Mallow tea.

Trillium is sometimes helpful for nosebleeds caused by dryness and airborne particles, and will predictably stop bleeding from hemorrhoids, piles, and diverticula, although the effect is mainly palliative and something else needs to be done to promote healing.

Uva Ursi

Arctostaphylos uva-ursi, A. nevadensis   (Ericaceae)
OTHER NAMES   Bearberry, Kinnikinnick, Pinemat Manzanita; *Coralillo*

APPEARANCE   Uva Ursi grows as a vine mat, along open areas and down slopes, with many small, shiny-leathery, spoon-shaped leaves along shredding, reddish-barked stems. The stems cross-root in the center of the plants, but around the edges, long runners may extend off downhill. In the spring the flowers are small, pinkish urns and mature into sporadic red berries; the flowers and berries look just like those of larger relatives (Manzanita), and the uses are the same. *Arctostaphylos nevadensis* is such a low-growing bush (also called Pinemat Manzanita) that, except for its more pointed leaves and larger stems, it is sometimes difficult to tell it apart from the more common *A. uva-ursi*. Its leaves are longer than Uva Ursi, but the latter plant, particularly in the northern coastal areas, has a number of forms that start to resemble *A. nevadensis*. I lump them together and gather them together. Up in British Columbia, Alberta, and Alaska, *A. alpina* (or *A. rubra*) is found in circumstances similar to that of circumboreal *A. uva-ursi*, which has less smooth and slightly toothed leaves, and little of the spoon-curl of the main plant; but I have been told that the only problem with its use is in the gathering of enough of it rather than its value. I grew up in California, and I tend to think of all these creeping plants as low Manzanitas. Folks from the East and North have told me they tend to think of Manzanita as a giant Uva Ursi.

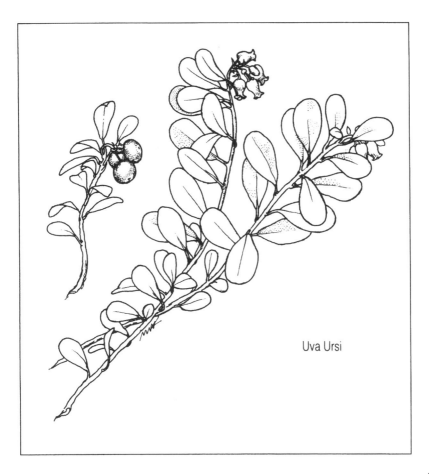

Uva Ursi

HABITAT *A. nevadensis* is found on dry slopes and mountains of the Sierra Nevada, the Panamints, and over into the high mountains of Nevada, growing from 5,000 to 10,000 feet; it then reappears in the coastal ranges of Oregon and Washington, usually at lower altitudes. The main plant, *A. uva-ursi,* is found from sea level to 11,000 feet, growing in the open on hillocks, in the mountains, on the dry sides of canyons, and in logged and burned forests—almost anywhere with somewhat acidic soil and sun.

CONSTITUENTS Uva Ursi is mainly arbutin and tannin, and most of its function can be reduced to those substances.

COLLECTING The easiest way to gather these plants is to find the long runners coming off of the matlike center, pull them up to the major central roots, and snip. They may be stuffed loosely in bags or bundled and dried Method A. *A. nevadensis* and *A. alpina* tend to form short, stubby stems with closely clustered leaves; and you usually aren't lucky enough

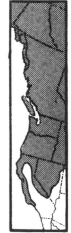

to find runners. These short stems should be dried loosely in bags. Trying to band and hang them is an extremely painstaking ritual. After drying, take the time to garble out the stems and dead leaves, and, if it is *A. uva-ursi,* the dead grass, feathers, and flotsam that come with the trailers. If you are going to collect the primary species, gather it from spring to late fall. *A. alpina* or *A. rubra* have thinner leaves and tend to wither and crinkle in off-season; gather these during the growing season.

STABILITY *A. uva-ursi* and *A. nevadensis* are good whole for three or four years; the structurally more delicate *A. alpina* and *A. rubra* are only good for up to two years at the most.

PREPARATION Dry Herb Tincture, 1:5, 50% alcohol, 30 to 60 drops in 8 ounces of warm water, up to four times a day; Standard Infusion, 3 to 4 fluid ounces, up to four times a day. For a sitz bath, the Standard Infusion, 8 to 12 fluid ounces in warm water, up to twice a day.

MEDICINAL USES The tea or tincture has one distinct and appropriate use—for cystitis and urethritis that occur after food or alcohol binging, with resultant alkaline urine. With a relatively stable diet and lifestyle, the number of hydrogen ions consumed (acids), minus the amount needed to digest proteins and butterfats in the stomach (normal alkaline-acid metabolism of the body being stable), leave enough hydrogen ions remaining to keep the urine slightly acid (6 to 6.5 pH) and antimicrobial against the normally present intestinal flora. With carbohydrate binging, and a short-term decrease in dietary proteins and therefore a decrease in the main food source of acids, the stomach will secrete its normal acids, and there will be a short-term deficit of hydrogen ions in the urine. Alkaline urine (above 7 pH) is more likely to allow coliform bacterial growth in the urethra and irritated mucosa resulting in pain on urination. The glycosides in Uva Ursi, especially arbutin, are metabolized and excreted in the urine as hydroquinone, an antimicrobial waste product that is most active in an alkaline pH. So: you drink several cups of the tea or take the tincture in water for a couple of days, drink a little cranberry juice (acidifying to the urine and also antimicrobial), and it should back off the infection and get things back to normal. If it doesn't help enough, change your approach.

Uva Ursi is so high in tannins that using the herb regularly for more than a couple or three days will start to irritate the stomach lining and even the kidneys. Shift to Yerba Mansa and Mallow tea or some Bidens and Redwood—even Yerba Santa will sometimes help the bladder infection that doesn't respond to Uva Ursi or its therapeutic and botanical relatives, Madrone and Manzanita. If the painful urination is getting better but the tannins are a problem, you can change to Blueberry or Pipsissewa, two relatives with similar but weaker effects and with little astringency.

The sitz bath is remarkably effective for birth recuperation, but I have been told by midwives that it is best to wait twenty-four hours after birthing to start the bath. It also helps alleviate hot, irritative inflammation in bacterial vaginosis, yeast infections, and vulvitis, as well as the acute pain in the initial outbreaks of genital herpes and venereal warts (either sex will be helped). The boiled tea is excellent as a wash for abrasions, infections, contusions, and burns. The astringency is high, shrinking, and cooling, and the other constituents are rather antiseptic for the broken skin. After a few washings or applications, the skin will be dry and tight and probably need a little salve, skin dressing, or oiling.

CONTRAINDICATIONS You shouldn't use the herb internally for more than about four days. It is astringent to the mucosa, and, especially in the last trimester of pregnancy, can decrease placenta-uterine membrane permeability; it is probably not a good idea to use Uva Ursi during pregnancy.

OTHER USES The dried, crushed leaves can be added to herbal smoking mixtures. They taste best if you brown them lightly in a frying pan before adding them to the blend.

Valerian

Valeriana dioica, *V. sitchensis*, *V. capitata*   (Valerianaceae)
OTHER NAMES   *V. sylvatica*, *V. californica*, *V. acutiloba*, etc.

APPEARANCE Valerians have similar appearances. They all form upright stems from 1 to 3 feet in height with one or two (or more) sets of opposite leaves along the stem, each group well separated from the next. The plants are root-perennial, and the aboveground growth is green, succulent, and new each year. The stems are for flowering and bear umbels of flowers that resemble those of both the Carrot and Mustard family. After flowering, the stem deteriorates, and basal leaves continue photosynthesis. In dry years, or in young individuals, there may be no flowering at all. This makes it very hard to identify Valerians. The roots are stout, succulent, usually yellow-brown in color, and have many transluscent rootlets descending below the main rhizome-root. Basal leaves may be whole but are usually dissected or irratically lobed, with the same plant bearing several variations.

 Valeriana dioica, a circumboreal plant, bears one or two pairs of bluntly divided leaves on a 12- to 18-inch flowering stem. The flowers are small and numerous, and form a rounded light pink umbel at the terminus. Several plants, some blooming, some sterile, may be attached to the same creeping root, with the various basal leaves being whole, lobed, or blunt-pinnate. The terminal leaflet of basal or cauline (stem) leaves is usually much larger than the lateral paired leaflets. The root has the usual perfumed, dirty tennis shoe smell of Valerian. *Valerian dioica* is also called *V. sylvatica* by some authors.

Valeriana sitchensis, or Sitka Valerian, is a delicate plant, often found in small but dense colonies. The warmer lowland variety, sometimes called var. *Scouleri*, sometimes *V. Scouleri*, has well-developed basal leaves and longer rhizomes, with smaller, more transitory flowering stems. The basal leaves have large terminal leaflets and much smaller lateral leaflets, often only one or two pairs, sometimes only the terminal leaflet (now called a leaf), and often long petioles. The stem leaves are also dominated by the terminal leaflet, and there may be only one or two pairs. The flowers are white to pink, and the umbel may expand laterally as the flowers mature. The stem dies, and the basal leaves persist; it has the same smelly root as other varieties. *V. sitchensis* intergrades with the variety, but in its pure, high mountain form it is a taller and more robust plant, with few persisting basal leaves and most of the foliage paired along the stem. With a shorter growing season than the lower variety, there is less emphasis on sterile basal leaf growth, and the sturdy 2- or 3-foot flowering stems are the main plant, often with five or six pairs of cauline leaves (usually larger than the basal leaves) bluntly and toothedly pinnate, with the terminal three leaflets being largest. There may be several flowering stems from the same root, and the root has less lateral rhizomatous growth, forming more of a fibrous semisucculent root mass.

Valeriana capitata is also called *V. acutiloba*, which is also called *V. capitata* ssp. *acutiloba*, or *V. capitata* ssp. *californica*, which is also called *V. californica* or *V. sylvatica* ssp. *glabra*. If you think that is bad, the same basic species is cross-divided into many more in the Rocky Mountains, Arizona, and Utah. This is our plant: it has many basal leaves, often forming a rosette, each leaf having a single large leaflet with one or more pairs of pinnate leaves. The big leaflet is the dominant one, and you may have to shuffle through the rosette to find any rudimentary pinnate leaflets. The persistent basal leaves will bear one or more succulent and ephemeral flowering stems, 1 or 2 feet high, with light pink, Mustardlike, umbelled terminal flowers that are rather distant from the small cauline leaves. After blooming in the spring, what is visible of the plants is their bright green basal rosettes; the dead flower stems are little more than a straw-colored twig. The basal and cauline leaves may be rounded or sharply pointed, the leaves may be smooth and glabrous or slightly downy, the stems may be 6 inches tall or 2 feet—it matters not. All these plants are variations of the same species, *V. capitata*. If I were talking about the Rocky Mountains, I would probably call the varieties *V. acutiloba*, only because that is the most widely used name in that area.

Valeriana occidentalis is a large plant, somewhat resembling a leafier version of *V. sitchensis*, with several 3-foot stalks from a single root mass,

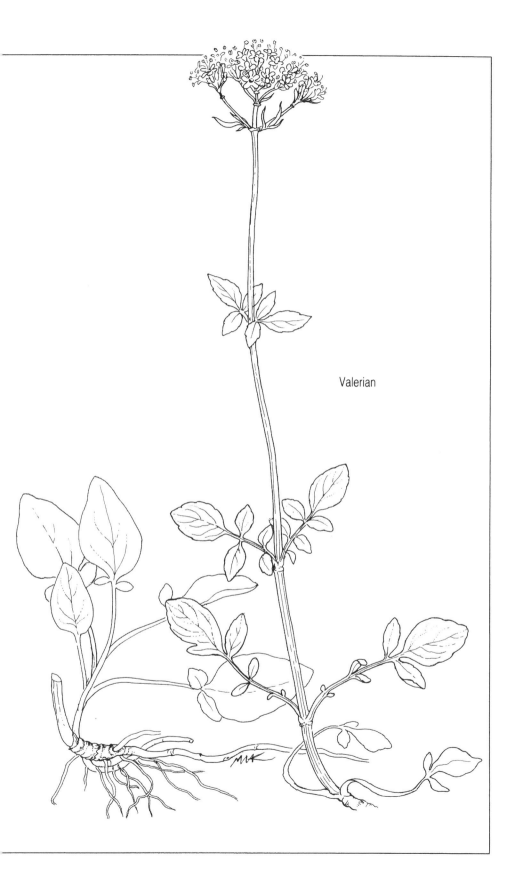

Valerian

and with pointed, linear pinnate leaves. *V. edulis,* or Tobacco Root, is another type, with many lanceolate and semipinnate basal leaves, bearing tall, thin-stemmed, wandlike flower stalks and many tiny flowered umbels, dispersed on the tips of an open, diaphanous panicle of opposite flowering stems. The basal leaves may stand upright from the atypical deeply buried, light brown tuber with yellow flesh. Both of these, although widespread, are inferior medicines. If you wish to use the roots of these two plants, the constituents are similar to the other varieties, just present in diminished amounts. Use twice the dosage.

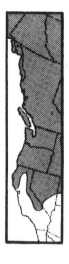

HABITAT *V. dioica* is found in wet mountain meadows where it gets really cold. That means the Cascades and Olympic Peninsula of Washington; the mountains of Idaho, northwest Montana, Alberta, British Columbia, and Alaska. The further north, the lower the altitude at which you'll find *V. dioica. V. sitchensis* is fond of moist forest clearings and shaded slopes, usually in the higher mountains, but not above timberline. It grows at the top of the coast range—Klamath crest in northern California; all up the Cascades in Oregon and Washington, on both sides; east to Idaho; and north to west-central Alaska. The variety *Scouleri* is found in California from Mendocino County northwards into coastal Oregon and lower altitudes of the Cascades in Washington and Oregon, but only the western slopes and riverside forest (what's left of it). It grows into southwestern British Columbia as well as northwestern Washington. *V. capitata* likes rich, shaded slopes towards the bottom of watersheds, where the canyons are moist but the wind coming up the valley is warm. It is found above the mouths of canyons in the Sierra Nevada from Tulare County northwards and across the Klamath Mountains to almost the coast in California; along the eastern slopes up through the Cascades; into the intermountain ranges in Nevada, Idaho, and Utah; and all along the mountains that ring (and form) the Great Basin. As *V. capitata,* var. *bracteosa,* Valerian is found through Alaska and much of British Columbia and western Alberta. *V. occidentalis* follows along the mountains that ring the Great Basin as well, but at higher, colder, and rockier moist places, from Modoc County, California, along the intermountain ranges west of the Rockies into eastern Oregon and Idaho. *V. edulis* is a high meadow plant, often growing in clayish, compressed soil, from New Mexico and Arizona up the Rockies through Montana; across Idaho into Alberta and British Columbia; south into the eastern Cascades of Washington and Oregon; and in the intermountain ranges of Nevada, Idaho, and Utah.

With all these Valerians to choose from, it is still hard to find them. They are widespread but erratic in distribution and can be infuriating to locate. They will be profuse in one valley or canyon and be missing from the next two . . . abundant on one slope for a half mile, disappear for two miles downstream, and reappear on the other side. Except for the peculiar Tobacco Root, all the varieties maintain great diversity in shape, height, and leaf structure. You need to look for the Valerian *stem* in the spring and early summer, and, with *V. capitata,* look for the Valerian rosette on shady slopes overlooking a creek.

CONSTITUENTS Isovaleric acid, valeric acid, valerine and chatinine alkaloids, and the distinctively scented volatile oil. Valepotriates and other compounds have been isolated in recent European studies, but the stuff above is mostly what Valerian is about.

COLLECTING Gather the roots in late summer through fall, and tincture fresh, or dry in flats. *V. capitata* has potent basal leaves, and you can include them in a fresh plant tincture along with the creeping roots. The tall variety of *V. sitchensis* needs to be picked when the leaves are starting to turn yellow and the plant is retreating back to the roots. The roots of all the Valerians are high in moisture, and you may expect to lose 80% to 90% of their fresh weight when dry.

STABILITY The dried root is strong for several years. I have seen ninety-year-old plant specimens pressed on herbarium sheets with partial root segments attached that still smelled faintly of dirty socks. Keep the roots in well-sealed jars, as the scent can be pernicious. Keep out of the reach of cats. One time I received a shipment of 10 pounds of Valerian roots, opened up the box to smell them after closing time at the store, gasped approvingly, reclosed it, and left. The next morning I returned, found the box pulled open, and a neighborhood cat in deep drugged slumber right in the middle of the roots. It took many minutes to arouse the animal, and its nervous system was completely scrambled for hours, as it stumbled, mewled, and drooled around the back of the store, a cartoon-furry junkie in extremis.

PREPARATION Fresh Root (or Whole Plant) Tincture, 1:2, ½ to 1 teaspoon in warm water as needed; Dry Root Tincture, 1:5, 70% alcohol, ¼ to ½ teaspoon as needed. Capsules, #00, 2 to 4, up to five times a day. Constant use of the dry root preparations can induce emotional agitation in some individuals.

MEDICINAL USES Valerian is a useful, safe, and reliable sedative and antispasmodic—for some people. It is most effective when you have been nervous, stressed, or become an adrenalin basket case, with muscular twitches, shaky hands, palpitations, and indigestion. You aren't hungry and you don't want a massage; you sit down or lie down, and jump up to do something five minutes later. You try to sleep, but go over in your mind all those zillion things that can go wrong: you didn't lock the door, left the light on in the garage, forgot to check on the kids, maybe left the terminal on at work, forgot to send off the check. You fix a cup of tea, lie down: did you turn off the burner? . . . And you wonder why your relationships go up in smoke?

Some people, on the other hand, find Valerian to be horrible, causing bad dreams and groggy awakenings with an emotional sock stuffed in the mouth. Here is why: Valerian is a stimulant to digestion, a stimulant to the lungs, and a stimulant to the cardiovascular output. If you are an adrenalin-stress person, with diminished intestinal tract function, have dilated and dry bronchial rings with shallow, guarded breathing and a rapid, thready adrenalin pulse, Valerian stimulates digestive functions, increases the depth and efficiency of respiration, slows and strengthens the pulse, and sedates the brain. It is a tonic sedative. It fits your metabolism. If, on the other hand, you are an adrenocortical-stress person, with a strong and demanding intestinal tract, good moist lungs, and the cardiovascular excess that accompanies moderate essential hypertension from increased blood volume and sodium retention, then Valerian will stimulate the functions that are already excessive, and leave you with both sedation and physical stimulation—not your herb.

Since this herb fits some people like a glove, there is the tendency to overuse it. The dried root preparations will, in time and with constant use, start to cause emotional shiftiness and lability. It is fine for occasional, even frequent, use but not for regular, daily doses. The fresh root has less of the stimulation and none of the accumulative effects, and, although weaker, is a reasonable sedative for more types of people. It is best to use the fresh root extract if you aren't sure, even if it is a bit less effective. If you like its calming effects, then the dry root, with its somewhat different chemistry, is probably going to be your sedative of choice.

Vanilla Leaf

Achlys triphylla   (Berberidaceae)
OTHER NAMES   Deer Foot; *Leontice triphylla*

APPEARANCE From spring to fall this plant sends up single fan-shaped leaves on sturdy little stems arising from masses of rhizomes. The leaf has three leaflets; the central one is bilateral, and the outside ones are irregularly formed. Colonies resemble little green umbrellas and may cover many square feet. The trifoliate leaves range in radius from 3 inches to more than a foot across, and the single wiry stem is short, from several inches to 1½ feet tall. In spring the roots send up the same type of stem, crowded with little white flowers on a spike that rises above the leaves. These form little rust-colored, curved seeds that fall off, after which the flower stem dies back and the leaves return to cheerfully making sugars for the root. The leaves die back in fall. Just imagine a chunky little shrub with all its branches buried horizontally in the ground, sending its leaves and flowers singly up into the air on skinny stems— Vanilla Leaf.

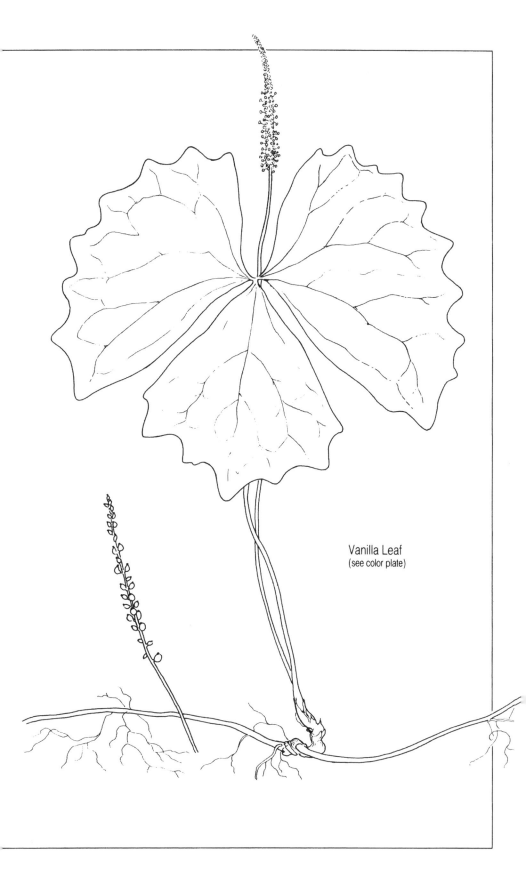

Vanilla Leaf
(see color plate)

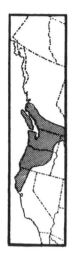

HABITAT Vanilla Leaf grows in shady, moist forests, from Mendocino County in California north in the coastal ranges to British Columbia; in the east Cascades to the ocean, down to central Oregon; and on the west side only from central Oregon to the California border. In the southern and drier areas, it is found near or by water; in rich, moist areas of the Northwest it can be found creeping around the edges of open meadows. It doesn't like logged forest too much (most of the Northwest), so look for it in shady sections of trees that are still standing.

CONSTITUENTS Coumarin, of course, which accounts for its vanilla scent. It is a member of the Barberry family, a group of plants rich in bioactive components, and the root has a strong, persistent taste; so Vanilla Leaf probably has a whole bunch of stuff, but I have been unable to find information about this plant or its single relative, *Achlys japonica* of northern Japan. Come on, Natural Products Chemistry Ph.D. candidates—strut yer stuff.

COLLECTING Snip off the stems at ground level and bundle the whole plant to dry, Method A. The leaves have no scent *until* they dry, so don't worry that you went and picked the wrong plant. If it is *dry* and there is no smell, you *did* pick the wrong plant. Bear in mind that a paper bag stuffed with alternating bundles of leaves dries down to zilch, maybe 10 parts to 1. When you get around to pulling the stems off, 2 pounds of green, fresh-bundled umbrellas will yield you a couple of ounces of dried leaves. Store the dried bundles in a plastic bag until you need some, then process the amount desired.

STABILITY When stored as above, it will last up to two years. If you process and garble immediately after drying, storing the leaves in a jar, they will stay aromatic for up to a year.

PREPARATION Nothing special, as it is not specifically a therapeutic agent.

MEDICINAL USES In recent years, coumarin has had much negative press, since it is the chemical base for several anticoagulant drugs and under some conditions can itself be absorbed into the bloodstream, although very poorly. In fact, a pinch of the herb added to tea gives it a very pleasant taste and fragrance. Early Oregon settlers used it freely as a vanilla substitute, crushing a little leaf into cake batter and cookie dough (with no known ill effect), and several native peoples in Washington used it as a tea to take away some of the pain from tubercular coughing.

CONTRAINDICATIONS It's probably best to avoid using Vanilla Leaf during pregnancy and with serious medication, especially anticoagulants.

OTHER USES The crushed leaf gives a lovely taste to pipe tobacco or rolling tobacco, and can be added to crude incense for burning or "smudging." Zubrovka nastoika (Polish sweet vodka) can be approximated very nicely by adding a handful of leaves to a fifth of regular stuff and steeping for at least a month. It gives a green color to the booze as well as a nice taste—perfect for a Russian-Irish person on St. Patrick's Day. You can make May wine with Vanilla Leaf instead of Woodruff, as well. Most of all, the bundles can be hung just for the pleasant scent, and the leaves can be used as a sachet, interleaved between layers of stored clothing or just tucked into your dresser.

Western Coltsfoot

Petasites palmatus (Compositae/Asteraceae)

OTHER NAMES Coltsfoot, Butterbur; *Petasites frigidus*, var. *palmatus*, *Tussilago palmatum*

APPEARANCE This chunky little plant starts off in March and April with flower stalks that grow to a foot tall, often the only thing blooming at that early season. The stalk is covered in green-purple clasping leaves, and the flowers form a white to purple rounded hood at the top. These flowers tend to be different sexes on different plants, but none of this is fixed. In fact, all of the five species of *Petasites* will gleefully hybridize; many of them form pure stands in large areas of the North, various forms occurring with bizarre irregularity hundreds of miles from similar populations.

Anyway, this isn't important to us, since the little leaves that start to erupt around the flower stalks are what we want—in two months. Long after the fertile parts have died back, large palm-shaped leaves cover the area; from ½ to 1½ feet across, they stand on succulent petioles from ½ to 1½ feet long. These rise directly from large colonies of lateral creeping roots, photosynthesizing for the rest of the growing season so the roots can grow and have the energy to flower next spring. The leaves are cheerful, bright green above, and densely fuzzy-light below. They look thick and robust but are really delicate and thin, with much of their thickness made up of the under-hairs; they are broad umbrellas for chlorophyll, and little else.

HABITAT There used to be a few stands in the mountains below Santa Cruz, California, nestled in rich, shady slopes. However, after the drought of the 1980s, I would not expect them to still be there; instead, look in similar localities along the coast, from Sonoma County northwards; across the Siskiyou Mountains; and up the Cascades through Oregon and Washington, usually at lower altitudes and mostly on the west side. *Petasites sagittatus* is exactly like *P. palmatus*, but with leaves that vary from saw-toothed-triangular to nearly the same palmate shape as the main

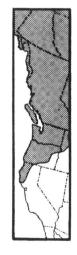

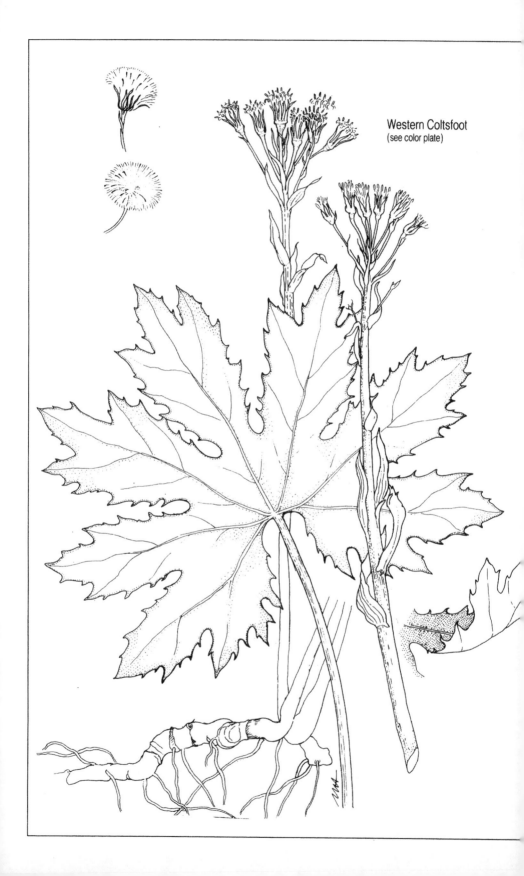

Western Coltsfoot
(see color plate)

species. *P. sagittatus* grows east of the Cascades in northeast Washington; over to western Montana; and up through Alberta. Both species and related hybrids (or is it the other way around?) grow up through British Columbia, the Yukon, and Alaska. In the lower forty-eight states, the plants hide in shady places between trees, in areas that have been clearcut, along roadside embankments, overlooking streams, and such.

Don't take that distribution thing too seriously, as I have found *P. palmatus* in northern Idaho and *P. sagittatus* in central Washington, on the west side of the Cascades (unless, of course, they were disjunct hybrids or something). All of the genus are found circumboreally, hybrid readily, and are sometimes lumped with the European Coltsfoot (*Tussilago farfara*); and the five *Petasites* species and the one *Tussilago* species have bandied back and forth. *Tussilago* is an escaped plant in the Northeast, but differs from the *Petasites* genus by having a Dandelionlike yellow flower and little of the antispasmodic effects of our genus. So, if you see *Tussilago* mentioned as a native plant, the source is wrong.

CONSTITUENTS The sesquiterpene petasin and related esters, saponins, and mucilage in the leaves; resins and volatile oils in the roots. The young leaves can contain a small amount of pyrrolizidine alkaloids, but these are nearly absent from mature leaves. The roots seem to be lacking these liver-damaging substances, and the small amounts found in the immature leaves (and perhaps the flowering stalks) are less toxic than they are in the *Senecio*-type alkaloids.

COLLECTING The leaves should be gathered from mid-June through late August, and the stems should be plucked at ground level. Form them into bundles, put rubber bands around them, and hang until dry. For the fresh plant tincture, you can use the whole leaf and stem without chopping; just weigh, stuff, and cover with alcohol. For storage, the dry herb can be crushed up without loss of strength. If you wish to use some for smoking, it is best to remove the stems and keep just the dried leaves, rubbing them down to a cigarette or pipe consistency. Make sure the leaf fragments are not too small, however; leaves that are reduced to a fuzzy wad make a very difficult draw. The roots are best gathered in the spring, cleaned of dirt and leaf scales, cut into small pieces, and dried. For use as a poultice the fresh root can be gathered whenever needed. Rinse the root if possible, lay it on a large, clean rock, and hammer it apart with a smaller rock.

STABILITY The fresh leaf tincture is stable for two or three years only, as it will take on an acrid scent and change chemistry after that. The crushed dried leaves are good for at least two years; the terpenes and mucilage constituents are quite stable. The root will last similarly.

PREPARATION A Standard Infusion, 2 to 4 fluid ounces sipped slowly, up to four times a day. You can also simply steep a wad of leaves as a regular cup of tea. The Fresh Herb Tincture, 1:2, 30 to 60 drops in a little water, up to five times a day as an antispasmodic. The dried root makes a Strong Decoction, 2 to 3 fluid ounces, up to three times a day. For the Fresh Root Poultice, just place a wad of the crushed root on the sore, cover with a leaf or cloth, and hold it in place with clothing—a scarf or whatever.

MEDICINAL USES The traditional use is still the best. The tea made of the dried herb is drunk for coughing and intercostal pain. The tea is soothing because of its mucilage, and the petasin acts as an antispasmodic and nerve sedative for the bronchial rings and pulmonary receptors. That means your throat doesn't feel as scratchy, your chest doesn't hurt as much, and you don't get into those paroxysmal coughing fits that make your loved ones cringe and the neighbors start dialing 911. Weak tea, with a little honey, is perfect for kids over the age of four or five. As with any such remedy, it quiets your cardiopulmonary excitability, makes you rest and calm down, makes you bearable—but it *doesn't* effect a change in any infection. It is palliative only, unless you are prone to wheezing and asthmatic consequences, in which case it may prevent the bronchial constrictions. It isn't really an asthma medicine, just something to keep it away if you have a chest cold.

The tincture, root tea, even the leaf tea will often help lessen painful spasms and cramps in the stomach, gallbladder, or colon. If you have an acute condition without any pattern, other approaches are usually better; but if you have a chronic problem—and whenever you are out of balance with your food, become emotionally stressed, don't get enough sleep, you have these early-warning pains—then the Coltsfoot approach is an excellent one. Just take the herb until the pains start to subside and you become relaxed enough to rest or sleep.

The herb can be smoked to aid simple lung irritability—if you are a smoker. Let's face it, smoke is itself an irritant, and if you don't smoke already, don't start smoking Coltsfoot if you have a problem. On the other hand, a smoker—already tolerant of the act—will find that some Coltsfoot will help. Coltsfoot leaves form a basis of many smoking mixtures.

The crushed root poultice (or even the moistened leaf) is an effective first aid for sprains, contusions, or damage from bumping into an unseen branch while hiking. It lessens the inflammation, decreases the pain by nerve sedation, and helps to inhibit bacteria if the skin is broken. It works best if the injury is to a part of the body with lots of sensory nerves, such as the arms, neck, head, or feet. It helps to limit the pain by depressing the rate of nerve firing and is a sedative to the nerves that are partially responsible for dilating the blood vessels near the injury. It is important to keep the poultice against the skin for at least one-half hour; otherwise the plant constituents will not be absorbed into the tissue.

Western Pasque Flower

Anemone occidentalis   (Ranunculaceae)

OTHER NAMES   Mountain Pasque Flower, Old Man in the Mountain; *Pulsatilla occidentalis* ·

APPEARANCE In the high mountain spring (May to early July), this little plant puts up its cream-colored, cup-shaped flowers, sometimes almost through the snow. The stems and feathery leaves are downy-silvery, and the (usually) six petals are actually sepals. The flowers, one to a stem, resemble a white rose with a yellow center filled with numerous stamens and pistils. By the time the plants are fully grown (1 to 2 feet tall), the flowers have become big, plumy, yellow-green, upturned mop heads, covered with hundreds of tasseled seeds waiting to be blown off into the wind.

HABITAT Western Pasque Flower grows on rocky and gravelly slopes of high coniferous forests, up to and above timberline. It can be found in California (usually above 8,000 feet) in the Sierra Nevada, from Tulare County northwards; the north coast range from Siskiyou and Trinity counties north to the Olympic Peninsula, Washington, and British Columbia; the Cascades from the California border up into Alberta; and in the high country of Idaho and western Montana. It is rare in Nevada and southern Idaho. Think high country, timberline, backpacking, Western Pasque Flower, and you'll get the idea.

CONSTITUENTS Anemonin, protoanemonin, "anemone camphor," and other little acrid surprises.

COLLECTING AND PREPARATION Gather the fresh seeding stems in late July or August when the seeds are ready to launch. To check, tug on several stems lightly and they should dislodge, exposing their attached seeds, already starting to harden. Clip off the seed heads with an inch or two of stem, tuck the stems under a rock so the seed plumes can catch the wind and fly away, and fresh tincture all the rest of the aerial parts, 1:2. The plant is stronger medicine in the late spring when it is 4 to 5 inches tall and flowering, but this collecting method allows seeding, adequate photosynthesis to feed and plump up the tubers, and is not likely to harm the little perennials. The chopped herb emits a strong acrid aromatic gas, so prepare the fresh tincture in a well-ventilated area. The dry herb is very feeble.

STABILITY The tincture is stable for several years.

MEDICINAL USES Western Pasque Flower is interchangeable with the former drug plant Pulsatilla. As the latter is seldom available in the proper form (fresh plant tincture), this is a valuable medicine for the Pacific Coast herb user. This *Anemone* is useful for insomnia, nervousness, and

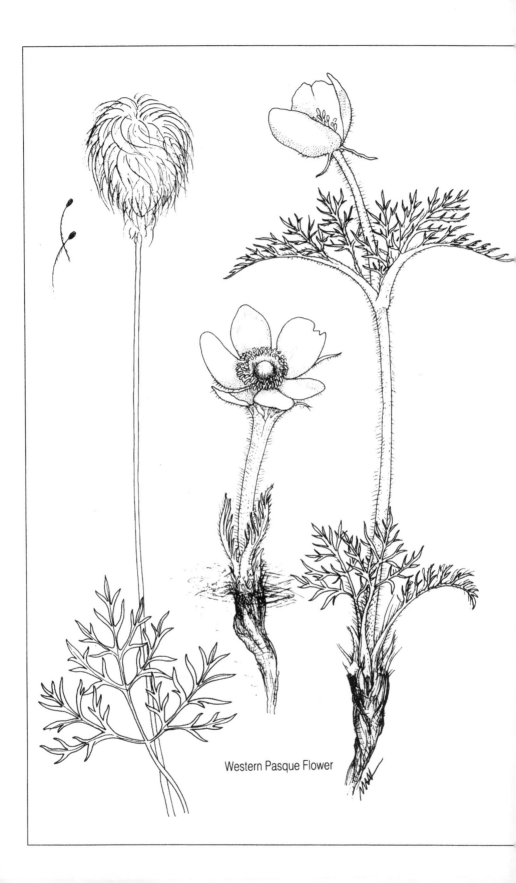

Western Pasque Flower

a generally agitated state of mind complete with a sense of doom, distress, and physical irritability. It is not for the red-faced, flushed person with feverish countenance, but the wan, chilly, and stretched-out person. If you are tired, overworked, tenuous, and overwrought, with a rapid and thready pulse, try some of the tincture. Women with bad PMS from time to time—irritable, gloomy, and uncentered, veritably yinned out— will often be helped, particularly when there are sharp pains in the abdomen or the skin feels overly sensitive to the touch. If you are tired, shaky, have clammy hands, and bags under your eyes, *need* to go to sleep and are so afraid that you won't be *able* to go to sleep that you end up *not* going to sleep, try some of the tincture.

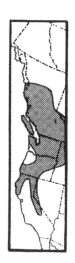

This Western Pasque Flower, along with Western Pulsatilla (*Anemone hirsutissima*) and Desert Anemone (*Anemone tuberosa*) all make fresh plant tinctures useful for the classic *Pulsatilla* of the Homeopaths, Eclectics, and the English Medical Herbalists. The *Pulsatillas* (including ours) are only active fresh; the Homeopaths that pioneered its use in the nineteenth century only used attenuations of the fresh mother tincture, and the Eclectic M.D.s only used the fresh plant as well. However, current use is of the virtually inert dried plant.

Dosage is important with this group; only use 5 to 15 drops of the tincture, and not in febrile, flushed, or excess conditions, not during pregnancy, and not with bradycardia. Otherwise, it is a safe antidepressant-sedative. In these proper low doses, the tincture will slow and strengthen the pulse and respiration, improve circulation and dispersal of blood to the central nervous system, dilate the peripheral blood vessels, and move the energy out to the edges of the body. Large quantities are inappropriate, acting as a parasympathomimetic and overstimulating the vagus nerve, with lowered blood pressure, nausea, salivation, and dizziness.

Anxiety attacks induced by overconsumption of today's faddish killer marijuana are helped by Western Pasque Flower; so is the clammy exhaustion with brain weavils experienced the day following overindulgence in the fluffed-out chunks on the mirror at that weird party the night before; multivitamins and 10 to 15 drops of the tincture every two or three hours are advisable in these cases.

CONTRAINDICATIONS Do not use during pregnancy or with bradycardia, and do not use in large quantities.

Western Peony

Paeonia Brownii   (Paeoniaceae/Ranunculaceae)
OTHER NAMES   California Peony, *Paeonia californica*

APPEARANCE Western Peony is a cheerful perennial plant, with ternately or biternately divided leaves. Its height is seldom over a foot, but a large plant may have hundreds of leaves, dozens of flowers, and cover a span of 2 or 3 feet. Stands of them may intersperse and form yards of lime green, succulent foliage, covering the ground between Oaks or Sage.

In the northern parts of its range and eastwards into the Great Basin and the western Rockies, the plants are sparser and less luxuriant, but the Dahlialike, dark-massed tubers are often larger. I have a hunch that the northern and eastern plants may have stronger roots, but frankly I have never run across them in large enough quantities to want to gather them, preferring, instead, to wait until I got to California or southern Oregon, where I know of large stands that I have harvested over the years. The flowers are terminal, one per stem, and nod over as if from great weight. Those of you who know the garden Peonies will probably not recognize these, as they have short, stubby, red, mauve, or chocolate petals that never extend much from the downturned calyx. They bloom in February and March in southern California, and as late as July in Washington, Idaho, and Wyoming. The mature seed capsules are usually nodding down to the ground. The distinguishing characteristics for Western Peony are the succulent, waxy green foliage (mostly basal), the odd flowers, and the bundles of dark brown-purple tubers found below ground.

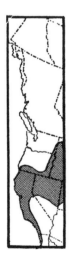

HABITAT The plants are common along the southern coast, from San Diego County north to Siskiyou County, California; in the Sierra Nevada from Tuolumne County northwards; in Oregon from Josephine County east, and up the eastern sides of the Cascades to northern Washington; across Nevada, Utah, Idaho, and the western edges of Wyoming, and probably on occasion in Montana and Colorado. In California and Oregon the Western Peony is a predictable plant, but it seems to be sporadic elsewhere, although local stands can be fairly extensive. I would suggest locating Western Peony on Washington and further east by way of herbarium specimens and their localities; in the Great Basin their habitat ranges from low Sagebrush flats to the middle Ponderosa forest—a vast area that includes as a potential most of the Great Basin, and could involve months of looking. Certainly, with such a tubered plant, gathering some pieces in the summer and leaving several tubers for the next year's growth will sustain the colonies for subsequent years.

CONSTITUENTS I have been unable to locate any analysis of this plant,

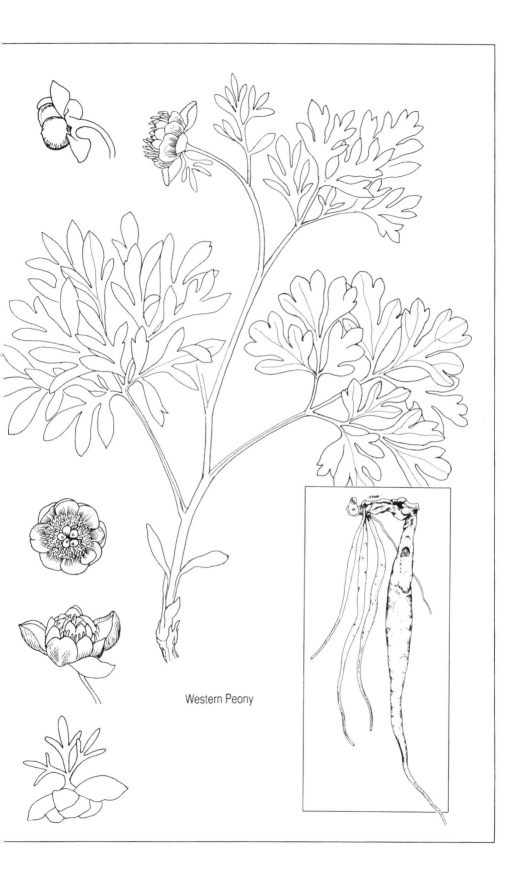

Western Peony

but it does the stuff that results from the usual Peony constituents, namely paeonol and paeoniflorin, and they should be present.

COLLECTING I have found the greatest strength in the tubers to be after flowering and before the foliage has started to die back. This means from late April to late June in California, and July through early September in the north country. Unfortunately, this necessitates digging the tubers before the seeds can fully mature, so be sure to properly replant some tubers or, with a large plant, take a bundle of them from the edge of the plant and leave as much foliage intact and as healthy as possible so that the remaining seedpods can mature properly. Since you need the dry root, and since they are very hard when dried intact and may deteriorate along the edges in the process, slice the tubers into thin cross-sections after letting them wilt whole for several days; dry the slices Method B.

STABILITY The dried slices will remain stable for several years. They should be stored sliced, and ground up when needed.

PREPARATION The Dry Root Tincture, 1:5, 60% alcohol, 10 to 25 drops, up to four times a day (acute problems), twice a day (tonic). The Cold Infusion can be taken, 1 to 2 fluid ounces at a time, or the root in capsules, 2 to 3 #00, both forms with similar frequency.

MEDICINAL USES Western Peony seems to have the same effects as the Asian and European plants, and can be useful in a variety of spasmodic crampy, irritative circumstances. It will help uterine cramping and fallopian cramping from mild endometriosis, although it works best if taken several times a day for the week previous to the beginning of menstruation. It acts as a menstrual stimulant for women with slow onset, clotty periods who are slender, dry-skinned, and frequently constipated, but for other women it simply reduces predictable cramping. In men it can be used for prostatic pain and testicular cramping after ejaculation, and I have seen it help hydroceles when combined with Red Root, both to reduce the pain and the actual swelling. Although I can't verify it, the same approach would probably be helpful for ovarian cysts.

All forms of the root are useful in spasmodic and hectic coughing, particularly when the cough reflex is followed by a period of barely suppressed, subcough tickling and irritation. It can be combined with Balsam Root or Osha to increase the effects, and, with moderate fever and aching in the chest, a little Baneberry or Black Cohosh can be added to further relax the muscles and sedate the irritability.

Western Peony by itself, or combined with Betony, is very effective for muscle pain and shakiness after excessive hiking, biking, or climbing, when the mind is tired but the somewhat abused muscular-skeletal system feels that it simply *must* twitch, cramp, and tremble until it has made the point to the brain that this sort of activity will *not* be easily tolerated. Western Peony helps prevent those shockingly drastic muscle discharges that can jolt you awake, just after nodding off, on the days you have been physically active. It also helps to relax you after you have driven ten hours, checked in at the Motel from Hell, and all you can feel is the wheel, the gas pedal, and the oncoming headlights while lying in the lumpy bed, staring at the picture of *Paris in the Rain* on the other wall, and listening to what sounds like a herd of clowns in rut in the parking lot. You know the feeling.

Finally, a couple of tonic doses a day are useful during times of emotional and intellectual stress for those people who get shaky hands or neck muscles towards evening—perhaps even to the point of seeing an aura and getting a migraine if they are not careful.

CONTRAINDICATIONS Western Peony is probably not appropriate during pregnancy—just to be on the safe side.

Western Skunk Cabbage

Lysichiton americanum   (Araceae)

OTHER NAMES   Yellow Skunk Cabbage, Swamp Cabbage; *Lysichitum americanum, L. kamtschatcense*

APPEARANCE There is no mistaking Western Skunk Cabbage. In the spring it sends up a foot-long, green flower stalk, covered in a bright yellow, enveloping leaf called a spathe. Eventually the flowers extend beyond the spathe, and it falls away; by this time the large cabbagelike leaves are well developed and on their way to their summer length of 2 to 5 feet. The leaves extend out from the root stalk and never from a stem, and the glaucous, green leaves (lighter underneath) have a large central vein. This makes it easy to distinguish from *Veratrum* (False Hellebore), which forms upright stalks, clasped by Lilylike, parallel-veined leaves, and forms a loose and branched mass of little cream flowers in the summer. This poisonous plant is also called Skunk Cabbage in some areas, and the spring spadix/spathe bloom of *Lysichiton* and the spring growth of *Veratrum* resemble each other. Wait until summer to dig and pick. By then the *Veratrum* is 4 or 5 feet tall and resembles a corn plant on steroids, growing next to a microwave relay station. If the carnivorous plant in *Little Shop of Horrors* were a biennial, then the *Lysichiton* resembles its first year's basal-leaf growth. Fanciful perhaps, but looking between the trunks of some Red Cedars in the Washington Cascades, into a bog filled with these arcane monsters, makes me look upwards and check for pterodactyls or King Kong fighting Tyrannosaurus rex.

The crushed leaves smell swampy-skunky, but the scent dissipates quickly. The root is large and octopoid, with a fleshy central bulb and many fleshy and crepey rootlets.

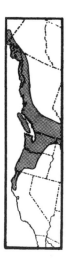

HABITAT Skunk Cabbage is found in swamps and bogs in forests from Kodiak Island in Alaska, south to Mendocino County and perhaps Sonoma County in California. In the Cascades it can be found from southern Oregon northwards, and east into northern Idaho and extreme northwestern Montana. It is more common at lower altitudes, but I have seen it up to 5,000 feet in Washington.

CONSTITUENTS Besides calcium oxalate crystals in the leaves and root, and anthocyanins and kaempferols in the foliage, the constituents are not known, although bioactivity is probably due to aromatic fractions of the essential oils, since old, nonsmelly roots have little therapeutic value.

COLLECTING Dig the roots in the summer or fall. This sounds simple enough, until you try to dig them. Insert a shovel into the ooze next to a plant, apply leverage, and observe that the plant doesn't move, but *you* sink into the muck. It takes patience, tolerance for gooey black silt on your hands, forearms, and knees, and a lack of aversion to the slugs that are often slithering around you. Wash the roots well, halve or quarter them from top to bottom, remove any remaining green stem flesh from the top of the root, rewash, and process into smaller pieces for fresh tincturing or to dry for tea or tincturing. The dried ripe seeds from its eastern relative *Symplocarpus foetidus* are supposed to be at least as strong a medicine as the root, but I have found little value from the seeds of our Western Skunk Cabbage.

STABILITY The dried root deteriorates unusually quickly, and it would be best, if you are planning tea or capsule use, to replenish the stock each year. The tincture is, of course, stable.

PREPARATION Fresh Root Tincture (central root, deprived of rootlets), 1:2, 30 to 60 drops, up to four times a day. Dry Root Tincture (entire root, recently dried), 1:5, 50% alcohol, 20 to 50 drops, up to four times a day. The tea is best made as a Cold Infusion, one scant teaspoon of the grated dry root, suspended in a muslin bag or tea bag overnight in a cup of water (or 4 teaspoons in a quart), up to four times a day. You can take the root in capsules if you powder the recent root, cap them up, and refrigerate or freeze to prevent deterioration; dose, 2 to 3 #00, up to three times a day, with warm water.

MEDICINAL USES Western Skunk Cabbage is less active than its eastern relative *Symplocarpus,* but, as that herb is so seldom available, or, if available, often old, our plant is excellent by comparison. It works best for spasmodic and painful cramps that are aggravated by stress and fear. It has a strong expectorant and bronchial antispasmodic effect and can

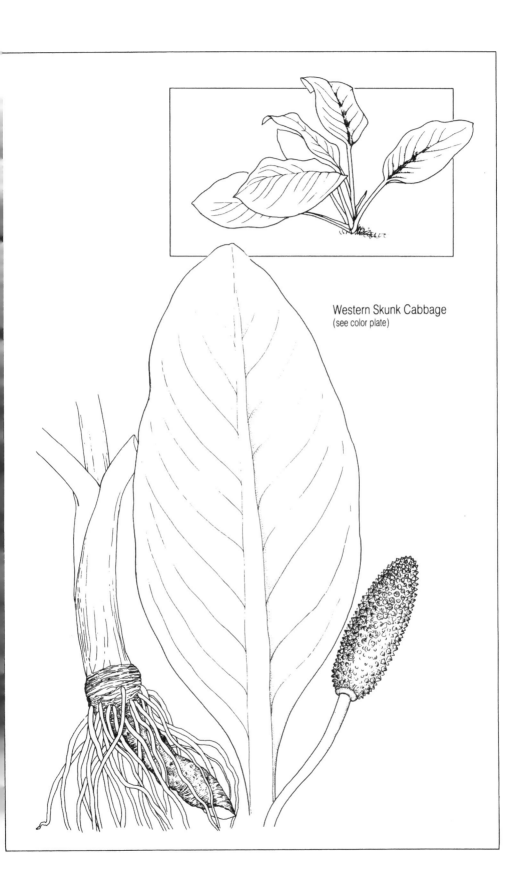

Western Skunk Cabbage
(see color plate)

be used by those with occasional bouts of moist asthma occurring under emotional duress and with a sense of panic or pain in the chest.

For bouts of coughing that culminate in semivomiting spasms and stomach pain, either from smoke inhalation or stress, nothing works better. An old-time preparation that is marginally palatable but very useful for kids that tend to this coughing/gagging syndrome is 1 part of the fresh chopped root simmered in 4 parts honey for a couple of hours, cooled, strained, and bottled. It smells nasty while simmering, so do it in an empty, ventilated house. *You* may not be able to take any (gag), but *they* didn't smell it happening, so they can take a teaspoon or two without the coaxing and threats usually needed for yucky stuff. Too much of Western Skunk Cabbage can cause nausea, moderate gastric irritation, and mild irritative diarrhea, so use it with a gentle hand.

OTHER USES The fresh leaves can be folded into cones for berry picking, and some folks use them like wax paper, interleaving fresh fruits and vegetables for short-term storage. The leaves apparently keep the foodstuffs fresh and slow spoilage until refrigeration or cooking is possible. Just make sure to pick off the slugs first.

White Sage

Salvia apiana　　(Labiatae/Lamiaceae)
OTHER NAMES　*Salvia Blanca; Audibertia polystachya*

APPEARANCE This can be one of our loveliest shrubs, or it can be a drab, lifeless patch of scruffy cabbages. In wet years the plants send up tall wands of silvery white flowers, and the plants, gracefully stretching towards the sky, may reach a height of 5 feet or more. These wands will seed and die back, leaving little more than long vertical sticks. The nontransitory, year-round parts are the many thick, sticky stems from which the flowers grow; they range in height from barely higher than the ground to 2 or 3 feet long and are surrounded with 1- to 4-inch-long, silvery white leaves. The leaves are paired, and the short, thick petioles tend to form a membrane around the stem. The leaves at the end of the evergreen stems form dense rosettes like an Aloe or Agave; the leaves along the stem may be fairly distant, presenting a jointed appearance. Smaller plants or plants that have had some severe drought may simply present a bunch of clustered basal rosettes, like Hen-and-Chicks (*Dudleya*). The leaves last through the winter, but can get frost-burned or die back from the periphery due to lack of water. The flowers have little of the popcorn-on-a-string appearance of most of the Sages; instead, they grow in pairs or from opposite stalks and form elongated and extended wand-panicles,

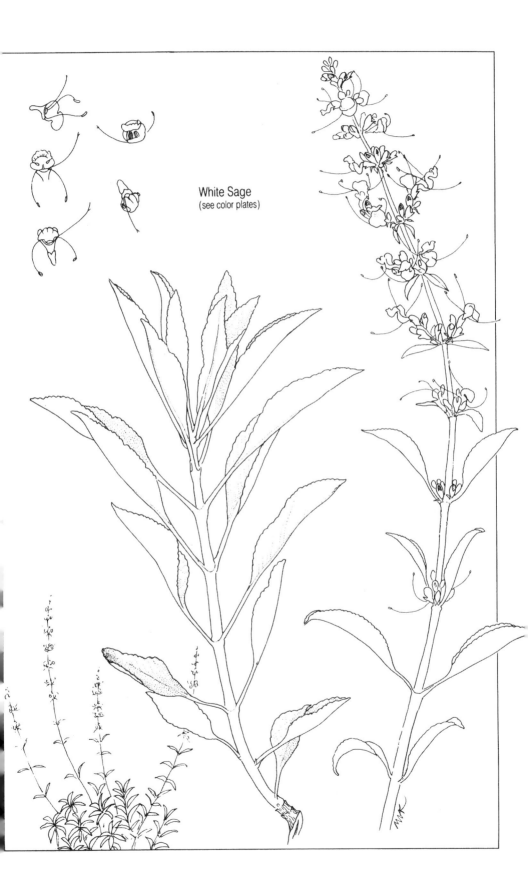

White Sage
(see color plates)

as ethereal as the foliage is stolid. The flowers have a conspicuous and elongated lower palate that gives the whole inflorescence a delicate visage.

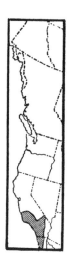

HABITAT White Sage grows in the foothills, on slopes and canyon walls, from northern Santa Barbara County south to northern Baja California; along the inner ranges to the edge of the Mojave and Colorado deserts; and as far east as Joshua Tree, the Tehachapi–San Gabriel crest, and the western border of Imperial County. It is found in San Diego, Imperial, Riverside, San Bernardino, Los Angeles, Ventura, Kern, and Santa Barbara counties, and as far south as Rosario in Baja California.

CONSTITUENTS The leaves contain up to 4% volatile oils, predominately camphor and eucalyptol; ursolic and oleanolic acids; alpha-amyrin; the abietane diterpenes 16-hydroxy-carnosic acid (approximately 1% or 2% of dry weight), and carnosic acid.

COLLECTING Gather the leaf rosettes or the whole leafing stem, discarding any flowering stem remnants; use fresh, or dry loosely in a paper bag. The best time for picking is after the flowers have seeded, from May or June to when the plant goes somewhat dormant, in October or November. Even in a rainy spring, many of the stems will not form flowering stalks, and these sterile stems can be harvested as early as February. The peak strength is early summer and midsummer, but the difference seems to be slight.

STABILITY Kept as whole leaves or whole leafing stems, the dry herb is strong for up to two years.

PREPARATION Fresh Herb Tincture, 1:2, or Dry Tincture, 1:5, 60% alcohol, 20 to 60 drops, up to five times a day; a teaspoon in a cup of warm water for a douche; full strength or diluted for topical use. The tea as a Standard Infusion, 2 to 4 fluid ounces, up to four times a day; or ½ ounce of crushed leaves in a quart of water for steam therapy or added to a sitz bath. The leaves can be ground and sifted to a medium powder for topical dusting.

MEDICINAL USES This plant is a dandy. It has been widely used throughout its area by native folks, both Anglo settlers and Spanish Californians. The diterpenes are effective against staph, candida, and Klebsiella pneumoniae—three bugs that cover a wide range of conditions; and the aromatics act as counterirritants to increase the depth of effect on tissues. The plant is best prepared as a tincture, since the carnosic acids are poorly water soluble. The tea is most effective if you fill a jar full of the leaves, add a tablespoon of alcohol on top of them, close the lid, and store the pickled leaves for tea use. The tea or tincture can be used for chest colds, and the leaves can be steamed for inhalation while you are at it. The douche is a good treatment for acute candidal vaginitis, and the sitz bath will help limit the yeast on the outside of the area. The tea, tincture, or powder is an excellent wash or dust for dirty scrapes and abrasions, and you can simply soak the area in the tea if it is a particularly nasty injury. Alternating the soak with a hydrogen peroxide wash will take care of almost anything.

OTHER USES The fresh rosettes can be wrapped in twine for a smudge stick, burned as a cleansing smoke after they have dried, or used in a sauna.

Wild Ginger

Asarum caudatum, A. hartwegii   (Aristolochiaceae)
OTHER NAMES   Canada Snakeroot

APPEARANCE The Wild Gingers have large, green, heart-shaped leaves that arise directly from creeping rootstocks. Healthy plants will cover several feet of ground with leaves, interspersed here and there between tree trunks, moss, and deadfall. The leaves smell like ginger when crushed; nothing else does, although the number of times I have mistaken Violets and Pyrolas for Wild Ginger because of similar leaf shape . . . is embarrassing.

Asarum caudatum grows from widespread, sprawling root stalks, with long leaf petioles (2 to 7 inches off the ground), sliding happily through leaf mulch. The roots are grey-brown and not much thicker than the petioles. The leaves are a dark bright green, often velvety, especially on the underside. The plant blooms in mid-spring, forming little, three-"petaled" cup-flowers, mauve to brown, with the petals (really sepals) having long tails. They grow at ground level off the leaf petiole and are hard to locate, as they are often obscured by leaf mulch.

Asarum hartwegii has similar shaped leaves, but on much shorter petioles, and they often just lay on the mulch or Redwood chuff. The leaves are frequently mottled with light green against the dark green. Other times the mottling is faint or even nonexistent. The flowers and roots are also similar, and, apart from different habitats, only the bicolored leaves and the petiole lengths distinguish the two species.

A third species, *Asarum lemmonii,* with delicate, smooth leaves and a flower with little stubby sepals (not long and graceful), is found in the northern Sierra Nevada, but I have never seen too much of it and would probably recommend against picking it.

HABITAT *Asarum caudatum* grows in the deep, dark deva places, from little ravines in the Santa Cruz Redwoods, north through the Redwoods and the coastal range to British Columbia. It doesn't grow quite as far

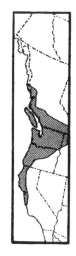

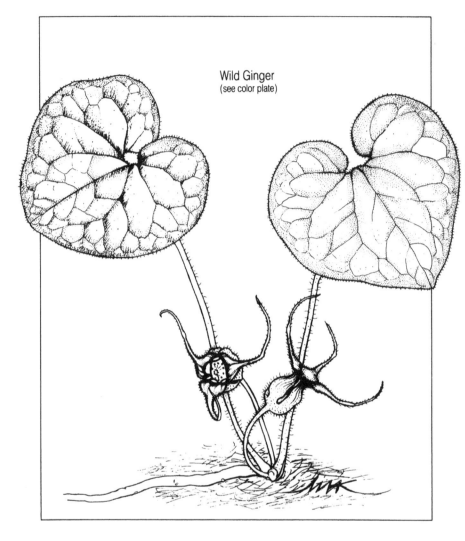

Wild Ginger
(see color plate)

north as to the Alaska Panhandle. From central Oregon north, it is found on both sides of the Cascades, and east through mountainous Idaho to western Montana. Although it probably grows in timbered areas, I have only seen it growing in old-growth forest. Presumably it needs the complex biosphere of old-growth forests, with deadfall, rotting logs, creeping fungus—all that stuff that makes a forest much different from stands of trees.

Asarum hartwegii is found in old-growth Yellow Pine and Red Fir forests, from Tulare County northwards in the Sierra Nevada; up across the Klamath Mountains into Oregon; and southwards into the north coastal range of California to Humboldt County. It likes sandy places in the higher mountains and grows at mostly from 3,500 to 7,000 feet, occasionally lower.

CONSTITUENTS Resin and volatile oils, with asarin, asarone (probably b-), and methyl-eugenol.

COLLECTING For tea, gather the leaves and dry loosely in a paper bag; band the leaves into little bundles (if *A. caudatum*) when appropriate. The roots should be cut or twisted into banded bundles 3 to 4 inches long and also dried loosely in a paper bag. Break the roots up only when you are going to use them.

STABILITY The dried leaves, if stored well, will last up to a year, or as long as the scent is present when crushed. The roots, stored whole, may last for several years. The ginger scent is the parameter of strength.

PREPARATION Fresh Root Tincture, 1:2, Dry Root Tincture, 1:5, 60% alcohol, either, 20 to 50 drops, up to three times a day; simple hot Leaf Tea.

MEDICINAL USES Wild Ginger makes you sweat. And not just from your skin. It makes you secrete from your tear glands, sinuses, mouth, and stomach; in fact, the main indication for using this spicy little friend is that some part of you is dry. For a slow onset, crampy, and clotty period, with poor progesterone buildup of endometrium secretions, it will stimulate the anticoagulant, antimicrobial, and thinning secretions of the uterus. With a simple hot, dry head cold, it will initiate secretions; with a hot and dry bronchial problem, it will initiate secretions; with a hot and dry *you*, it will initiate sweating. Drink the leaf tea hot, or use the root tincture in hot water. A few drops for kids and babies will stop some colic, particularly with belly gurgles and demon farts. If you need to stimulate the eruptions of measles or chicken pox, the hot tea or tincture works as well as anything I have run across.

If you get a fever, start to sweat and get chilled, or can't seem to get to the sweating stage at all (maybe you started with a headache and took too much aspirin), take some Wild Ginger. I am not saying that sweating works miracles, but let's face it: if you have a fever (even in a membrane like your sinuses), the sweat signals that you are over the acute phase—usually.

CONTRAINDICATIONS If you use too much Wild Ginger with gastric irritation, a red-tipped tongue and moist mouth, you may get nauseous. Its stimulation of the uterine mucosa makes it not advisable to use during pregnancy.

OTHER USES Like Ginger Root.

Yarrow

Achillea Millefolium   (Compositae)

OTHER NAMES   Millefoil; *Plumajillo; A. lanulosa*

APPEARANCE Yarrow is a perennial, tending to form large mats of interconnected roots and feathery basal leaves, from 2 to 5 inches long. From May to August it sends up tall, flowering stalks, topped with flat umbels of snow-white flowers, sometimes tinged with pink. In wet years or wet localities the stalks are numerous, crowded with leaves, and several feet tall. In dry years there are few flower stalks with fewer leaves, and the height may be only a foot or two, the energy being kept in the roots and basal leaves. The plant is highly aromatic, reminding me of a cross between Chamomile and Pine. As I have always lived in the Southwest, the scent is highly evocative of cool summers in the mountains, afternoon rains at 9,000 feet in July, rolling around in Pine chuff and Yarrow . . . sigh. If you live in Vancouver, the scent probably brings memories of clearing the edges of the lawn with the weed-eater. In any case, it is a handsome plant in flower, with its white flower heads, dark green feather-foliage, and evocative scent.

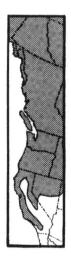

HABITAT In southern California look for it in the high mountains where the Pines grow and skiers doggedly drive up in the winter hoping for some natural snow but (four years out of five) settling for what has been spit out by a sno-cone-maker on steroids. This means places like Big Bear, Arrowhead, and Mount Pinos. It is common in the Yellow-Pine forests of the Sierra Nevada, the north coastal range, and down to the river valleys of Oregon. In Washington, British Columbia, and Idaho it can be found at any altitude, in Nevada only in the higher conifer areas.

CONSTITUENTS Primarily sabinene, isoartemisin ketone, 1,8-cineole (eucalyptol), camphor, and bornyl acetate, with a wide range of secondary aromatics that vary wildly in the different chemical races of this amorphous species. Unlike some variable relatives like Tansy and *Parthenium*, the main effects of Yarrow are not altered by its subtle differences. The flowers are highest in aromatics, the foliage is higher in tannins, and the roots hold their aromatics in complex resins. Although useful in aromatherapy, the lovely blue distilled oil of Yarrow manufactured in Europe is otherwise inferior to the whole plant.

COLLECTING Gather the recently flowered stalks and dry Method A. If you want to save the stalks for use in the I Ching, remove the flowers and strip off the leaves after drying; otherwise combine the upper half of the stems with the flowers and leaves. Roots should be washed and dried in bundles or in flats, Method B. Leave the plant in fairly large pieces and store in jars; the aromatics are lost quickly if the dried herb

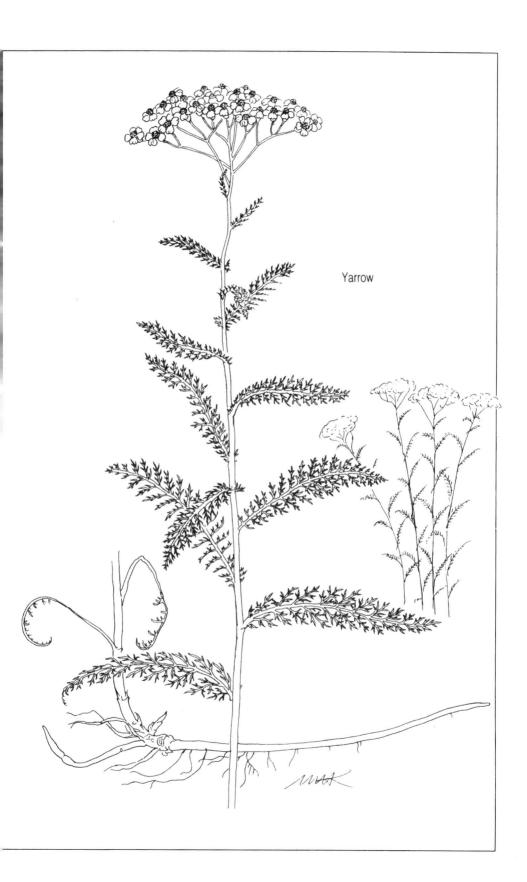

Yarrow

is overprocessed or left in bags for storage. You may encounter Yarrow with malformed or bulbous flowers (insect galls). There is nothing particularly wrong with them as medicine (they have a bit more tannin than usual and some protein from the larva), but they look weird and I avoid them.

STABILITY Flowers and leaves last 18 to 24 months; roots are good for several years.

PREPARATION Tincture of the fresh plant in flower, 1:2, tincture of the recently dried plant in flower, 1:5, 50% alcohol, 10 to 40 drops in warm water, up to five times a day for either form. As a tea, the herb in a Standard Infusion, 2 to 4 fluid ounces, up to four times a day. The dried root, broken into toothpick lengths, is simply chewed. A traditional down-home, good-timey method (redolent with images of cured ham, Asafetidy bags, and road-kill possum) is to fill a small jar with the root sections, pour 2 or 3 tablespoons of corn whiskey or rum over them, shake them up, and cap well. This makes them softer and (for some) tastier to chew on.

MEDICINAL USES Yarrow has many and subtle uses, but the simplest is its benefit for acute fevers, particularly those that begin a head cold or flu. Drunk as a hot infusion or used as tincture in hot water, it stimulates sweating and moderately lowers the temperature, both directly and by heat loss resulting from the perspiration. For children who seem to glow infrared when they get sick from anything, a teaspoon of Yarrow, a teaspoon of Chamomile, and a little Anise or Fennel works wonders, particularly if you have vague dread about aspirin, find that Tylenol doesn't lower their fever, and can't remember how to pronounce ibuprofen. Brew up the tea and have them sip it until they feel better or fall asleep.

Yarrow is an effective hemostatic and sometimes helps bleeding hemorrhoids and nosebleeds (especially from allergies); I have also seen it help bleeding stomach ulcers, using two or three doses a day for a couple of weeks. Topically, the fresh plant or the powdered leaves will stop or slow bleeding from cuts or scraped knees or elbows. The whole plant has rather strong anti-inflammatory effects, particularly in the skin and mucosa (innate immunity), and will help in recovering from gastroenteritis (intestinal flu) and from the lingering irritability of dysentery and diarrhea. Yarrow is antimicrobial against *Shigella* and should be combined with generous amounts of Echinacea to modify and help turn around shigellosis.

Its anti-inflammatory effect can be useful topically as well. A poultice of the fresh or moistened dry plant helps reduce muscle pain and joint inflammation. A bath made of an ounce of the herb steeped in 2 quarts of water, and the resultant tea added to the bathwater is helpful in the joint inflammation of rheumatoid arthritis and other low-level autoimmune or allergic conditions that settle in the joints. Poultices are also helpful in aggravated or recent varicose veins, especially during pregnancy.

Yarrow has a long history of use for menstrual problems, often with conflicting recommendations. It aids women with a long cycle and slow, congested, and extended menses with chronic dull pain, helping to tonify the uterus and promote more regular flow. Its effect on inflammation is more important here than its hemostatic astringency. Conversely, in women with orderly cycles, short and well-defined menses, and none of the aches and pains, it will act as a hemostatic for the occasional abnormal flow, even to the extent of being a reasonable tea for postpartum bleeding. In general, moderate use aids in stabilizing endometrium blood supply. Large amounts can increase blood supply, so it probably is not appropriate for extended use during pregnancy.

Being both anti-inflammatory and astringent/hemostatic, it lends itself well to low-level chronic cystitis and urethritis, with irritated urethra and prostate; take two cups a day for a couple of weeks.

The root is good to chew on for toothache and gum problems, especially when steeped in whiskey or rum.

CONTRAINDICATIONS Not appropriate for extended use during pregnancy.

OTHER USES The stalks are used in throwing the I Ching. The flowers can be simmered in water and the face held over the steam for improving the complexion. I am all beard and forehead, but I have been told it helped the complexion of my scalp. The tea is a dandy hair rinse.

Yellow Pond Lily

Nuphar polysepalum   (Nymphaeaceae)
OTHER NAMES Yellow Water Lily, Cow Lily, Spatterdock, Indian Pond Lily; *N. luteum*, var. *polysepalum, Nymphaea polysepala*

APPEARANCE There is little mistaking this lovely friend. The large floating, heart-shaped, waxy green leaves are borne on long, round petioles that arise from submerged rhizomes. The rhizomes are thick, covered with regular leaf scars, and attached to the mud with long, fleshy roots. The flowers are single, floating, and, like the leaves, at the ends of long peduncles that arise from the rhizome. The petals (actually sepals) and the columnar pistil are bright yellow; the ring of stamens around the base of the pistil is purple or greenish red. If the stamens are yellow, then you have found the closely related *Nuphar variegatum,* which has flattened leaf petioles and slightly smaller flowers—and no difference in use.

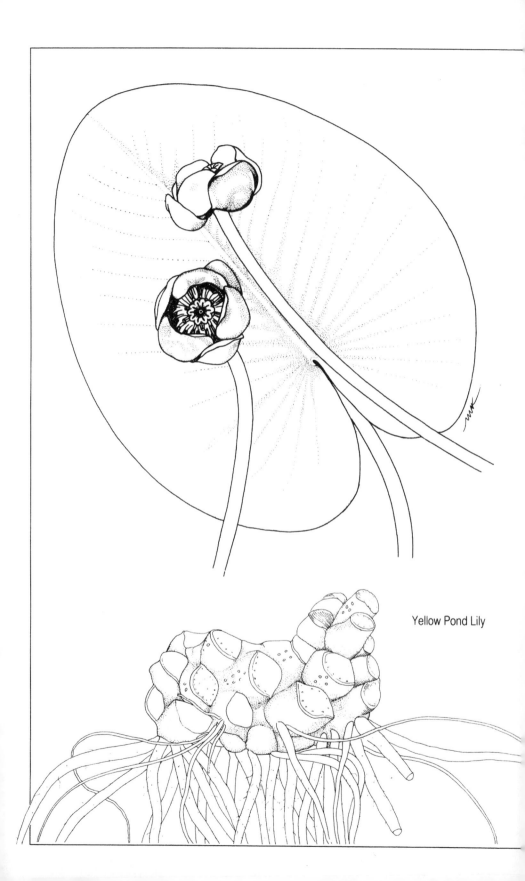

Yellow Pond Lily

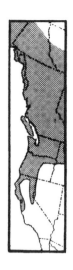

HABITAT Yellow Pond Lily is found in cold or cool marshes, bogs, ponds, and natural lakes (the shallow ends), from Santa Cruz County (north coastal range) and Mariposa County (Sierra Nevada), north through most of Alaska and British Columbia; east and south into the Rocky Mountains; and in most any of our cool, high mountains. It is most common in or near natural ponds, lakes, and swamps with standing water; but it is not common in dams and man-made circumstances.

CONSTITUENTS The alkaloids nuphacristine, nupharidine, thiobinupharidine, pseudothiobinupharidine, allothiobinupharidine, thiobidesoxynupharidine, phytosterols, two gallotannins, two ellagitannins, and mucilage.

COLLECTING This is the fun part. You are supposed to be able to dig up the root with a shovel (giggle). If it's summertime, strip down to swimming gear, or nongear (nekkid), make your way to the open water, swim over, dive down, pull, grunt, come up for air, go down again, try to find the thick roots, grab, apply leverage with your feet, and sink deep into the glurch. Come up with the root shard, look at it, go down, and get some more. What feels big underwater is not much at all, in reality. The only time I have ever *seen* a leech was diving for some roots in western Ontario, and I found it on my *body* (grimace, groan, shiver)! The best way to collect Yellow Pond Lily is to find some growing by the edge of a lake, with a sharp drop-off from the bank; then you will only get muck to your knees, not hypothermia from diving in north country water. Wash the rhizomes, scrap off junk with a brush, slice, and dry, Method B. The seedpods mature in early or mid-fall, and are usually a bit aloft from the water. They are about the size of a fig, with a pig snout, and are the texture of green fruit leather when ripe. Dry Method B and rub out the small seeds from the pulp.

STABILITY Not pertinent.

PREPARATION Fresh Root Tincture, 1:2, 10 to 20 drops, up to three times a day. Weak Decoction of the dried root, 2 to 4 fluid ounces, also up to three times a day. The ground seeds, 1 to 2 #00 capsules, morning and evening. The fresh or dried root can be mashed or mixed with water for a local Poultice or boiled up and added to bathwater.

MEDICINAL USES The plant is an effective astringent and anti-inflammatory for the intestinal tract and particularly the urinary tract. The seeds and the dry root are best used for this purpose; if using the seeds in capsules, swallow with some pleasant tea, such as Peppermint or Lemon Balm. For the intestinal tract, the best use is for inflamed, hot, and painful membranes, ranging from esophagus and stomach pain, to acute colitis or the jalapeño syndrome with itching rectal heat. The seeds and root tea also soothe lower urinary tract heat, either from too much sex, three days driving in a subcompact in the summer—or the jalapeño syndrome.

The fresh root has a peculiar effect on the reproductive organs and is one of the few herbs I have seen cool or suppress the structure. That means if you have vaginal, uterine, or ovarian irritation (female) or prostate or penis irritation (male), use the fresh root tincture internally; and, for women, I recommend a douche of 4 ounces of the root tea, with water added for convenience, or a sitz bath made with 8 ounces of the weak decoction added to the appropriate water for the container. For testicular or scrotal hydroceles or local inflammation, use the tincture combined with Trillium and Red Root; the same is true for painful ovaries and mittelschmerz, especially when painful to pressure. Remember that the root is for cooling and shrinking hot, inflamed, and sharply painful conditions; it is not for dull, congested, subacute and achy conditions that need stimulation.

The root poultice or bath is sometimes startling in its effect, but only if you have an inflamed and swollen joint, or an acute episode of osteo- or rheumatoid arthritis.

CONTRAINDICATIONS The fresh root is not for dull, congested, subacute and achy conditions that need stimulation.

OTHER USES Janice Schofield, the Alaska herb-maven, suggests making Pond Lily Popcorn, by using ¼ cup of seeds popped in 2 tablespoons of oil, with the usual suspects rounded up for flavoring (butter, nutritional yeast, and so forth). This sounds a lot more palatable than the old Assiniboin and Micmac tradition of frying them in bear fat.

Yerba Buena

Satureja Douglasii (Labiatae/Lamiaceae)

OTHER NAMES California Yerba Buena; *Micromeria chamissonis, M. Douglasii, Satureia Douglasii*

APPEARANCE This lovely little plant is a trailing evergreen perennial, creeping through thickets, between trees, by streams, and down (or up) moist gullies. The stems are thin and wiry, and because they root anytime they can, what otherwise might be a 4-foot-long runner may send down three or four roots along its length, with stems in turn growing off at angles from the rooted sections . . . well, it's a mess. Sometimes the stems travel along grass and across the base of thickets or down a rocky slope from a patch of rich soil above, where they don't root; here you have your premium, high-grade gathering circumstance, with dozens of yard-long stems that can be bundled, dried, and stripped of leaves and flowers in twelve seconds.

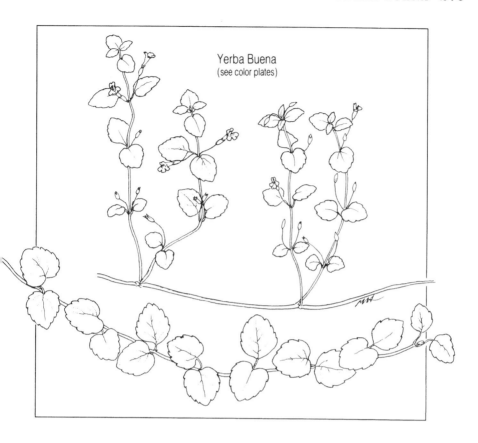

Yerba Buena
(see color plates)

The leaves are beautiful tiny blunt-toothed pairs, ½ to ¾ an inch long, on short little petioles, with little solitary flowers sprouting from each leaf axil. The opposite leaves stand out from the stem at right angles, the flowers at a 45-degree angle. They are up to ½ inch long, little-lipped tubular flowers, and have a color from white to purple-tinged. The stems are the usual four-sided ones you expect from the Mint family. The crushed plant gives off that delicious musky-mint scent that sets this plant apart from any other. Sometimes you become aware of Yerba Buena because the scent wafts up from the ground and you find you have been walking all over a patch of the plants. A warning is in order for pickers, however. Along the coast it is often found in competition with Poison Oak, and care must be taken not to gather Yerba Buena that may have come in recent contact with it. The oils from the leaves of Poison Oak can rub off on its intimate neighbors and create problems for sensitive individuals who handle the herb or drink the tea.

HABITAT It is found in the circumstances mentioned above, from the Santa Monica Mountains of California (sparingly, these days) up the coast all the way to southwestern British Columbia; along the western

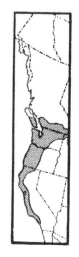

sides of the Cascades; and over into northern Idaho. A small amount makes it over the Bitterroots of Montana; and it is protected in that state. By and large, it is most abundant from Santa Barbara County north to southern Oregon, a stretch of coastline where it can be expected to grow in any appropriate circumstance. In the rest of the habitat it is abundant but unpredictable.

CONSTITUENTS Volatile oils that contain at least one monoterpenoid; the plant has had little constituent analysis otherwise.

COLLECTING Gather the runners from April through August (or September along the coast). As mentioned, long, unbranching stems are the ideal, but you do what you have to. If you gather long stems, bundle and dry them; if you collect many short stems, break them and dry them loosely in a paper bag. After drying, the leaves and flowers (if there are any) can be stripped off the stems and stored for tea. The stems can be used if needed, but they are less aromatic and tend to be a shade bitter.

STABILITY Stored in whole leaf form, the herb is strong for a year and can still make a decent cup of tea after two years, although the breadth of the patina is diminished (it gets stale in time).

PREPARATION Put a few leaves in a cup, boil water, pour the water over the leaves, steep for ten minutes, sip the tea, and sigh. (That's right folks, order right now, operators are standing by. . . .) It makes a complementary herb to add to Catnip to lessen the somewhat gross aftertaste, or to add to Chamomile when the taste gets tiring; and an incredibly delicious mixture can be made with equal parts of Yerba Buena, Lemon Mint, Spearmint, Brook Mint, Hummingbird Sage, or Lemon Balm. You may not want to drink it, only smell it, but it makes a righteous tea—if you can get your nose out of the jar long enough.

MEDICINAL USES It can be drunk as a diaphoretic if you have a mild fever with bloodshot eyes and dry skin; and it can be added with safety to other less elegant leaf teas to flavor them without detracting from their effect. It has been used as a skin wash for rashes and prickly heat, but with so many other herbs for that purpose—stolid and proletariat plants that work better (but taste worse)—I wouldn't bother wasting Yerba Buena. In summer months try 3 parts Yerba Buena and 1 part Hibiscus with a dollop of honey, and make a sun tea to which you add some ice. If you have children, you know that one will always flee in terror when a therapeutic tea is in the offing; add a little tincture of whatever noxious stuff is due them to Yerba Buena tea, and they won't even notice the taste in this lovely context. Yerba Buena was the old name for San Francisco, by the way.

Yerba del Lobo

Helenium hoopesii   (Compositae)
OTHER NAMES   Mountain Sneezeweed, Golden Sneezeweed

APPEARANCE Yerba del Lobo is a stout, thick-stemmed colony plant with Irislike root masses, dark brown skin, and light grey flesh. These give rise to many basal leaves—light green, glabrous, somewhat succulent, and narrow. They may be a foot or more in length. The root is aromatic, the leaves only slightly. The flowering stems are mature by late summer, and are 2 or 3 feet high, thick, and with only a few leaves that become progressively smaller towards the top. Most Sneezeweeds have stem leaves with a membrane or wing extending down the stem from the leaf attachment; this species does not. The flowers are yellow to orange, 2 to 3 inches across, and have a raised, spherical yellow disk, drooping ray flowers up to an inch long, three-toothed at the tip, and one or two dozen in number. The flower resembles a cross between a Coneflower, Sunflower, and Daisy. The light green stems may have only a single flower, or three or four on small terminal branches. The whole plant may have from one to a dozen stems, and in dense stands it may be difficult to tell where one plant begins and another ends. Like Yarrow or Arnica, in dry years many plants will not bloom, and you'll have to look for the massed basal leaves without any flower stems. Dig these up and leave the individuals with flowers to spread seed.

HABITAT Yerba del Lobo grows in the high mountains of the Sierra Nevada, from Tulare County in California, north to the Steen Mountains and southeastern Cascades in Oregon; the Warner Mountains in northeastern California; the highest ranges of Nevada; and the Rocky Mountains. It grows in creeks, in moist meadows, and in alluvial valleys above 6,000 feet and below 10,000 feet. As it is toxic to livestock and avoided by them, it benefits from high country overgrazing. In such conditions it is found in abundance with False Hellebore, Aconite, and *Senecios*, other perennials associated with too many cattle.

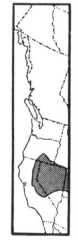

CONSTITUENTS Hymenoxon (a sesquiterpene lactone), other pseudoguaianolides, phenols, and probably *Senecio*-type alkaloids.

COLLECTING Gather the whole plant, roots, stems, and, if appropriate, the flowers, in late summer. If it is too late in the season for the foliage and floral parts, gather just the roots. The roots, however, often take weeks to dry whole; so clean them, remove the dead sections, slice lengthwise, and dry Method B. Dry the foliage and stems Method A.

STABILITY The aerial parts are good for a year, the roots for two, even if powdered.

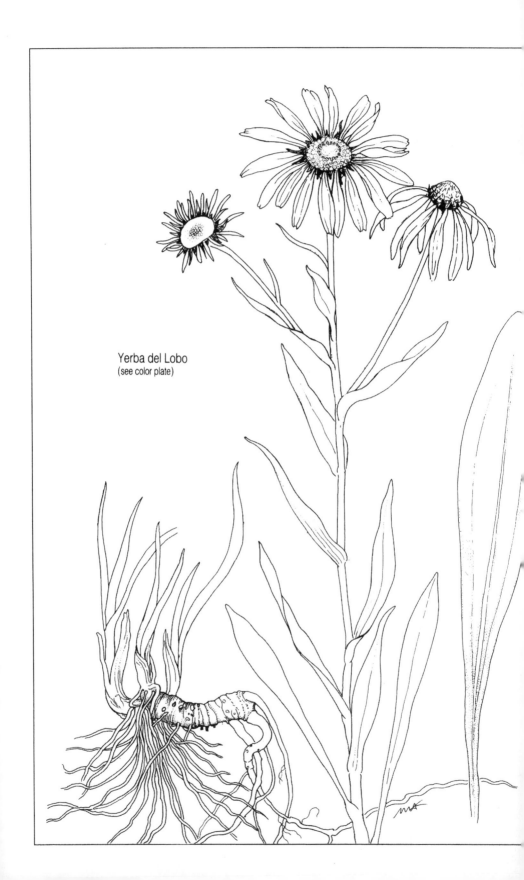

Yerba del Lobo
(see color plate)

PREPARATION For an External Liniment, make a 1:5 tincture of the dried herb, using 50% vinegar and 50% rubbing alcohol (90% strength). For internal use, make a simple Hot Infusion with ½ teaspoon of the ground root in hot water, drinking the suspended particles along with the tea.

MEDICINAL USES The liniment, bizarre though it smells, is effective when applied to sore joints, sprains, muscle bruises, and arthritic joints. If the pain is aggravated by cold and damp weather, your liniment needs 1 teaspoon African Bird Peppers (*Capsicum*) or 2 teaspoons of ground Ginger to each pint of liquid. Rub the liniment into the flesh until evaporated, and do not wash it off (unless it irritates). This is a traditional New Mexican Spanish remedy. It is similar in effect to Arnica, although feebler; but it has the advantage of not having the potential for skin reactions, and will not cause the subcutaneous inflammation that Arnica can cause if it comes in contact with broken or scratched skin.

The mild tea of the root is distinctly effective for internal bruises and dull aching, although I would not recommend more than two or three cups a day, and only use it for a couple of days. A single cup of the tea will break most fevers with a strong sweat and will subsequently lower temperature. For fevers that manifest with chills, add a little ginger to the ½ teaspoon of ground root. Because of its constituents (known) and its botanical closeness to the *Senecios,* and the possibility that it contains some of their more liver-toxic alkaloids (not known), this is an internal medicine for the strong and durable individual—not those with liver problems, a history of hepatitis, or chronic disease. Although most pregnant women are also strong and durable, the second person involved is not, so don't drink the tea during pregnancy.

CONTRAINDICATIONS Do not use during pregnancy or for those with liver problems, hepatitis, or chronic diseases.

Yerba Reuma

Frankenia grandifolia   (Frankeniaceae)
OTHER NAMES   Alkali Heath

APPEARANCE Yerba Reuma is a low-growing shrublet, upright and somewhat prostrate. It is grey-green in color, usually has many branches, and has small Rosemarylike leaves, about ½ inch long, opposite, lighter on the underside, and stem-clasping. The flowers are small, bright pink, and peek out from leafy branches and in axils of the upper foliage; they are usually five-petaled and emerge from a tubular calyx. The plants are normally about a foot tall, grow in stands, and from a distance are

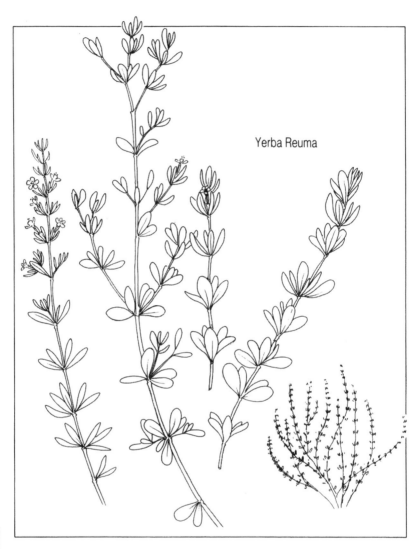

Yerba Reuma

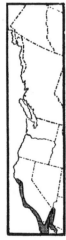

drab and insignificant; up close, they are still drab and insignificant, except for the bright little flowers—and the fact that you have now found them. The foliage usually has a salty, astringent taste.

HABITAT Yerba Reuma grows solely in salt marshes and on beaches. It is found from Marin County in California south to the tip of Baja California, and all along the coast of the Sea of Cortez. A smaller variety is found along the Colorado River and inland salt flats of the Mojave and Imperial deserts; in the Central Valley of California; and in the Panamint Basin, over into southwestern Nevada. A smaller species, *F. palmeri*, with little white flowers, and growing as barely more than grey tufts, is found in San Diego salt marshes and on both sides of Baja California, south to Kino Bay in Sonora.

CONSTITUENTS Catechol tannins, other polyphenols such as frankenic acid (similar to krameria red) and gallic acid; it has a high ash (mineral) content.

COLLECTING Gather the aboveground plant and dry in paper bags.

STABILITY The dried herb, stored properly, is good for several years.

PREPARATION Cold Infusion, 2 to 6 fluid ounces, up to three times a day; it may be used freely externally. For a Douche, use ¼ ounce of herb in 12 ounces of water. Make a Hot Infusion, cool to body temperature, and use. For an Eyewash, make ½ cup of strong tea and use, bathing the eyelids as well. Make a fresh batch each time. Because the plant itself is salty, you don't need to add salt for either the douche or eyewash. The Vinegar Tincture is made 1:5 with apple cider vinegar.

MEDICINAL USES Yerba Reuma is a remarkably effective astringent and antimicrobial. Originally manufactured by Parke-Davis as a fluid extract and a glycerate in 1880, it was rather widely used in medicine up until the First World War. As we don't have Witch Hazel or Rhatany growing in the Pacific West, it is fortunate that we have this little equivalent. It is an excellent wash for any skin irritations, from infections, to rashes, to sunburn or windburn; use either the tea or the vinegar tincture. If the tincture stings too much, just dilute it to a comfortable strength. Yerba Reuma, with its complex tannins, effective for most of the intestinal tract as an astringent, is quite reliable for diarrhea, dysentery, and vomiting. It can be used as well for gargling for a sore throat and as a mouthwash for sore gums. For vaginitis or vulvitis, use the douche once every other day until symptoms subside. For rhinitis and conjunctivitis, use the eyewash up to four times a day, making the tea fresh each time.

OTHER USES A few branches added to the brine in pickling increases the crispness of the finished product.

Yerba Santa

Eriodictyon californicum, E. crassifolium, etc.   *(Hydrophyllaceae)*

OTHER NAMES Mountain Balm, Consumptive's Weed; *Yerba Blanca; E. glutinosum*

APPEARANCE *Eriodictyon californicum* is the species that was the former official drug plant. It is a handsome, sticky-shiny, dark green shrub, up to 8 feet in height, but usually around waist to chest high. The leaves are long, tapered lance-shaped, and crowded in varnished profusion along the upper lengths of the branches. The upper surfaces are resinous and shiny, dark green, almost verging on black; the undersides are yellowish and felty, with a single prominent central vein and small weblike side veins. The edges are marked with small unequal teeth. The leafy stems are varnished yellow-green and are flexible; the lower branches are somewhat woody and brittle. The blossoms are borne at the ends of the leafing stems, on their own short peduncles, an unfurling scorpion panicle of small, blue, tubular flowers.

Eriodictyon crassifolium resembles the previous in shape and size, but the leaves are broad, oval, flattened, and covered in fur on both sides. The shrubs look grey-green, even silvery, and lack the overt surface resins of *E. californicum*. In some localities they have less leaf hair and look a bit blue-green, but most of the time the foliage looks like greygreen felt. The shrub shape is often broader than the other, and the flowers are white to light blue-pink, with the same unfurling scorpion shape. *Eriodictyon trichocalyx* has the same broad leaf and shrub form of the previous, but with the upper surface a sticky blue-green, the lower surface lighter, and with very little leaf fuzz. The flowers are the same shape and color as the previous. The two interbreed.

Eriodictyon angustifolium resembles *E. californicum* in that it has a sticky-resinous cover on all parts of the foliage and stems; but it has very thin leaves and white to pale lavender flowers.

All Yerba Santas like roadsides; drive up into lower foothills, and if there is a stand nearby, it will have spread down to the edge of the road and can be clearly seen at 45 mph.

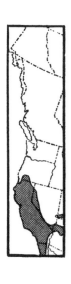

HABITAT *Eriodictyon californicum* grows on ridges and slopes, from the north coastal range of California as far south as Monterey County, up into southern Oregon, and down the west side of the Sierra Nevada from near Mount Lassen to almost as far as Tehachapi. It is also found in the San Bernardino Mountains. It grows at an altitude of from 1,000 feet to 5,000 feet.

Eriodictyon crassifolium occurs in lower mountains, from 2,000 to 5,500 feet, between the Santa Lucia Mountains of Monterey County, California, south to Baja California, and inland from Kern County south. *E. trichocalyx* follows the chaparral belt from Santa Barbara County to Baja California; and the inland mountains that ridge the Los Angeles Basin, from the San Gabriel Mountains, south through the Santa Rosa Mountains, and down into the Anza-Borrego Desert. *E. angustifolium* is a plant of the Mogollon Rim in Arizona that also occurs in southern Nevada in the mountains around Las Vegas, and in California in the higher reaches of the Providence and New York mountains at the northeastern edge of the Mojave Desert.

CONSTITUENTS Eriodictyol, homoeriodictyol, chrysoeriodictyol, xanthoeriodictyol, eriodonol, eriodictyonic acid, ericolin—all in a base of volatile oils and resins. The plants contain high levels of flavonoids, and the

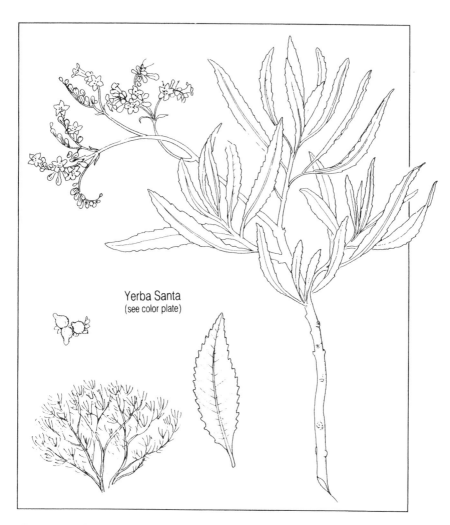

Yerba Santa
(see color plate)

chemistry of the genus is deep, profound, and quirky. A friend of mine got his doctorate from the University of Arizona isolating some strange flavanones from *E. angustifolium,* and he said he could have gone on forever if his committee had let him.

COLLECTING The two sticky species, *E. californicum* and *E. angusti-folium,* are best gathered in the spring and early summer, when the foliage is green and fresh. Break off the leafy stems and band them, making sure they are not piled together. They can melt into a sticky, amorphous wad and ferment in the center, so keep the bundles apart from each other, separating the individual stems within a bundle once a day so *they* don't wad up. When dry, strip off the leaves and flowers (if any), discarding the stems. The other two large-leaved species can usually be picked, dropped into a paper bag, and left until dry. The foliage is more dispersed in these species, and they seldom form the intensely compacted, leafing stems of the others, so just pick the leafing and blooming tips. These also are best picked early in the year. Any Yerba Santa growing in a sheltered locality may have good, healthy leaves almost any time of the year, but spring and early summer are the most likely times for a good herb.

STABILITY Yerba Santa is often stable for two years, although *E. crassifolium* deteriorates the quickest and should be replaced yearly. Always leave Yerba Santa whole until using.

PREPARATION The Fresh Tincture, 1:2, the Dry Tincture, 1:5, 65% alcohol, both 20 to 30 drops in hot water, up to five times a day. The tea is made as a Standard Infusion, 3 to 4 ounces, up to four times a day. The two broad-leaved species, *E. crassifolium* and *E. trichocalyx,* tend to be more soluble in water, and I have had better luck with them as a simple tea or in tea formulas made for decongestants. In making the Dry Tincture, I have had to increase the alcohol percentage to 80% in years when the herb is so fecund that the leaf varnish resembles epoxy resin, decreasing it to 65% in drier years. I percolate tinctures, and the solvency is a bit more critical using this method; if you are macerating the tincture, 65% alcohol should be adequate.

MEDICINAL USES Yerba Santa is one of our best decongestants, used for any lung or sinus condition that is juicy, hypersecretory, and gaggy. It decreases the secretions and lessens the underlying inflammation. If you are coming down with bronchitis, have early symptoms of moist, humid asthma, or are starting to get a runny nose from a head cold or sinus allergy, the tea or tincture will start to decrease the drool very quickly. If you do too much, it can start to dry up the membranes excessively, so many herbalists throw in some expectorant or secretory stimulant along with it. It might seem weird to mix a membrane drier with a membrane moistener, but Yerba Santa acts to decrease the puffy thickening of the mucosa, and if you add some Balsam Root, Grindelia, or Lomatium, you are increasing the fluid secretions from the same tissues that Yerba Santa shrinks—squeezing the sponge, as it were. With its decongestant effects and its high level of flavonoids, Yerba Santa is very useful for chronic gastritis and chronic urethral irritation. The flavonoids help to strengthen the fragile, irritated membrane capillaries that are distended and leaky from the chronic irritation that underlies the problem. As a general cold and allergy tea, Yerba Santa, especially the broad-leaved species, can be combined with equal parts of Horehound, Mormon Tea, Western Coltsfoot, California Bayberry, and Balsam Root. Boil up a scant tablespoon of the finely chopped mixture in a cup of water for ten minutes, let it cool to a bit warmer than body temperature, strain, add some honey, and drink. Remarkably effective, yes?

APPENDIX A: SUPPLEMENTAL HERB LIST

This is a brief list of some of the other herbs to be found in the Pacific Coast region, together with general geographic distribution, the parts used, preferred preparations, therapeutic effects, and comments where appropriate; these are all my personal observations. Finally, when possible, I have made reference to the five books that I feel are useful in the Pacific region for further plant identification and other uses: Edible and Medicinal Plants of the Rocky Mountains and Neighboring Territories *by Terry Willard;* Discovering Wild Plants *by Janice Schofield;* A Field Guide to Medicinal Plants *by Steven Foster and James Duke; and* Medicinal Plants of the Mountain West *and* Medicinal Plants of the Desert and Canyon West *by the author. These are referred to as Willard, Schofield, Foster, Moore (Mountain), and Moore (Desert). There are some excellent older, out-of-print books, and perhaps a current text or two that I haven't seen, but these five books and this current one are pretty much the whole ball game in western North America. Two of them deal substantially with edible plants, and the third (Foster) is intended mostly as a field guide that covers the eastern half of North America, doing so in a gentlemanly and academically restrained fashion.*

Herbs are listed by the common name first but by alphabetical order of the scientific name.

FIR (1. *Abies lasiocarpa.* 2. *A. grandis.* 3. *A. concolor.* 4. *A. amabilis.* 5. *A. procera.* 6. *A. magnifica*). *Distribution* 1. Cold, wet mountains from the central Yukon south through the Rocky Mountains, Olympic Mountains, and Cascades, almost to the California border; 2. coastal ranges from northern California to southwest British Columbia, and along the Cordillera from southeast British Columbia through northern Idaho and northwest Montana; 3. high mountains from southern Oregon into the northern coastal range, California, and down the Sierras to the southern California mountains; 4. coastal ranges from northern California to the Alaska Panhandle, Victoria Island, and the western slopes of the Cascades; 5. western slopes of the Cascades; 6. southern Oregon, down the Sierras and into western Nevada. *Parts Used* Bark, pitch, and needles. *Preparation* Weak Decoction f͟ ͟ ͟ ͟rnal wash, 1 to 3 fluid ounces, up to five times a day internally; Salve ͟ ͟ ͟ d B; strong cup of tea, up to three times a day; dried needles for smudge ͟ ͟ ͟ se. *Herb Uses* Bark: disinfectant astringent externally, stimulating astr͟ ͟ ͟ internally, for GI, lungs, and skin/mucosa deficiency. Pitch: similar to Po͟ ͟ ͟ ud oil. Needles: diuretic and expectorant tea; nice incense. *References* F ͟ ͟ ͟ Willard.

ACACIA (*Acac ͟ ͟ ͟ eggii*). *Distribution* Southern California to southern Nevada and eastwards ͟ ͟ ͟ e middle deserts. *Parts Used* Pods, leaves, twigs, roots, and gum. *Preparat ͟ ͟ ͟ eaves, stems, and pods powdered for tea or topical dusting; the gum as a r͟ ͟ ͟ ͟ge (1 ounce of gum dissolved in 3 fluid ounces of water); the root made ͟ ͟ ͟ ͟ Cold Infusion, drunk as needed. *Herb Uses* Astringent, emollient, disi͟ ͟ ͟ ͟nt, anti-inflammatory, for mucous membranes of upper respiratory, int͟ ͟ ͟ d tract, and so forth. *References* Moore (Desert).

YERBA DEL CA ͟ ͟ ͟ ͟R (*Acalypha californica*). *Distribution* Rocky hills and arroyos from San ͟ ͟ ͟ go County, California, through most of Baja California. *Parts*

289

Used Whole plant. *Preparation* Powdered plant applied to skin or made into tea for topical wash. *Herb Uses* Anti-inflammatory, astringent, and antimicrobial for rashes, bites, burns, and skin infections; applied to gums for inflammation. *Comments* Also called California Copperleaf, this is a low-growing, copper-red shrub used widely by Mexicans and Native Americans. It works remarkably well for all topical uses and is also used internally, although I have not utilized it this way. Some members of the Euphorbia family are potentially toxic, so it is probably best to only use the herb topically.

CALAMUS or SWEET FLAG (*Acorus calamus*). *Distribution* Swamps, bogs, and shallow lakes from northwestern Montana through Alberta, the Yukon, and eastern British Columbia. *Parts Used* Rhizome and reedlike leaves. *Preparation* Fresh Root Tincture, 1:2, Dried Root Tincture, 1:5, 60% alcohol, 15 to 45 drops, up to three times a day. Dried leaves to flavor tea or use for smudging. *Herb Uses* An aromatic bitter, one of the best herbs for indigestion, gas, hiatus hernia pain, and colon cramps; has an antihistaminelike effect for head colds and hay fever. *References* Foster.

GIANT HYSSOP (*Agastache* spp.). *Distribution* East side of the Cascades in Oregon and Washington, into British Columbia; east to Alberta and south to Nevada; north coastal range and Sierras of California; middle mountain slopes. *Parts Used* Whole plant, dried Method A. *Preparation* Standard Infusion, 2 to 4 fluid ounces or a strong cup of tea, up to four times a day. *Herb Uses* Astringent, diaphoretic, moderate sedative; very similar to Hedge Nettle in use. *Comments* Some strains do not taste good, but some Giant Hyssop can taste lovely, sort of anise-minty. *References* Foster.

AGAVE (*Agave* spp.) *Distribution* Mojave and Colorado deserts south into all of Baja California; the southern edge of the Great Basin in Nevada. *Parts Used* Leaf and root. *Preparation* Dry Leaf Tincture, 1:2, ¼ teaspoon in water; dried leaf as a simple tea; Dried Root Tincture, 1:5, 50% alcohol, ¼ teaspoon in warm water, up to three times a day. *Herb Uses* For foul burps from stomach fermentation, chronic constipation, or as a simple diuretic for water retention, use the leaf preparations; use the root tincture as an antiarthritic when joints hurt from barometric pressure changes. *References* Moore (Mountain), Moore (Desert).

AGRIMONY (*Agrimonia striata, A. gryposepala*). *Distribution* A streamside plant in California and Oregon; a meadow plant further north in southeast British Columbia across into Alberta, and south into the Rockies. *Parts Used* Whole plant, dried Method A. *Preparation* Standard Infusion, 2 to 4 fluid ounces, as needed. *Herb Uses* Astringent, anti-inflammatory, used for GI irritation, diarrhea, irritated gallbladder or bile ducts. *References* Foster, Moore (Mountain).

COUCH GRASS (*Agropyron repens*). *Distribution* Urban and rural weed, erratic and frustrating. *Parts Used* Lateral rhizomes, sometimes the stems (inferior). *Preparation* Cold Infusion, 2 to 4 fluid ounces, up to four times a day. *Herb Uses* A simple diuretic to increase volume of urine by stimulating sodium excretion. *References* Foster.

TREE OF HEAVEN (*Ailanthus altissima*). *Distribution* Naturalized tree found in urban and rural ditches and near streams, often growing as a dense thicket of large shrubs. *Parts Used* Bark, fruit (samaras). *Preparation* Cold Infusion, 1 to

2 fluid ounces, up to five times a day (preferably lower doses, since large amounts can cause dizziness). *Herb Uses* An effective antiprotozoa agent for amebiasis and giardiasis; inhibits pinworms; somewhat antiviral against pulmonary echoviruses. *Comments* A relative of *Castela* and *Quassia*, but native to China; thought by some to have been planted by Chinese settlers, as it is a widely used TCM medicine. We might use *Quassia* for "Montezuma's revenge" when traveling far south; I imagine that Chinese immigrants might have wanted *Ailanthus* for "white barbarian's revenge" on this continent. The main thing is, the further from home you travel, the more alien the bugs are on your food. Traveler's diarrhea is a kinder, less xenophobic term. *References* Foster.

LADIES MANTLE (*Alchemilla occidentalis*). *Distribution* From southern British Columbia to central California, eastern Washington and eastern Oregon, in lower meadows. *Parts Used* Whole annual plant, dried. *Preparation* A tea as needed. *Herb Uses* Simple Rose family astringent, for GI inflammation, diarrhea, heavy menses, or as a douche, enema, or eyewash.

ALDER (*Alnus* spp.). *Distribution* Waterways, streams, and seeps (everywhere there is water and forest) from coastal Alaska to southern California. *Parts Used* Leaves, bark. *Preparation* Strong Decoction, 1 to 2 fluid ounces, up to four times a day; dried leaf for a simple tea (blech!); both for external washes. *Herb Uses* Astringent, mildly heating; like Yellow Dock or Walnut, it helps tonify the small intestinal lining to improve food absorption and fat metabolism. *References* Foster, Schofield, Willard.

HOLLYHOCK (*Althea rosea*). *Distribution* Cultivated plant gone wild. *Parts Used* Leaves, roots. *Preparation* Cold Infusion of root, as needed; leaves as infusion. *Herb Uses* Emollient and demulcent for all membranes; leaves as a soothing poultice; root for urethral irritation and as immunostimulant for GI and lungs. *References* Moore (Desert).

RAGWEED or BURSAGE (*Ambrosia* spp.). *Distribution* Mostly weeds of waste places, from southern British Columbia to Baja California and everywhere else. *Parts Used* Herb in flower, dried Method A. *Preparation* Standard Infusion 1 to 2 fluid ounces, up to five times a day. *Herb Uses* For head colds, allergies, and moderate histamine reactions, replacing Eyebright (*Euphrasia*) in most circumstances. A very efficient astringent where there are copious secretions with inflammation. *References* Foster.

SCARLET PIMPERNEL (*Anagalis arvensis*). *Distribution* Gardens and vacant lots from Vancouver Island south and east. *Parts Used* Whole plant, dried Method B. *Preparation* Standard Infusion, 1 to 2 fluid ounces, up to three times a day. *Herb Uses* A simple laxative for water retention and poor fat digestion. *Comments* Short-term use.

YERBA MANSA (*Anemopsis californica*). *Distribution* Saline seeps, swamps, and hot springs through California and the southern half of Nevada; formerly common in the Central and Imperial valleys, but unusable because of agribusiness pollution—only use from clean localities! *Parts Used* Roots and leaves, dried Method B. *Preparation* Fresh Plant Tincture, 1:2, Dry Plant Tincture, 1:5, 60% alcohol, 30 to 60 drops, up to five times a day; or a tea made in any fashion. *Herb Uses* Use for mouth, gum, and throat inflammations, stomach ulcers, urinary tract irritation, arthritis aggravated by diet, and as a douche, enema, or topical wash. Anti-inflammatory, antimicrobial, both astringent and heating like Bayberry. It is a substitute for Goldenseal with mucous membrane problems and would deserve a major monograph in this book except for the fact that most of its California range has been polluted by agribusiness. The last time I was in the Kestersen Wildlife Refuge in California (to get some Yerba Mansa) was in 1981, and I found the birds dead, the plants dying, and the people sick and moving away. *References* Moore (Desert).

DOGBANE (*Apocynum* spp.). *Distribution* Middle British Columbia and Alberta, south and east in agricultural areas, irrigation ditches, alongside rivers and streams, and in rural waste places. *Parts Used* Dried rhizomes and roots. *Preparation* Ground root for topical use, Dry Root Tincture, 1:5, 50% alcohol, 5 to 20 drops, up to three times a day, used with care. *Herb Uses* Vasodilating diuretic with dry skin, constipation, *and* water retention. Topical for sweat-inducing counterirritant. The tea for stimulation of scalp. *Comments* Use internally with care. *References* Foster, Moore (Mountain), Willard.

BURDOCK (*Arctium* spp.). *Distribution* Eurasian weed spread by burrs, found in waste places with rich but compacted alluvial sediment, and with livestock now or in the past. *Parts Used* Roots and seeds. *Preparation* Root as Cold Infusion, 2 to 4 fluid ounces, up to four times a day; Fresh Root Tincture, 1:2, Dry Root Tincture, 1:5, 50% alcohol, ¼ to ½ teaspoon, up to four times a day. Seeds as tincture, 1:5, 60% alcohol, 10 to 30 drops, up to five times a day. *Herb Uses* Use the root preparation for IgE allergies, elevated uric acid, water retention, and "blood purifying." Use the seeds for water retention with high blood pressure from sodium retention, also for pre-eclampsia in the last trimester. *References* Foster, Moore (Mountain), Willard.

ASPARAGUS (*Asparagus officinalis*). *Distribution* Old farms, hedgerows, and alluvial meadows, from southern British Columbia to central California eastwards, wherever it has become an escaped plant from cultivation. *Parts Used* Rhizomes and roots. *Preparation* Fresh Root Tincture, 1:2, Dry Root Tincture, 1:5, 50% alcohol, ¼ to ½ teaspoon in a cup of water, up to three times a day. *Herb Uses* Use as a simple diuretic, especially for high blood pressure, as a sodium remover, and for anabolic mesomorphs with overacidic urine. *References* Foster, Moore (Mountain).

ASTRAGALUS (*Astragalus americanus*). *Distribution* Old-growth spruce forests from northern Wyoming through Montana, Alberta, eastern British Columbia, the Yukon; into central Alaska, on both sides of the Cordillera; northeast Asia. *Parts Used* Roots and stems. *Preparation* Cold Infusion or Standard Decoction, 2 to 3 fluid ounces, up to three times a day; Fresh Root Tincture, 1:2, 30 to 60 drops, up to four times a day. *Herb Uses* As immune tonic, antimicrobial, and tonic for hyperglycemia and hypertension. *Comments* This species of *Astragalus* is identical or nearly identical to *A. membranaceus*, the main cultivated species used in Chinese herbal medicine, and TLC (thin-layer chromatography) tests have shown it to have the same general constituents as the Chinese plant. *References* Willard.

WILD OATS (*Avena fatua*). *Distribution* A European weed grain found in all farming and waste areas, from inner cities to old Hutterite homesteads, from the Alaska Panhandle, south into Baja California, and eastwards. *Parts Used* Fresh unripe seeds, filled with latex not yet turned to starch. *Preparation* Fresh Seed Tincture, 1:2, 10 to 20 drops, up to six times a day. *Herb Uses* Nervous exhaustion from adrenalin stress, intoxicant overuse. *References* Moore (Desert).

BIRCH (*Betula* spp.). *Distribution* Found in wet localities in the southern Sierras and Siskiyou Mountains of California, central and eastern Nevada, southeastern and northeastern Oregon; the Washington Cascades; and the deep forests of British Columbia and Alberta. Paper Birch *owns* the north country, from the Bitterroots, northern Idaho, to northeastern Washington, and to the Aleutians. *Parts Used and Preparation* See Alder (*Alnus* spp.). *Herb Uses* See Alder, with the addition of anti-inflammatory and analgesic effects from the salicylates found in Birch. *Comments* The two birches interbreed. *References* Foster, Moore (Mountain), Schofield, Willard.

PRODIGIOSA (*Brickellia grandiflora*). *Distribution* Mountains and moist lower slopes of the East Cascades in Washington and Oregon, east and south through the Rockies, intermountains, coastal ranges, and the Sierras in California, and so forth. Widespread in clean localities. *Parts Used* Whole plant, dried Method A. *Preparation* Standard Infusion, 2 to 4 fluid ounces, up to three times a day. *Herb Uses* Type II diabetes. *Comments* Morning and afternoon doses are widely used by Mexicans, New Mexicans, and Native Americans. Also called *Hamula*. *References* Moore (Desert).

BUPLEURUM (*Bupleurum americanum*). *Distribution* High mountains even above timberline in north Idaho, northwestern Montana; in grasslands in Alberta, eastern British Columbia, up through the Yukon into most of Alaska. Stunted in lower forty-eight states, tall in the north country. *Parts Used* Whole plant, especially root. *Preparation* Fresh Plant Tincture, 1:2, 30 to 60 drops, up to four times a day; Standard Infusion 2 to 4 fluid ounces, up to four times a day. *Herb Uses* Bile-stimulating laxative, antihistaminic, to lower fever, and as a tonic for high blood pressure and Type II diabetes in the chunky mesomorph. *Comments* Chinese medicine uses a close relative in many tonics, and the constituents of the two Bupleurums are virtually identical.

ELEPHANT TREE (*Bursera microphylla*). *Distribution* A little bit in southeast California; southwest Arizona, and *all* the way down both sides of Baja California. A desert tree. *Parts Used* Twigs, foliage, and gum. *Preparation* Tincture of Resin, 1:5, 75% alcohol, Fresh Twig Tincture, 1:2, 10 to 20 drops, up to four times a day. *Herb Uses* As an immunostimulant for lungs and lower urinary tract; applied to gums and skin abrasions as its relative Myrrh. The gum makes a fine incense. *References* Moore (Desert).

SHEPHERD'S PURSE (*Capsella bursa-pastoris*). *Distribution* Vacant lots, suburbs, pastures, grazing pastures, and city parks from central Alaska, south and east. *Parts Used* Whole herb. *Preparation* Fresh Plant Tincture, 1:2, 30 to 60 drops, up to four times a day; recent Dried Herb Tincture, 1:5, 50% alcohol, similarly. *Herb Uses* Urinary tract astringent, uric acid diuretic for hyperuricemia; hemostatic for hematuria, excess menses, and so forth; oxytocin agonist for postpartum bleeding or difficult placenta delivery. *References* Foster, Moore (Desert), Schofield, Willard.

CENTAURY (*Centaurium/Erythraea* spp.). *Distribution* The various species are widespread along the east side of the Cascades; through Nevada, Arizona, California, Baja California, usually in moist places, seeps, and alkaline bogs. *Parts Used* Whole plant, dried Method A. *Preparation* Fresh Plant Tincture, 1:2, 10 to 20 drops, Cold Infusion, 1 to 2 fluid ounces, both ten minutes before meals. *Herb Uses* Bitter tonic, same as Gentian.

EPAZOTE or AMERICAN WORMSEED (*Chenopodium ambrosioides*). *Distribution* In Oregon and Washington, a city and agricultural weed; in California and Baja California, common near coasts and valleys in all circumstances. *Parts Used* Dried herb, cleaned from stems. *Preparation* Standard Infusion, 2 to 3 fluid ounces, up to three times a day, no more than one day at a time. *Herb Uses* The tea for suppressed, crampy menses; as a spice for bean dishes, dark chile powders. *Comments* A purported abortifacient, it seldom works and is dangerous. The use of the seeds for roundworms can be effective; such a use is not a trivial matter, and it is necessary to take great care. *References* Moore (Desert).

DESERT WILLOW (*Chilopsis linearis*). *Distribution* Inland deserts of California, Nevada, Arizona, and Baja California, always along water drainage where there is underground moisture. *Parts Used* Leaves, twigs, bark, flowers, and pods. *Preparation* Standard or Cold Infusion, 3 to 6 fluid ounces, up to three times a day; powder for topical use. *Herb Uses* Reliable antifungal and general antimicrobial; substitute for Pau D'Arco in candidiasis; can be used as a douche, enema, skin remedy, or first aid. *Comments* An effective, little-known herb. *References* Moore (Desert).

PIPSISSEWA (*Chimaphila umbellata*). *Distribution* Old-growth or second-growth forests in shady chuff, from the San Bernardino and San Jacinto mountains in southern California to coastal Alaska, eastwards. *Parts Used* Aerial parts, spring through fall. *Preparation* Fresh Herb Tincture, 1:2, 20 to 50 drops, up to four times a day; Standard Infusion, 4 to 8 fluid ounces, up to three times a day. *Herb Uses* Fresh tincture for chronic dry skin, inability to sweat, and suppressed eruptions. The tea for concentrated urine with urethritis and cystitis, mucus in the urine, or chronic ache on urination or BPH. *References* Foster, Moore (Mountain).

CHICORY (*Cichorium intybus*). *Distribution* Eurasian weed widely established in many areas from southern British Columbia to southern California, eastwards. *Parts Used* Dried roots. *Preparation* Strong Decoction, 3 to 6 fluid ounces, up to four times a day. *Herb Uses* Like Dandelion root, for sodium retention; to stimulate bile secretions in constipation, without irritating liver. *Comments* Spring roots can be split, dried, roasted, and ground for mixing with coffee or as a substitute. The diuretic effects remain after roasting. *References* Foster, Moore (Mountain), Willard.

CLEMATIS (*Clematis* spp.). *Distribution* Rural and forested areas and thickets from Alaska to Baja California. *Parts Used* Whole leafing vine. *Preparation* Fresh Plant Tincture, 1:2, 10 to 20 drops, as needed; Standard Infusion, 2 to 6 fluid ounces, up to three times a day. *Herb Uses* Fresh poultice for bad joints; take internally for migraines not responding to vasoconstriction. *References* Foster, Moore (Desert), Willard.

CANADIAN FLEABANE (*Conyza/Erigeron canadensis*). *Distribution* Widespread from coastal British Columbia to Baja California, in pasture and grazing areas; also urban weed. *Parts Used* Flowering plant, dried Method A. *Preparation* Standard Infusion 2 to 4 fluid ounces, up to four times a day. *Herb Uses* Use as an astringent hemostatic, especially in chronic conditions, ulcerative colitis, and so forth; otherwise use the same as Oxeye Daisy. *References* Foster, Moore (Desert), Willard.

CORAL ROOT (*Corallorhiza* spp.). *Distribution* Moist chuff, coniferous forests throughout the West, from southeast Alaska to southern California eastwards. *Parts Used* Roots and lower stems. *Preparation* Fresh Plant Tincture, 1:2, ½ to 1 teaspoon; Cold Infusion, 4 to 8 fluid ounces, reheated, both up to four times a day. *Herb Uses* Sedative diaphoretic in fevers with hot, moist skin; a first aid in bacterial infections with fever, to keep the temperature down through sweating until medical attention is possible. *References* Foster, Moore (Mountain).

RED OSIER or DOGWOOD (*Cornus* spp.). *Distribution* From central Alaska to southern California in moist mountains, along streams. *Parts Used* Leaves, bark, roots, and stems. *Preparation and Herb Uses* Same as Bunchberry (*Cornus canadensis;* see main text). *Comments* The bark of Red Osier (*C. stolonifera*) is the Red Willow used in Native American ceremonial smoking mixtures. *References* Foster, Schofield, Willard.

JIMSON WEED (*Datura* spp.). *Distribution* Weed found in central valleys of Washington and Oregon occasionally; common in California, Nevada, Arizona, Baja California, and so forth. *Parts Used* All parts potent (and potentially toxic); dried leaf most practical. *Preparation* Powdered herb topical, Salve, Method A: Dry Herb Tincture, 1:10, 60% alcohol, 3 to 12 drops, up to five times a day (*use with care*); crushed leaves mixed with Western Coltsfoot for smoking in bronchial spasms. *Herb Uses* Topical poultice for local analgesic; tincture for liniment; internally *with care* for hay fever, really bad intestinal cramps (see Silk Tassel); smoked as mentioned; salve for hemorrhoids. *Comments* Nasty stuff. *References* Foster, Moore (Mountain).

WILD CARROT or QUEEN ANNE'S LACE (*Daucus carota*). *Distribution* Frequent weed in moist localities, along roadsides, and in pastures. Unpredictable. *Parts Used* Dried roots, ripe seeds. *Preparation* Root: Standard Infusion, 2 to 6 fluid ounces, up to four times a day; Dry Seed Tincture, 1:5, 60% alcohol, 20 to 60 drops, up to four times a day. *Herb Uses* Tea and tincture as simple diuretic, for fluid retention, especially after weather or air pressure changes; tincture as a menstrual stimulant. *References* Foster.

TEASEL (*Dipsacus sylvestris*). *Distribution* River valleys and coastal areas from southern British Columbia to the Sacramento Delta, eastwards. Eurasian native. *Parts Used* Dried flowering herb. *Preparation* Standard Infusion, 2 to 4 fluid ounces, up to four times a day. *Herb Uses* The tea is a bitter tonic when indigestion is accompanied by dry skin and constipation. Take twenty to thirty minutes before meals and before retiring.

SUNDEW (*Drosera* spp.) *Distribution* Low nitrogen bogs and snow ponds. Sundew is very sporadic in the western lower forty-eight states but common in Canada and Alaska. *Parts Used* Whole fresh plant, cleaned as well as possible. This sounds easy, but imagine trying to wash off a huge, wet Gummi Bear covered in sand. *Preparation* Fresh Herb Tincture, 1:2, 5 to 15 drops, up to five times a day. *Herb Uses* For dry, spasmodic, and explosive coughing, with dry and sensitive membranes. *Comments* If Sundew were not so scarce in the western U.S., it would be a full monograph in this book. *References* Foster, Schofield, Willard.

HORSETAIL or SCOURING RUSH (*Equisetum* spp.). *Distribution* Wherever there is water, from Alaska to Baja California. *Parts Used* Whole herb, dried. *Preparation* Standard Infusion, 2 to 4 fluid ounces, up to five times a day. *Herb Uses* As a diuretic and kidney tonic; to strengthen the mesenchyme in the kidneys, lungs, and the liver. The tea is a good hair rinse. *References* Foster, Moore (Mountain), Schofield, Willard.

TURKEY MULLEIN (*Eremocarpus setigerus*). *Distribution* Baja California, north to southern Washington; east to the Mojave Desert and southwest Nevada; usually in lower, dry areas, especially along roadsides. *Parts Used* Whole plant, dried Method B. *Preparation* Fresh Vinegar Tincture, 1:2, Standard Infusion, 2 to 3 fluid ounces, up to three times a day or as a bath. *Herb Uses* Vinegar as liniment for sore intercostals, pleurisylike pain; applied to forehead for sick headaches, hangovers. A partial bath with some tea will break any fever. *References* Moore (Desert).

STORKSBILL or ALFILERILLO (*Erodium cicutarium*). *Distribution* Valleys, foothills, and desert roadsides, from southeast British Columbia to Baja California; widespread. *Parts Used* Whole plant, dried. *Preparation* Standard Infusion, 4 to 6 fluid ounces, or a simple strong tea. *Herb Uses* Systemic astringent, mild hemostatic, and diuretic; useful for stomachache, diarrhea, menstrual hemorrhage, and water retention. *References* Foster, Moore (Mountain).

EUCALYPTUS (*Eucalyptus globulus*). *Distribution* California, southern Nevada, and so forth; out of major frost, wherever it has been planted and naturalized. *Parts Used* Young leaves from new branches or suckers. *Preparation* Standard Infusion, 2 to 4 fluid ounces, or as a bath. *Herb Uses* Diaphoretic, disinfecting diuretic; for any respiratory distress, either drunk, steam-inhaled, or as a bath. *References* Moore (Desert).

BURNING BUSH or WESTERN WAHOO (*Euonymus occidentalis*). *Distribution* Lower, clean river drainage west of the Cascades, from southern Washington through Oregon; coastal range to Santa Cruz, California; disjunct in the San Bernardino Mountains; and elsewhere in southern California. *Parts Used* Bark of larger stems, and roots. *Preparation* Cold Infusion, 2 to 3 fluid ounces, up to three times a day. *Herb Uses* Bile stimulant for nonstone gallbladder pain; for steatorrhea with looseness or light-colored constipation. Use with care, as it may cause nausea in excess. *References* Foster (on related species), Moore (Mountain).

EYEBRIGHT (*Euphrasia mollis, E. sibirica*). *Distribution* Coastal and inland meadows; semiparasitic, usually on grasses, from Siberia, across Alaska, the Yukon, down through inland British Columbia; some around Puget Sound; through Alberta, sparingly. *Parts Used* Whole plant, fresh or dry. *Preparation* Fresh Plant

Tincture, 1:2, 30 to 90 drops, up to four times a day. Dry herb for tea (inferior), as needed. *Herb Uses* For acute head cold, hay fever, with lots of acrid secretions and red eyes. The tincture is best taken internally; the eyewash is no better than that of a hundred other plants and a waste of this little dainty. Internally it is an anti-inflammatory, antihistaminic, and hepatic astringent. *References* Foster, Schofield.

FENNEL (*Foeniculum vulgare*). *Distribution* Common escapee along the coast from Puget Sound to San Diego County. *Parts Used* Seeds and foliage. *Preparation* Fresh Seed Tincture, 1:2; dried seeds for tea; leaves for spice, tea, or flavor additive. *Herb Uses* Indigestion, dyspepsia, simple stomachache, colic, as needed, in whatever form appropriate; an aromatic anesthetic and antispasmodic. *References* Foster.

OCOTILLO (*Fouqueria splendens*). *Distribution* Baja California, southern California desert hillsides, eastwards to Texas. *Parts Used* Stem bark. *Preparation* Fresh Bark Tincture, 1:2, 10 to 20 drops, up to four times a day. *Herb Uses* Lymphagogue, especially for impaired fat absorption with pelvic congestion, hemorrhoids, and so forth. *References* Moore (Desert).

WILD STRAWBERRY (*Fragaria* spp.). *Distribution* Moist places with acid soil, the mountains in California, descending to lowlands as far north as the Aleutian Islands. *Parts Used* Leaves and stems, dried Method B. *Preparation* A simple tea or a Standard Infusion as an isotonic wash for eyes, or as a douche, or enema. *Herb Uses* A simple Rose family astringent, with the same uses as Raspberry, Potentilla, Rose, and so forth. *References* Foster, Moore (Mountain), Schofield, Willard.

ASH (*Fraxinus* spp.). *Distribution* Ashes are found along streams and river bottoms from southern Washington, south to northern and central Baja California; east into southern Nevada and southern Utah. Mostly coastal. *Parts Used* Bark and leaves. *Preparation* Bark, Cold Infusion, 2 to 4 fluid ounces, up to three times a day. Leaves, Standard Infusion for topical use. *Herb Uses* The bark is tonic to intestinal tract secretions when deficient and when digestion is slow and generally inefficient; astringent to structure; stimulating to circulation. Leaf tea is astringent, antifungal, and stimulating, and is used for skin washes and baths. *References* Foster, Willard.

FREMONTIA or CALIFORNIA SLIPPERY ELM (*Fremontia californica*). *Distribution* Dry hillsides between 3,000 and 6,000 feet, along the Sierras and inner ranges of southern California mountains; Mogollon Rim in Arizona; Baja California; east side of the San Pedro Martirs. *Parts Used* Bark, all year; leaves before summer. *Preparation* Simple poultice; Cold Infusion of bark; Standard Infusion of leaves, all as needed. *Herb Uses* Major-league emollient-demulcent; use wherever Slippery Elm or Marshmallow is called for—for sore throat, vomiting, colitis, gastric ulcers, douche, enema, and so forth. *References* Moore (Mountain).

CLEAVERS (*Galium aparine*, etc.). *Distribution* Anywhere, from early spring in the lowlands to midsummer in the high mountains. Spread by little burrs, this naturalized plant can occur in many areas, from Alaska, south and east. *Parts*

Used Whole, matted herb. *Preparation* Fresh Plant Juice, 1 to 2 fluid ounces, up to four times a day; dried recent herb; lots of tea as needed. *Herb Uses* Fresh juice for gastric, mouth, or skin ulcers; tea as a simple diuretic. *References* Foster, Moore (Mountain), Schofield, Willard.

GENTIAN (*Gentiana* spp.). *Distribution* All high mountains. *Parts Used* All parts. *Preparation* Fresh Plant Tincture, 1:2, Dry Plant Tincture, 1:5, 50% alcohol, 10 to 20 drops before meals. *Herb Uses* The bitter tonic. *References* Foster, Moore (Mountain).

GERANIUM or CRANESBILL (*Geranium* spp.). *Distribution* Meadows, open forests, and in disturbed soil throughout our area, as far north as Alaska and south Yukon. *Parts Used* Herb, roots. *Preparation* Dry Plant Tincture, 1:5, 50% alcohol, 10% glycerin, ½ to 1 teaspoon, as needed; Strong Decoction, 1 to 4 fluid ounces, as needed. Powdered plant for topical first aid, hemostatic. *Herb Uses* For ulcers, diarrhea, bleeding gums, excess uterine bleeding, as a gargle, and so forth. The tea can be used as a douche for simple vaginitis. Use the powder as indicated. *References* Foster, Moore (Mountain), Schofield, Willard.

AVENS (*Geum* spp.). *Distribution* Meadows, moist woods, and alluvial flats, from Alaska to Baja California. It doesn't like pollution too much, so look away from cities and agribusiness. *Parts Used* Whole herb, dried as needed. *Preparation* Standard Infusion, as needed. *Herb Uses* A simple Rose family astringent, used like Raspberry, Rose, Potentilla, Agrimony, and so forth. *References* Foster, Moore (Mountain).

LICORICE ROOT (*Glycyrrhiza lepidota*). *Distribution* Alluvial gravel, river- and drainage-banks, even waste places, from southeast British Columbia, mostly east of the Cascades and Sierra Nevada, and to the Rockies. *Parts Used* Roots and rhizomes, dried. *Preparation* Strong Decoction, 1 to 3 fluid ounces, up to three times a day. *Herb Uses* For adrenalin-stress individuals with frequent urination, dry constipation, frequent dry bronchial and sinus mucosa, and dry mouth. For gastric ulcers, due to its well-documented anti-inflammatory effects on lining. Use roots chewed for sore throat. *Comments* This species is seldom sweet like the Eurasian and Chinese Licorice roots, but it is also less likely to cause the degree of sodium retention they can induce. *References* Foster, Moore (Mountain), Willard.

RATTLESNAKE PLANTAIN (*Goodyera* spp.). *Distribution* G. *repens* grows from central Alaska, through British Columbia and Alberta, down the Cordillera. G. *rotundifolia* grows down the coast to Monterey and Tulare counties in California and eastwards. Found in lower, shaded, old-growth forests, often with Pipsissewa. *Parts Used* Whole plant, especially the roots. *Preparation and Herb Uses* Fresh plant; rehydrated dry plant as soothing topical poultice; tea drunk to soothe sore throat, coughing. *References* Foster, Moore (Mountain).

GRINDELIA (*Grindelia* spp.). *Distribution* Widespread from the Alaska Panhandle to northern Baja California and eastwards, usually at lower altitudes. *Parts Used* Upper flowering branches. *Preparation* Fresh Plant Tincture, 1:2; Dry Herb Tincture, 1:5, 70% alcohol; Standard Infusion, 2 to 3 fluid ounces. *Herb Uses* For any bronchial conditions with thick viscous mucus, difficult expectoration; bronchial asthma with tachycardia. Fresh plant tincture for poison ivy/oak, diluted topically. *References* Foster, Moore (Mountain), Willard.

ESCOBA DE LA VIBORA (*Gutierrezia sarothrae*, etc.). *Distribution* East Cascades through to Cordillera; plains, Central Valley, coastal flats, and inland desert in California, eastwards. If the area is dry, flat, overgrazed, and boring, you'll probably find Escoba. *Parts Used* Flowering stems, bundled and dried. *Preparation* A bundle, steeped for tea in a quart or two of water. *Herb Uses* Use the tea, added to a bath, for arthritis and muscle-tendon pain. *References* Moore (Mountain), Moore (Desert).

AMERICAN PENNYROYAL (*Hedeoma* spp.). *Distribution* Eastern Mojave Desert, into Nevada, Utah, Arizona, north and east. *Parts Used* Flowering stems. *Preparation* Fresh Plant Tincture, 1:2; dried herb for Standard Infusion. *Herb Uses* See European Pennyroyal in main text. *References* Foster, Moore (Mountain).

COW PARSNIP (*Heracleum lanatum*). *Distribution* Cold, wet areas, either high mountains and creeks in southern areas or seasides in the northwestern areas; commonplace to Alaska, eastwards. *Parts Used* Fresh seeds and fresh roots. *Preparation* Fresh Seed or Root Tincture, 1:2. *Herb Uses* Use the seed tincture for toothache, gum abcess, applied topically. The fresh root tincture is used to stimulate nerve growth after injury. *References* Moore (Mountain), Schofield, Willard.

CAMPHOR WEED or MEXICAN ARNICA (*Heterotheca subaxillaris*). *Distribution* Native plant usually growing as a weed, mainly in the southern half of California and Baja California, east to Arizona; southern Nevada. *Parts Used* Whole flowering plant. *Preparation* Fresh Plant Tincture, 1:2, Dry Plant Tincture, 1:5, 60% alcohol, both external; Standard Infusion, 2 to 4 fluid ounces or topical. *Herb Uses* The tea is anti-inflammatory, antifungal, and antimicrobial externally; it is used like Arnica for injuries. *References* Moore (Desert).

HOPS (*Humulus lupulus, H. americanus*). *Distribution* The first is the European plant of commerce, frequently found growing wild in the Northwest. The second is native to wet canyons and streams, from Nevada, Utah, and Arizona eastwards. *Parts Used* Ripe "flowers" (strobiles) and the whole last yard of summer branches. *Preparation* Fresh Flower Tincture, 1:2, 30 to 90 drops as needed; *very* recent dried strobiles, Cold Infusion, 2 to 4 fluid ounces as needed; whole vine ends, dried, powdered as Salve, Method A or dusted on skin. *Herb Uses* Sedative for insomnia with GI pain and physical agitation; also for nervous stomach. The herb is an efficient antimicrobial (as well as the flowers) but lacks the sedative kick, so use on the skin. *References* Foster, Moore (Mountain).

HENBANE (*Hyoscyamus niger*). *Distribution* Sporadic naturalized plant found in pastures, and along hedgerows and roadsides in Oregon, Washington, and southern British Columbia; common in Idaho, Montana. *Parts Used* Upper plant, including seeds and flowers. *Preparation and Herb Uses* Same as Jimson Weed (*Datura*).

JEWEL WEED or TOUCH ME NOT (*Impatiens* spp.). *Distribution* Some naturalized, some native, they are found in moist places, usually in swamps, and along lakesides and waterways, from the north half of Oregon to central Alaska, and eastwards. There is a little in California, but the stands are threatened. *Parts Used, Preparation, and Herb Uses* Fresh juice, leaves for poison ivy and skin rashes. *References* Foster, Schofield.

BLUE FLAG (*Iris missouriensis*). *Distribution* Cool mountain meadows with water near the surface in the big southern California ranges, Sierras, and Cascades; through inland British Columbia; the Great Basin; and the Rocky Mountains. *Parts Used* Rhizomes, dried and cleaned. *Preparation* Tincture, 1:5, 80% alcohol, 5 to 10 drops, up to four times a day. *Use with care:* best in formulas; 1 to 2 #00 capsules, three times a day. *Herb Uses* A stimulant to liver bile, pancreatic, and intestinal membrane secretions; best for GI dryness, with light, marbly feces, poor fat digestion, and overprocessed diet inducing labile blood sugar. Good preparation for dietary changes. *References* Foster, Moore (Mountain), Schofield.

CALIFORNIA WALNUT (*Juglans californica, J. hindsii*). *Distribution* The first occurs along moist waterways from Santa Barbara to San Diego counties; the second occurs around the Sacramento Delta; planted extensively elsewhere. *Parts Used* Leaves. *Preparation* Fresh Leaf Tincture, 1:2, ½ to 1 teaspoon, up to four times a day; Standard Infusion, 2 to 4 fluid ounces, similarly. *Herb Uses* Astringent and tonic to ileum and colon, helping to improve mucous membrane absorption of digested nutrients; ileocecal congestion, steatorrhea. *References* Foster.

JUNIPER (*Juniperus communis*). *Distribution* This prickly mat-bush is found from northern California and northern Nevada to central Alaska and southern Yukon, as well as parts in between and east, usually in the higher and middle mountains. In the rest of California, there are California and Sierra Junipers, moderately sized, scaly trees. *Parts Used* Ripe berries and dried needles. *Preparation* Berry Tincture, 1:5, 75% alcohol, 20 to 40 drops, Standard Infusion of crushed berries or needles, 2 to 3 fluid ounces, both up to four times a day. Chew the berries before meals for achlorhydria or in place of a snack to lower blood sugar from adrenalin hyperglycemia. *Herb Uses* Besides chewing berries, other uses are as a urinary tract disinfectant/diuretic for urethritis in acid pH urine (usually sexually transmitted) and in combination with Yerba Santa. *References* Foster, Moore (Mountain), Schofield, Willard.

RHATANY (*Krameria Grayi, K. parviflora*). *Distribution* Both are found as semi-parasitic shrubs in the Mojave, Colorado, and Baja California middle deserts; Nevada and further east. *Parts Used* Roots and blooming stems. *Preparation* Fresh Plant Tincture, 1:2, Dry Tincture, 1:5, 50% alcohol, 10% glycerin, both 20 to 50 drops, up to five times a day; Strong Decoction, 1 to 3 fluid ounces; or all used topically. *Herb Uses* World-class disinfectant astringent on any skin distress; use topically on gums; gargle for pharyngitis; use internally for chronic indigestion, moist mouth, or soft stools. *References* Moore (Desert).

WILD LETTUCE (*Lactuca* spp.). *Distribution* Anywhere in waste places and pastures from southern British Columbia, south and east. *Parts Used* Flowering stems, dried Method A. *Preparation* Standard Infusion as needed. *Herb Uses* Safe, feeble, but usable sedative and cough-suppressor for kids and sensitive adults. *References* Foster, Moore (Mountain).

CHAPARRAL or CREOSOTE BUSH (*Larrea tridentata*). *Distribution* The most common low desert shrub in the Colorado, Mojave, and Arizona deserts; Baja California. *Parts Used* Healthy leafy branches, dried Method A, garbled. *Preparation* Tincture, 1:5, 75% alcohol, 20 to 60 drops, up to three times a day; 1 to 2 #00 capsules, up to three times a day; Salve, Method B. *Herb Uses* Arthritis, allergies, and IgE-type conditions where diet aggravates notably; free-radical therapy when there are distinct problems in liver-fat metabolism. The salve is a strong antimicrobial and moderate sun block. *References* Moore (Desert).

MOTHERWORT (*Leonurus cardiaca*). *Distribution* Escaped garden herb, locally abundant in Oregon, Washington, and further east along the Cordillera. *Parts Used* Flowering herb. *Preparation* Fresh Tincture, 1:2, Dried Tincture, 1:5, 60% alcohol, 30 to 60 drops, up to four times a day; Standard Infusion of *recent* herb, 2 to 4 fluid ounces. *Herb Uses* Neuralgia, skin hypersensitivity, shingles, and herpes; crampy amenorrhea; thyroid stress, with rapid pulse and hypertension. *References* Foster.

OSHA or LOVAGE (*Ligusticum* spp.). *Distribution* Several species occur along the coastal ranges of California and the western slopes of the Sierra Nevada, but most of our *Ligusticums* ring the Great Basin, on the east side of the Sierras and Cascades, including the Blues, Selkirks, the major Nevada ranges, and all along the Rockies. *L. scoticum* is a circumboreal species, growing down into British Columbia and Alberta, but is an inferior medicine. *Parts Used* Roots, dried. *Preparation* Tincture, 1:5, 70% alcohol, 20 to 60 drops, up to five times a day; Cold Infusion of grated root, 2 to 6 fluid ounces, similarly. *Herb Uses* For dry, irritative cough; acute chest cold with dry membranes and fever; obstinate respiratory virus that doesn't peak properly. *References* Moore (Mountain), Schofield, Willard.

TOADFLAX (*Linaria vulgaris, L. dalmatica*). *Distribution* Both are widespread aliens but unpredictable. Spring moisture, cold winters, and disturbed land are their requirements. They are not common in California, and are more common in the Great Basin than the coastal drainage areas. *Parts Used* Whole herb, dried Method A. *Preparation* Standard Infusion, 2 to 4 fluid ounces, Tincture, 1:5, 50% alcohol, 20 to 40 drops, both up to three times a day. *Herb Uses* Liver stress from diet, malabsorption, alcohol, stress, or posthepatitis wobbles. By itself for short-term use, with other herbs for tonic use. *References* Foster, Moore (Mountain).

DESERT THORN or WOLF BERRY (*Lycium* spp.). *Distribution* Widespread in the California, Nevada, Baja California, and Arizona deserts. *Parts Used* Green branches in bloom. *Preparation* Fresh Plant Tincture, 1:2, 30 to 60 drops, up to four times a day; Standard Infusion, 2 to 3 fluid ounces, up to four times a day. *Herb Uses* Decongestant for head colds, hay fever. A Nightshade alkaloid plant, it is feebly active, good for colds, not appropriate for long-term use, and has no toxicity in the recommended amounts.

BUGLEWEED (*Lycopus* spp.). *Distribution* Major waterways throughout the West, usually in diverse plant communities, with Willows, Mints, Nettles, and so forth, from southern California to southern British Columbia, and along the Cordillera, both east and west drainages. *Parts Used* Whole aerial plant in bloom. *Preparation* Fresh Plant Tincture, 1:2, 15 to 40 drops, up to four times a day; almost inert after drying. *Herb Uses* Tachycardia; rapid GI transit time; arrhythmias and palpitations, often causing insomnia; all due to a mixture of adrenalin and subclinical thyroid stress. *References* Foster, Moore (Mountain).

MALLOW (*Malva neglecta*). *Distribution* Everywhere that has spring weeds. *Parts*

Used Whole herb, dried. *Preparation* Standard Infusion, as needed; powdered herb for poultice. *Herb Uses* Same as Hollyhock (*Althea*). *References* Foster, Moore (Mountain), Willard.

ALFALFA (*Medicago sativa*). *Distribution* Rich pastures, meadows, and so forth. Widespread escapee from cultivation. *Parts Used* Plant in flower, dried Method A and cleaned of large stems. *Preparation* Standard Infusion, as needed. *Herb Uses* A nutritional tea, high in usable, soluble electrolytes, helpful in inflammatory states, overly acidic urine, metabolic stress, and during recuperation from illness. *References* Foster, Moore (Mountain), Willard.

MARAVILLA or WILD FOUR O'CLOCK (*Mirabilis* spp.). *Distribution* Dry places in California and Baja California, usually in mountain rain shadows; from Kern County, California, east through the high and middle deserts of Nevada and Arizona; always in full plant communities, not waste places. *Parts Used* The large, tuberous roots. *Preparation* Fresh Root Tincture, 1:2, 30 to 60 drops before meals; a pea-sized chunk of the fresh or dry root chewed before meals. *Herb Uses* An appetite suppressant to lessen stomach capacity in early stages (one to two weeks) of a serious weight reduction program. It is mildly anesthetic to stomach lining and mildly stimulating. *References* Moore (Mountain).

CATNIP (*Nepeta cataria*). *Distribution* A garden escapee, often well established in canyons and along streams, secluded waste places, old gardens, and so forth. *Parts Used* Flowering herb, stem and all, dried Method A. *Preparation* Fresh Plant Tincture, 1:2, recent dried plant, 1:5, 50% alcohol, ¼ to 1 teaspoon, up to five times a day; Standard Infusion, 2 to 8 fluid ounces, or as needed. *Herb Uses* Flatulent colic, mild gastralgia with red-tipped tongue, general stomachache; combines well with Fennel seed for children; an often effective sedative for sick folks. *References* Foster, Moore (Mountain).

EVENING PRIMROSE (*Oenothera Hookeri*). *Distribution* This and several other upright, yellow-flowered biennial *Oenotheras* are found in nearly all middle and lower mountain slopes and meadows, from southern British Columbia to northern Baja California, and eastwards. *Parts Used* Roots and ripe seeds, dried. *Preparation* Strong Decoction, 2 to 6 fluid ounces, up to three times a day. The seeds, 1 to 2 teaspoons a day in food, ground to use, refrigerated whole. *Herb Uses* The root is an unpredictable tea; for some women with regular menstrual cramps it is a sustainable, long-term remedy for acute cramps; for others it has little value. The seeds are the easiest to gather of our natural GLA (gamma-linoleic acid) sources and will help prostaglandin imbalances in chronic dysmenorrhea, rheumatoid, or IgE-mediated allergies, as well as dry, eczematous skin. *References* Foster, Moore (Mountain), Willard.

PRICKLY PEAR CACTUS (*Opuntia basilaris*, etc.). *Distribution* Central California to Baja California; eastwards into southern Nevada, Arizona, and so forth—the predictable dry localities. *Parts Used* The skinned pads, juiced; the flowers, dried. *Preparation* Fresh juice, 2 to 4 fluid ounces, up to two times a day; flowers as infused tea, 2 to 3 per cup, up to three times a day. *Herb Uses* The juice for Type II diabetics (insulin-resistant), especially for plump individuals with dimply, edemic fat under the arms and between the thighs; for urethritis from irritation; flowers for flavonoids in treating capillary fragility. *References* Foster, Moore (Desert).

PINE (*Pinus* spp.). *Distribution* What can I say? Wherever there are forests. *Parts Used* Pitch and dried needles. *Preparation* Pitch or resin in Salve, Method B; the tea, Standard Infusion, 2 to 4 fluid ounces, up to three times a day, but not for more than several days. *Herb Uses* The salve is used as a stimulating dressing for splinters, foreign-body responses, and superficial, pus-forming infections. A piece of the resin can be chewed as a simple expectorant, and the tea is a pleasant diuretic and expectorant, although extended use can irritate weak kidneys. New-growth spring needles, shorter, juicier, and lighter-colored, are a good source of vitamin C. *References* Foster, Moore (Mountain), Willard.

PLANTAIN (*Plantago major, P. lanceolata*). *Distribution* A nearly universal weed from urban lawns to high mountain meadows. Streamside and meadow plants are large and upright, lawn Plantains are flattened, low enough to escape the lawn mower. *Parts Used* Fresh leaves and fresh juice. *Preparation* Fresh leaves as a poultice; juice internally, 1 to 2 teaspoons, up to three times a day, preserved with 30% alcohol, 35% glycerin, or simmered for twenty minutes with an equal volume of honey (Weiss). If using regularly for gastric ulcers, juice a bunch and freeze into cocktail-sized cubes; dose: one cube, melted, three times a day. *Herb Uses* Antimicrobial and anti-inflammatory topically (*P. lanceolata* is better); as an anti-inflammatory healer for gastric or skin ulcers (*P. major* is better). *References* Foster, Moore (Mountain), Schofield, Willard.

BISTORT ROOT (*Polygonum bistortoides*). *Distribution* Snow meadows from 10,000 feet in California to sea level in northern Alaska and the Yukon, and all points between and eastwards. *Parts Used* Roots and lower stems, dried. *Preparation* Strong Decoction, 1 to 4 fluid ounces; Tincture, 1:5, 50% alcohol, 10% glycerin, 30 to 90 drops, either up to four times a day. Both forms for topical use. *Herb Uses* See Alum Root in main text. *References* Foster, Moore (Mountain), Schofield, Willard.

ASPEN (*Populus tremuloides*). *Distribution* All forests from southern California (sporadic) to northern Alaska and the Yukon (sporadic), and everywhere in between (abundant). *Parts Used* Bark, dried. *Preparation* Strong Decoction, 2 to 4 fluid ounces, up to five times a day in acute conditions. *Herb Uses* Same uses as aspirin, but, since absorption is slower and more dispersed, it is frequently better tolerated (tastes terrible, however). *References* Foster, Moore (Mountain), Schofield, Willard.

POTENTILLA (*Potentilla* spp.). *Distribution* Widespread in meadows, along streams, and in forests throughout our area. *Parts Used* Whole herb, dried. *Preparation* Any infusion, as needed, internal and external. *Herb Uses* A Rose family astringent, used in the same way as Agrimony, Ladies Mantle, Raspberry leaves, and so forth. *References* Foster, Moore (Mountain), Schofield, Willard.

SELF HEAL (*Prunella vulgaris*). *Distribution* A ubiquitous worldwide wetlands plant. In California and Baja California, it is more likely to be in canyons and woods; further north, it can be a weed; but wherever it grows, it is wet. *Parts Used* Aerial parts in bloom. *Preparation* Fresh plant as a poultice; fresh juice for bites, gums sores, and so forth. *Herb Uses* Same as for Hedge Nettle. *References* Foster, Moore (Mountain), Willard.

WILD CHERRY or CHOKECHERRY (*Prunus virginiana*). *Distribution* Rivers and creeks from San Diego County, northwards to southern British Columbia, and eastwards. *Parts Used* Bark of larger stems and trunk, from summer to late fall. *Preparation* Cold Infusion, 2 to 6 fluid ounces, up to three times a day; Tincture, 1:5, 60% alcohol, 10% glycerin, 30 to 90 drops, up to four times a day. *Herb Uses* Respiratory sedative for acute conditions, with heat, rapid breathing, hectic coughing, and rapid pulse. *References* Foster, Willard.

CALIFORNIA TEA (*Psoralea physodes*). *Distribution* Open hillsides and forest clearings from central Washington to Orange County, coastal California. *Parts Used* The leaves, dried. *Preparation and Herb Uses* A lovely tea for taste, also an antispasmodic for cramps.

WAFER ASH or HOP TREE (*Ptelea crenulata*). *Distribution* Lower canyons and foothills of the coastal range north and south of San Francisco; the western slopes of the Sierra Nevada, from Shasta to Kern counties. *Parts Used* Bark and leaves. *Preparation* Fresh Tincture, 1:2, Dry Tincture, 1:5, 65% alcohol, 10 to 20 drops, up to four times a day. *Herb Uses* A bitter tonic that also stimulates secretions of the stomach and small intestines; a general stimulating tonic for those recuperating from illness. *References* Foster, Moore (Mountain).

PYROLA (*Pyrola* spp.). *Distribution* A plant of shady, chuff-covered, old-growth forests from northern San Diego County to Alaska and the Yukon, and eastwards. *Parts Used* The aboveground part of the plant. *Preparation and Herb Uses* Same as for Pipsissewa (*Chimaphila*). *References* Foster, Moore (Mountain), Schofield, Willard.

OAK (*Quercus* spp.) *Distribution* From Vancouver Island to Baja California, and eastwards. The varieties are many, but Oak is Oak. *Parts Used* Leaves, stems, and bark. *Preparation* Strong Decoction or Cold Infusion, 1 to 4 fluid ounces, up to four times a day, or topical as needed. *Herb Uses* Same as for Alum Root (see main text). *References* Foster, Moore (Mountain).

CASCARA SAGRADA (*Rhamnus purshiana*, etc.). *Distribution* Coffeeberry (*R. californica*) and Hollyleaf Buckthorn (*R. crocea*) are widely dispersed in the lower scrub woodlands and chaparral of California, Baja California, southern Nevada, and Arizona. Cascara Sagrada grows from northern California almost to the Alaska Panhandle; west of the Cascades; and down the Rockies to central Idaho. It is especially common in heavily timbered forests. *Parts Used* Bark of limbs and the small trunks. Let it age for one year, heat at 180 degrees for twenty-four hours or in a dehydrator at 140 degrees for twelve hours—or buy it commercially. *Preparation* Cold Infusion 2 to 6 fluid ounces at night; Tincture, 1:5, 50% alcohol, 1 to 2 teaspoons at night. *Herb Uses* An occasional laxative for chronic constipation, without organic cause, taken before retiring for morning effect. *References* Foster, Moore (Mountain), Willard.

SUMACH (*Rhus* spp.). *Distribution* Usually found in lower canyons, foothills, and on sheltered slopes; the many Sumachs range from southern British Columbia to coastal Baja California and inland. *Parts Used* Leaves and ripe red berries, dried. *Preparation* Cold Infusion, 1 to 2 fluid ounces, as needed; dried leaf powder for topical application; ripe berries as "Rhusade." *Herb Uses* A good, gentle astringent; for intestinal inflammations; as a douche or enema; topically for herpes sores, ulcerations, and even diaper rash; a good but slow hemostatic. *References* Foster, Moore (Desert), Willard.

WILD ROSE (*Rosa* spp.). *Distribution* A rose is a rose is a rose, from the Brooks Range in Alaska to northern Baja California, and eastwards—in forests, thickets, logged wastelands, canyons, and so forth. *Parts Used* Dried flower buds, dried leaves, and hips after a *good* frost. *Preparation and Herb Uses* Standard Infusion of buds in isotonic water for eyewash; leaves the same as other Rose family astringents like Agrimony or Ladies Mantle; the hips as an infusion for vitamin C, flavonoids. *References* Foster, Moore (Mountain), Schofield, Willard.

RASPBERRY or BLACKBERRY (*Rubus* spp.). *Distribution* Same as above. *Parts Used* Dried leaves from sterile (nonflowering) canes; root bark. *Preparation* Standard Infusion of leaves, as needed; root bark, a Strong Decoction, 2 to 4 fluid ounces, up to four times a day. *Herb Uses* Use the leaves as for Ladies Mantle, the root bark as for Alum Root. *References* Foster, Moore (Mountain), Schofield, Willard.

YELLOW DOCK (*Rumex crispus*). *Distribution* Waste places anywhere, from Alaska to Baja California, and eastwards. Plants in running water are too feeble to use; the best roots come from some environmental stress. *Parts Used* Dried roots, yellow to orange in pith color. *Preparation* Tincture, 1:5, 50% alcohol, 30 to 75 drops, up to three times a day; #00 capsules, 1 to 2, up to two times a day. *Herb Uses* Sluggish digestion, malabsorption, steatorrhea, or constipation, often with dry skin. *References* Foster, Moore (Mountain), Schofield, Willard.

WILLOW (*Salix* spp.). *Distribution* Wet places from Alaska to Baja California, and eastwards. *Parts Used* Bark, dried. *Preparation and Herb Uses* The same as for Aspen (*Populus tremuloides*). *References* Foster, Moore (Mountain), Schofield, Willard.

ELDERBERRY (*Sambucus* spp.). *Distribution* Southwest Alaska to the middle of Baja California, and eastwards. *Parts Used* Flowers and leaves, dried. *Preparation* Flowers, Standard Infusion, 2 to 4 fluid ounces; leaves, Standard Infusion, 1 to 2 fluid ounces, either up to four times a day. *Herb Uses* A simple alterative diaphoretic, especially when combined with Peppermint or Pennyroyal; with no fever, it is an excellent diuretic for simple water retention to dilute urine in cystitis. *References* Foster, Moore (Mountain), Schofield, Willard.

SKULLCAP (*Scutellaria lateriflora, S. galericulata*). *Distribution* The first Skullcap is a transcontinental species, sometimes growing in rich woods and thickets, but usually found in bottomlands. Growing by creeping roots, it may form large pure stands. It is found from the north Central Valley in California, north to central British Columbia; sporadic in the Great Basin. The second Skullcap grows in cold, clean stream and river basins, usually with Nettle, Brook Mint, and Willow. California Skullcap, a unique yellow-flowered species, can be locally abundant in lower forests from Alameda County north to the Klamath Mountains, down the Sierras to Yosemite National Park. *Parts Used* Flowering herb. *Preparation* Fresh Plant Tincture, 1:2, 30 to 90 drops; the dried herb loses so much strength that this is the only proper form. *Herb Uses* A nerve sedative for any condition characterized by oversensitivity of the peripheral nerves, from sciatica to shingles to facial pain to acupuncture or bodywork sensitivity; insomnia from sensory irritability. *References* Foster, Moore (Mountain), Willard.

MILK THISTLE (*Silybyum marianum*). *Distribution* In Oregon, from Eugene to Portland in the Willamette Valley; in the Central Valley of California; and from San Diego County to southern Oregon, along coastal strands and in upland pastures. *Parts Used* Ripe seeds. *Preparation* Freshly ground seeds, 2 to 3 #00 capsules, up to three times a day; Tincture, 1:5, 60% alcohol, ½ to 1 teaspoon, up to four times a day. *Herb Uses* Early treatment for chronic liver problems; rehabilitation from alcohol, solvent, or IV recreational abuse; protects hepatocytes from heavy metal, chemical, and alcohol injury; limits fatty degeneration and speeds up hepatitis recovery, slowing or reversing cirrhosis. *References* Foster, Moore (Desert).

YERBA DEL NEGRO or SCARLET GLOBEMALLOW (*Sphaeralcea* spp.). *Distribution* From southern British Columbia, south into the Great Basin; southeast into the Rockies; comes into California and Baja California from the east and is found throughout the lower valleys and deserts. *Parts Used* Upper stems in bloom. *Preparation* The powdered plant for poultice; the infusion as needed. *Herb Uses* The foliage, especially in warmer areas, is remarkably slimy; the powder can be applied dry or mixed with water as a protective and drawing poultice. The tea is used the same as for Hollyhock (*Althea*) *References* Moore (Mountain).

CHICKWEED (*Stellaria media*). *Distribution* Usually an urban or suburban garden weed, although native Chickweeds work fine as well. *Parts Used* Whole fresh plant. *Preparation* Crushed whole or juices from the fresh plant. *Herb Uses* Topical and upper GI anti-inflammatory and analgesic; the juice for painful urination. *References* Foster, Moore (Desert), Schofield, Willard.

GREEN GENTIAN (*Swertia radiata*, etc.). *Distribution* Southeastern British Columbia, south and east through the Cordillera into New Mexico, Arizona, and the California Sierra Nevada. A middle and high mountain plant found in meadows and on open moist forest slopes. *Parts Used, Preparation, and Herb Uses* Same as Gentian (*Gentiana* spp.). *References* Moore (Mountain).

DANDELION (*Taraxacum officinale*). *Distribution* Better than the *Wall Street Journal, New York Times,* and *USA Today* combined—what can I say? *Parts Used* Roots, preferably gathered in late summer and fall. *Preparation* Fresh Root Tincture, 1:2, ½ to 1½ teaspoons, up to four times a day; Strong Decoction, 2 to 6 fluid ounces, up to four times a day. *Herb Uses* A tonic or adjunct therapy for anabolic-stress individuals, with acidic urine, high blood pressure, sodium retention, and elevated uric acid. The fresh root tincture is good as an anti-inflammatory for hives, arthritis, and other extended allergic reactions. The root stimulates bile, and is both a laxative and a liver tonic, but without the irritation induced by most bile stimulants. *References* Foster, Moore (Mountain), Schofield, Willard.

SALSIFY (*Tragopogon* spp.). *Distribution* Moist waste places throughout the temperate West, but more common east of the Sierras and Cascades. *Parts Used* Dried roots, fall first year or spring second year. *Preparation* Strong Decoction, 3 to 6 fluid ounces, up to three times a day. *Herb Uses* The same as for Chicory (*Cichorium*).

PUNCTURE VINE (*Tribulus terrestris*). *Distribution* Dry, warm, gravelly waste places, from the Great Basin in eastern Washington, south into California, Nevada, Baja California, and the warm Southwest. *Parts Used* Dried herb and seeds. *Preparation* In tea, ½ to 1 teaspoon of the powdered plant, up to two times a day. *Herb Uses* A reliable therapy for elevated blood fats and elevated uric acid, usually in bullnecked mesomorphs with high blood pressure. *References* Moore (Desert).

BLUE CURLS or CALIFORNIA ROMERO (*Trichostema lanatum*). *Distribution* The coastal range and inland coastal foothills, from Monterey County to northern Baja California; usually grows with Sage, Buckwheat Bush, and Yerba Santa. *Parts Used* Flowering stems, dried and stripped for tea, Method A. *Preparation* As a tea to taste, as needed. *Herb Uses* The tea is sour-sweet-piney and delightful. It is an aromatic stomach soother, like Chamomile, stimulates sweating, and is a mild emmenagogue for late, crampy periods. *References* Moore (Mountain).

RED CLOVER (*Trifolium pratense*). *Distribution* A widely naturalized pasturage plant, it grows in cool, moist meadows, pastures, and vacant places, from central California to central Alaska, as well as in other appropriate locations throughout North America. *Parts Used* Terminal leaves with flowers. *Preparation* Standard Infusion or Strong Decoction, 4 to 6 fluid ounces, up to three times a day—i.e., a good, stiff cup of tea. *Herb Uses* Although all kinds of claims are made for this herb, it is a sound and efficacious tea, supplying essential minerals in free ion form, as well as small amounts of sedative constituents. Combines well with Alfalfa (*Medicago*) and Nettle. This is further delineated in Nettle. *References* Foster, Moore (Mountain), Schofield, Willard.

MULLEIN (*Verbascum thapsus*). *Distribution* Still another European plant, Mullein grows in higher areas in southern California, especially in the San Bernardino Mountains; in the pine forests of the Sierras; in open, dry forests north to south British Columbia; and in the Great Basin. *Parts Used* Dried roots, dried leaves, and fresh or dried flowering stalks. *Preparation* Root, Strong Decoction, 2 to 3 fluid ounces, up to four times a day. Leaves, Standard Infusion, 2 to 4 fluid ounces, up to four times a day or cleaned of stems and used as a smoking mixture base. Fresh Flower Tincture, 1:2, 30 to 90 drops, up to four times a day; dry flower heads as a steeped oil; Salve, Method A, without beeswax. *Herb Uses* Root tea for incontinence, from bladder weakness, birthing, or catheterization. Leaf tea for mild sore throat, coughing, and raspiness. Flower tincture for the same uses, but it is *much* stronger; the oil as a skin emollient and analgesic. *References* Foster, Moore (Mountain), Willard.

BLUE VERVAIN (*Verbena* spp.). *Distribution* The upright species grow in forests from British Columbia along the western edges of the Great Basin, with some in the higher mountains of southern California. The spreading, decorative *Verbenas* grow in the low and desert parts of our range. *Parts Used* Dried herb. *Preparation* Standard Infusion, 2 to 5 fluid ounces, up to three times a day. *Herb Uses* A sedative and diaphoretic for the early, agitative stages of a virus. *References* Foster, Moore (Mountain), Moore (Desert).

VIBURNUM or HIGHBUSH CRANBERRY (*Viburnum edule, V. opulus*). *Distribution* Woods, riverbanks, and thickets from northeastern Alaska and the Yukon south to the central Cascades of Oregon, and into Alberta. *V. opulus* grows from central British Columbia to the Columbia River Gorge, eastwards into northern Idaho, western Montana, and Alberta. *Parts Used* The trunk and root bark. *Preparation* Fresh Bark Tincture, 1:5, ½ to 1 teaspoon, up to four times a day. Cold Infusion or Strong Decoction, 3 to 4 fluid ounces, up to four times a day. *Herb Uses* Uterine cramps, intestinal cramps, leg pains derived from pelvic cramps, orchitis, even fallopian endometriosis pain. Also use for threatened miscarriage with rhythmical cramps, but little or no spotting in the last trimester. *References* Foster, Schofield, Willard.

PERIWINKLE (*Vinca Major*). *Distribution* Suburban and rural areas (escaped plant) from Seattle to Los Angeles, usually in the shade. *Parts Used* Leafing stems. *Preparation* Fresh Herb Tincture, 1:2, Dry Herb Tincture, 1:5, 50% alcohol, both 20 to 40 drops morning and evening. *Herb Uses* A hemostatic in functional uterine bleeding, bleeding hemorrhoids; the tincture, mixed with 5 parts glycerine for rectal application. For migrainelike headaches, with pounding in temples, occurring after adrenalin stress from circumstances or a rebound reaction to low blood sugar from skipping meals. *Comments* An incredibly complex alkaloid plant, its safe use mentioned here is for acute, short-term need. If you get many such headaches that need Periwinkle, it's time to do more than take an herb. *References* Moore (Desert).

VIOLET (*Viola* spp.). *Distribution* The shady, wooded places where you would expect to find violets, from Alaska to Baja California, and eastwards. *Parts Used* Whole plant in flower. *Preparation* The plant is *good* food. Otherwise, Fresh Plant Tincture, 1:2, 30 to 90 drops, the recent dried plant, Standard Infusion, 2 to 3 fluid ounces, both up to four times a day. *Herb Uses* The fresh plant is remarkably high in vitamin C and beta-carotene. The tincture or tea is a laxative and sedative, and helps eczema in kids and old folks. *References* Foster, Schofield, Willard.

COCKLEBUR (*Xanthium strumarium*). *Distribution* Waste places, usually with poor drainage; seasonal seeps, pastures. *Parts Used* Whole plant in flower. *Preparation* Fresh Plant Tincture, 1:2, 30 to 60 drops, up to four times a day. The herb as a Strong Decoction, 2 to 3 fluid ounces, up to four times a day. *Herb Uses* Cocklebur is a peculiar but useful diuretic, increasing the volume of urine, helping to pass acidic gravel, and acting as an astringent and hemostatic to the bladder and urethra. It also helps decrease excess sweating, bilious yellow diarrhea, and copious respiratory secretions. Use it short-term for resolving acute conditions, as it can become a liver irritant if taken constantly. *References* Foster, Moore (Mountain).

YUCCA (*Yucca baccata*). *Distribution* Mojave and Colorado deserts, from east San Bernardino County into southern Nevada; most of Arizona. *Yucca glauca* is found in the Great Basin, usually at higher elevations, from Montana south to Arizona. *Parts Used* Dried roots. *Preparation* Take 2 to 4 #00 capsules morning and evening. *Herb Uses* The capsules are a reliable anti-inflammatory for both major types of arthritis, and for individuals with IgE atopy, it lessens uterine, prostate, and colon inflammation started by idiosyncratic allergies. It combines well with Figwort. *References* Foster, Moore (Mountain), Willard.

I have only included vascular plants in this list, and only those I have personal experience with. I have not included lichens, such as Usnea and Lung-wort, or the fungi, such as Ganoderma (Reishi).

Finally, and most importantly, these are brief thumbnail sketches. I have tried to give the general information that might indicate to you if the plant is of interest, whether it is in your area, and so forth. Some of these plants have contraindications, side effects, or should not be used during pregnancy. *You will need more information!*

APPENDIX B: THERAPEUTIC USE LIST

This is an index only. Please refer to the main text for specific information before using any herb.

ALCOHOLISM

Gastritis, acute
Matilija Poppy
Oregon Grape
Red Root

Gastritis, chronic
Bunchberry
California Bayberry

Hangovers
Buckwheat Bush
Hedge Nettle
Labrador Tea

Liver/Portal congestion
California Buckeye
California Mugwort

ALLERGIES

Hay Fever/Respiratory
Bidens
Mormon Tea
Oxeye Daisy
Pearly Everlasting
Yerba Santa

IgE/Atopic/Rheumatoid
Bittersweet
Blueberry
Devil's Club
Figwort
Licorice Fern
Nettle
Oregon Grape

ALTERATIVE
Bittersweet
Bleeding Heart
Buckbean
California Bayberry
California Spikenard
Devil's Club
Figwort
Oregon Grape
Red Root

ANTIDEPRESSANT
California Spikenard
Devil's Club
Hypericum
Lemon Balm
Stream Orchid
Western Pasque Flower

ANTIFUNGAL

Candidiasis
Red Cedar
Sweet Root
White Sage

General, external
Amole Lily (Scalp)
California Bay
California Bayberry
California Mugwort
Labrador Tea
Oregon Grape
Oxeye Daisy
Red Cedar
Sweet Root
White Sage

General, internal
Balsam Root
Red Cedar
Sweet Root
White Sage

ANTI-INFLAMMATORY

General, systemic
Baneberry
Black Cohosh
Bunchberry
Figwort
Hawthorn
Hedge Nettle
Licorice Fern
Pearly Everlasting
Red Root
Yarrow

Mucous membranes
Hedge Nettle
Oxeye Daisy
Pitcher Sage
Salal
Yellow Pond Lily
Yerba Santa

Topical
Balsam Poplar
Figwort
Hedge Nettle
Oxeye Daisy
Pearly Everlasting
Pitcher Sage
Western Coltsfoot
Yarrow
Yerba Reuma

ANTIMICROBIAL/ ANTISEPTIC
Arnica
Balsam Poplar
Bidens
California Bay
California Mugwort
Goldthread
Hedge Nettle
Lomatium
Matilija Poppy
Oregon Grape
Oxeye Daisy
Red Cedar
White Sage
Yerba Reuma

ANTIOXIDANT
California Mugwort
Pitcher Sage

ANTISPASMODIC
Angelica
Baneberry
Black Cohosh

Lemon Balm
Matilija Poppy
Prickly Poppy
Silk Tassel
Stream Orchid
Valerian
Western Coltsfoot
Western Peony
Western Skunk Cabbage

ANTIVIRAL

Hypericum (?)
Lemon Balm
Lomatium
White Sage

ARTHRITIS

External

Arnica
Balsam Poplar
California Bay
Prickly Poppy
Yarrow
Yellow Pond Lily
Yerba del Lobo

Internal

Balsam Poplar
Baneberry
Bittersweet
Black Cohosh
Buckbean
Figwort
Nettle
Yarrow

ASTHMA

Dry, adrenergic

Angelica
California Spikenard

Moist, congested

Bidens
Horehound
Oxeye Daisy
Yerba Santa

Preventative

Horehound
Mormon Tea
Western Coltsfoot

ASTRINGENT

Internal

Bidens
Buckwheat Bush
California Bayberry
Hedge Nettle
Madrone
Maidenhair Fern
Manzanita
Oxeye Daisy
Pearly Everlasting
Pitcher Sage
Red Root
Salal
Uva Ursi
Yellow Pond Lily
Yerba Reuma

Topical

Alum Root
Bidens
California Bayberry
Hedge Nettle
Madrone
Manzanita
Mormon Tea (resin)
Salal
Uva Ursi
Yerba Reuma

BACK PAIN

Hypericum
Prickly Poppy
Western Coltsfoot

BATH HERBS

Bittersweet
California Bay
Pearly Everlasting
Yarrow

Sitz bath

Goldthread
Madrone
Manzanita
Uva Ursi
White Sage
Yellow Pond Lily
Yerba Reuma

BIRTHING

Partum muscle relaxant

Betony

Prepartum varicosities

Yarrow

Prepartum water retention

Nettle

Postpartum bleeding

Buckwheat Bush
Trillium
Yarrow

Postpartum sitz bath

Buckwheat Bush
Madrone
Manzanita
Uva Ursi

Postpartum urinary problems

Prickly Poppy

BLOOD PRESSURE

High, essential

Hawthorn

High, labile

Baneberry
Black Cohosh

BRONCHITIS

Early, dry, inflamed

Balsam Poplar
Balsam Root
Desert Milkweed
False Solomon's Seal
Horehound
Lomatium
White Sage

Later, congested, phlegmy

Balsam Poplar
Balsam Root
Pearly Everlasting
Red Root
Redwood
Wild Ginger

BRUISES/CONTUSIONS
Arnica
Betony
Bleeding Heart
California Mugwort
Pearly Everlasting
Yerba del Lobo

BURNS
Balsam Poplar
Balsam Root
Hypericum
Matilija Poppy
Pearly Everlasting
Prickly Poppy
Yerba Reuma

CFS/EBV/CMV/HIV
For general resistance
Lomatium
Red Cedar
Red Root
Sweet Root
White Sage

COLITIS
Chronic
Bunchberry
California Bay
For cramps
Angelica
Lemon Balm
Peppermint
Salal
Silk Tassel
Mucus colitis
Goldthread
Oregon Grape
Oxeye Daisy
Ulcerative
Bidens
Oxeye Daisy
Yellow Pond Lily

COUGHING
Congested, but improving
Arnica

Bidens
Horehound
Hummingbird Sage
Maidenhair Fern
Salal
Disinfectant-expectorant
Balsam Poplar
Balsam Root
Lomatium
White Sage
Dry, hot, irritated
Desert Milkweed
Devil's Club
False Solomon's Seal
Pearly Everlasting
Red Root
Western Coltsfoot
Western Peony
Western Skunk Cabbage
Painful
Balsam Poplar
Western Coltsfoot
Western Peony
Western Skunk Cabbage
Subacute, chronic
Arnica
California Bayberry
California Spikenard
Western Coltsfoot
Vanilla Leaf

DECONGESTANT
Bidens
Buckwheat Bush
California Mugwort
Horehound
Inside-Out Flower
Mormon Tea
Nettle
Oxeye Daisy
Pitcher Sage
White Sage
Yerba Santa

DIABETES
Type I
Blueberry

Type II
Devil's Club

DIAPHORETIC
General
Brook Mint
California Mugwort
Desert Milkweed
European Pennyroyal
Lemon Balm
Wild Ginger
Yarrow
Yerba Buena
With nausea
Angelica

DIARRHEA/DYSENTERY
Astringent
Alum Root
Fireweed
Pearly Everlasting
Yarrow
Yerba Reuma
Cramps/Tenesmus
California Bay
Silk Tassel
Recuperation
Bunchberry
Oregon Grape

DIURETIC
Buckwheat Bush
Mormon Tea
Nettle
Oxeye Daisy

ECZEMA/PSORIASIS
Bittersweet
Nettle
Oregon Grape

ENEMA HERBS
Alum Root
Buckwheat Bush
Fireweed
Goldthread
Madrone
Manzanita

Nettle
Oxeye Daisy
Pearly Everlasting
Uva Ursi
White Sage
Yerba Reuma

EXPECTORANT
Balsam Poplar
Balsam Root
Devil's Club
Horehound
Hummingbird Sage
Pearly Everlasting
Red Cedar
Redwood
Wild Ginger

EYE PROBLEMS
Conjuctivitis, eyewash
Buckwheat Bush
Nettle
Oregon Grape
Oxeye Daisy
Yerba Reuma

Conjuctivitis, internal
Bidens
Hedge Nettle
Inside-Out Flower
Nettle

Opthalmalgia
Hedge Nettle

FAINTNESS/DIZZINESS
California Bay

FAT, FAULTY METABOLISM
California Mugwort
Devil's Club
Oregon Grape
Red Root

FEVERS
General
Bunchberry
Lemon Balm
Lomatium
Wild Ginger

Yarrow
Yerba Buena

With chills
Bunchberry

With hypersecretions
Oxeye Daisy

With nausea
Angelica

With pain, irritation, red eyes, tachycardia
Aconite

FIRST AID
California Bayberry
California Mugwort
Composition Powder
(see California Bayberry)
False Solomon's Seal
Goldthread
Hedge Nettle
Lomatium
Matilija Poppy
Mormon Tea (resin)
Oregon Grape
Yerba Reuma

GALLBLADDER PAIN
Silk Tassel

GASTROENTERITIS
Matilija Poppy
Oregon Grape
Oxeye Daisy
Peppermint
Silk Tassel
Spearmint
Yarrow
Yellow Pond Lily
Yerba Reuma

HEADACHES
General
Bunchberry
Hedge Nettle

With muscle stress, pained eyes
California Bay

With nausea, coated tongue, orbital pain
Buckwheat Bush

With nausea, red eyes
California Mugwort
European Pennyroyal
Licorice Fern
Oregon Grape
Red Root

With TMJ pain
Hypericum

HEART/ARTERIAL
Atherosclerosis
California Mugwort

General cardiotonic
Hawthorn

Mild cardiac edema
Nettle

HEMATURIA
Bidens
Nettle
Oxeye Daisy
Trillium

HEMORRHOIDS
Balsam Root and
Hypericum
Buckbean
California Buckeye
Goldthread
Red Root
Trillium
Yellow Pond Lily

HEMOSTATIC
Internal
Buckwheat Bush
Hedge Nettle
Maidenhair Fern
Nettle
Trillium
Yarrow
Yerba Reuma

Topical
Alum Root

Mormon Tea (resin)
Yarrow
Yerba Reuma

HERPES ZOSTER/ SHINGLES

Pain

Aconite
Hypericum

IMMUNOSTIMULANT

Arnica
Balsam Root
California Snakeroot
Lomatium
Red Cedar
Red Root

INFLUENZA

Balsam Root
Lomatium
Red Cedar
Wild Ginger
Yarrow

Recuperation

Redwood

IRRITABLE BOWEL SYNDROME (IBS)

Goldthread
Matilija Poppy
Pearly Everlasting
Peppermint
Silk Tassel

JOINT PAIN

Arnica
Balsam Poplar
Bleeding Heart
California Mugwort
Hedge Nettle
Western Coltsfoot
Yarrow
Yellow Pond Lily
Yerba del Lobo

LAXATIVE

Oregon Grape
Prickly Poppy
Sweet Root

LIVER DEFICIENCY

General

California Snakeroot
Oregon Grape
Sarsaparilla

Antioxidant in hyperlipidemia

California Mugwort

With arthritis

Buckbean

With portal congestion, hemorrhoids

California Buckeye

LYMPH SYSTEM

General

California Bayberry
Red Root

Lymphadenitis

Figwort
Red Root

MOUTH AND GUM SORES

Alum Root
California Bayberry
Goldthread
Lomatium
Matilija Poppy
Nettle
Oregon Grape
Yerba Reuma

MUSCLE PAIN

Dull, achy

Black Cohosh

External

Arnica
Balsam Poplar
Baneberry (liniment)
California Mugwort
Yerba del Lobo

Internal

Arnica
Balsam Poplar
Betony

Bleeding Heart
Western Peony
Western Skunk Cabbage
Yarrow

NARCOTIC/ANALGESIC

Bleeding Heart
California Poppy
Matilija Poppy
Prickly Poppy

NAUSEA/VOMITING

Angelica
Oxeye Daisy
Peppermint
Silk Tassel
Spearmint
Western Skunk Cabbage
Yerba Reuma

NEURALGIA

Aconite
Balsam Poplar
Hypericum
Western Peony

PAIN

With inflammation and heat

Aconite

Muscle and joint

Balsam Poplar
Baneberry
Black Cohosh
Bunchberry
Western Coltsfoot

Nerve-derived

Aconite
Hypericum
Western Pasque Flower

Whole body

California Poppy
Matilija Poppy
Prickly Poppy
Stream Orchid

POULTICE HERBS

False Solomon's Seal

Figwort
Hedge Nettle
Pearly Everlasting
Western Coltsfoot
Yarrow

*REPRODUCTIVE
SYSTEM—FEMALE*

**GENERAL ANTI-
INFLAMMATORY**
Lemon Balm
Oxeye Daisy
Yellow Pond Lily

MENOPAUSE

Depression
Western Pasque Flower

*With episodes of terminal
munchies*
California Spikenard
Devil's Club

Excessive sweating
Oxeye Daisy

Hot flashes
Black Cohosh

MENSES

Cramping
Lemon Balm
Silk Tassel
Stream Orchid

*Excessive, prolonged
bleeding*
Buckwheat Bush
Nettle
Oxeye Daisy
Trillium
Yarrow

*Painful, slow onset,
clotty*
Baneberry
Black Cohosh
California Mugwort
European Pennyroyal
Maidenhair Fern
Western Peony
Wild Ginger

**PELVIC
INFLAMMATORY
DISEASE**
Pitcher Sage

**PREMENSTRUAL
SYNDROME**
With breast tenderness
Figwort (external)
Red Root

*With constipation,
Pelvic congestion*
Angelica
Oregon Grape

With morbidity, chills
Stream Orchid
Western Pasque Flower

*With oily skin, acne,
constipation*
Oregon Grape

*With simple water
retention*
Buckwheat Bush
Nettle

VAGINITIS/VAGINOSIS
Douche
Alum Root
Bidens
Buckwheat Bush
Fireweed
Goldthread
Lomatium
Nettle
Oregon Grape
Oxeye Daisy
Red Cedar
White Sage
Yellow Pond Lily
Yerba Reuma

External
Goldthread
Oregon Grape

Internal
Bidens
Oxeye Daisy
Sweet Root

*REPRODUCTIVE
SYSTEM—MALE*

**BENIGN PROSTATIC
HYPERTROPHY**
Bidens
Pitcher Sage
Red Root
Sarsaparilla
Trillium
Western Peony
White Sage
Yarrow

**GENERAL ANTI-
INFLAMMATORY**
Yellow Pond Lily

**ORCHITIS,
EPIDIDYMITIS**
Baneberry
Black Cohosh
Red Root
Western Peony

SCIATICA
Aconite
Hypericum

**SEBORRHEA/
DANDRUFF**
Amole Lily
Oxeye Daisy
Red Cedar

SEDATIVE
Baneberry
Betony
Black Cohosh
California Poppy
Hedge Nettle
Labrador Tea
Lemon Balm
Matilija Poppy
Prickly Poppy
Stream Orchid
Valerian
Western Pasque Flower
Western Skunk Cabbage

SINUSITIS/HAY FEVER
General
Mormon Tea

Nettle
Oxeye Daisy
Wild Ginger
Yerba Santa

With heavy discharge

Bidens
Composition Powder
(see California Bayberry)
Inside-Out Flower
Pearly Everlasting

With red eyes, frontal headache

California Mugwort
Lomatium

SKIN DRESSING

Balsam Poplar
Balsam Root
Figwort
Fireweed
Goldthread
Lomatium
Oregon Grape
Prickly Poppy
White Sage

SKIN POWDERS

Alum Root
California Bay
California Bayberry
Goldthread
Lomatium
Matilija Poppy
Oregon Grape
Oxeye Daisy
Red Cedar
White Sage
Yarrow
Yerba Reuma

SKIN WASH

Goldthread
Matilija Poppy
Mormon Tea (resin)
Oregon Grape
Oxeye Daisy
Pearly Everlasting
Red Cedar
Salal

White Sage
Yerba Reuma

SORE THROAT

Antimicrobial

White Sage

Astringent gargle

Alum Root
Salal
Yerba Reuma

Congested, subacute

Arnica (gargle)
California Bayberry

Painful inflammation

False Solomon's Seal
Hedge Nettle
Hummingbird Sage
Lomatium
Pearly Everlasting
Red Root

SPRAINS

Bleeding Heart
Western Coltsfoot

STOMACH

Achlorhydria

Desert Milkweed
Wild Ginger

Chronic gastritis

Bunchberry
California Mugwort
False Solomon's Seal
Hypericum
Silk Tassel
Spearmint
Yerba Santa

Dyspepsia, acid indigestion

Angelica
Brook Mint
Peppermint
Spearmint
Yerba Buena

Hypersecretion

California Mugwort
Oxeye Daisy

Ulcer astringent

Alum Root
Bidens
Pearly Everlasting

Ulcer pain

Hypericum
Yarrow

Ulcer preventative

California Mugwort
Hypericum

STRESS PREVENTION

California Spikenard
Devil's Club
Hypericum

SUNSCREEN

Pitcher Sage

TONICS

Anabolic excess

Nettle

Bitter tonic

Buckbean
California Snakeroot
Goldthread
Oregon Grape

Cardiac

Hawthorn

Catabolic excess

Sarsaparilla

Digestion

California Snakeroot
Goldthread
Oregon Grape

Lung/Pulmonary

Devil's Club
Maidenhair Fern
Red Cedar
Redwood

Reproductive deficient

Black Cohosh
Devil's Club
Western Peony

Reproductive excess

Yellow Pond Lily

Skin
Bittersweet
Oregon Grape
Sarsaparilla

TONSILLITIS
Acute
Red Root
Chronic, obstinate
Arnica and Red Root

TOOTHACHE
Bleeding Heart
California Poppy
Prickly Poppy

TRANQUILIZER
With aching muscles
Betony
Cold, shaky, nervous
Bleeding Heart
Western Pasque Flower
With skin, sensory, muscle excess
California Poppy
Hypericum
Stream Orchid
Western Pasque Flower

URIC ACID EXCESS/GOUT
Bidens
Nettle

URINARY TRACT
Cystitis/Urethritis
Alkaline pH
Blueberry
Madrone
Manzanita
Uva Ursi
Chronic
Red Cedar
Yerba Santa
Pain
Bidens
Hedge Nettle
Nettle

Prickly Poppy
Redwood
Simple astringent
Buckwheat Bush
Nettle
Oxeye Daisy
Yarrow
Yellow Pond Lily

UTERINE FIBROIDS
Trillium
Yarrow
Yellow Pond Lily

VARICOSE VEINS
California Buckeye
Red Root

VASCULAR
Vasoconstriction
Maidenhair Fern
Vasodilation
Arnica
Baneberry
Black Cohosh
California Bayberry
Wild Ginger

VENEREAL WARTS
Manzanita
Red Cedar
Uva Ursi

OTHER USES

FOOD
Balsam Root
Bunchberry
Madrone
Nettle
Salal
Yellow Pond Lily

HAIR TONIC
Amole Lily
Maidenhair Fern
Nettle

INCENSE
Red Cedar
Vanilla Leaf

INSECT REPELLENT
Oxeye Daisy

MOISTURIZER
Lomatium

MOXIBUSTION
California Mugwort

PICKLING
Alum Root
Yerba Reuma

SHAMPOO
Amole Lily

SMOKING
Hummingbird Sage
Manzanita
Pearly Everlasting
Uva Ursi
Vanilla Leaf
Western Coltsfoot

SMUDGING
California Mugwort
Hummingbird Sage
Red Cedar
White Sage

SPICES
Angelica (leaf)
California Bay
Vanilla Leaf

TEAS, FOR TASTE
Bergamot Mint
Brook Mint
California Bayberry
Hummingbird Sage
Labrador Tea
Lemon Balm
Peppermint
Pitcher Sage
Spearmint
Sweet Root
Vanilla Leaf
Yerba Buena

"WAX PAPER"
Western Skunk
Cabbage (leaves)

GLOSSARY

These definitions apply to uses within the context of this book. They may be narrower or broader than when used in medicine, botany, chemistry, and so forth.

ACHENE A dry, one-seeded fruit, without a predictable opening and formed from a single carpel, usually one of many, like an unshelled Sunflower seed.

ACHLORHYDRIA The lack of free hydrochloric acid in the stomach; more broadly, inadequate or suppressed secretions. The causes vary from stomach ulcers, alcoholism, adrenalin stress, and old age to a stomach carcinoma. Without enough acid, pepsin is inactive, proteins are poorly digested, and the prolonged contact with foreign, intact proteins increases food sensitivities in the upper intestinal mucosa.

ACUTE A type of disease or disorder having a sudden onset, severe symptoms, and a generally short duration (e.g., a head cold or knee sprain). The opposite of chronic.

ADRENAL CORTEX The outer covering of the adrenal glands, the two triangular endocrine glands that rest atop the kidneys. Formed in fetal development from the same tissue that becomes the gonads, the adrenal cortex secretes a number of steroid hormones that regulate carbohydrate use, salt balance, reproductive functions, anabolism, catabolism, and inflammation. In Chinese Medicine these functions relate to kidney yang. Inside the cortex is the adrenal medulla, modified nerve tissue that is the source of epinephrine (adrenalin) and relates to kidney yin.

AERIAL The parts of plants growing aboveground.

ALKALINE In our context, a substance having a pH above that of neutral water (7.0) when in solution. Signified as pH (potential of Hydrogen), alkaline fluids, such as the blood (pH about 7.4), have the ability to neutralize acids (solutions below pH 7.0). Metabolic wastes are acids, and the alkaline reserve of the blood neutralizes them until they are excreted.

ALKALOID One of a varied family of alkaline, nitrogen-containing substances, usually plant-derived, reacting with acids to form salts. Normally intensely bitter, alkaloids form a body of substances widely used in drug and herbal therapy. They are usually biologically active and have a toxic potential. (Examples: caffeine, morphine, berberine). The term is more pharmaceutical and medical than chemical since alkaloids come from a variety of otherwise unrelated organic compounds.

ALTERATIVE A term applied in naturopathic, eclectic, and Thomsonian medicine to those plants or procedures that stimulate changes of a defensive or healing nature in metabolism or tissue function when there is chronic or acute diseases. The whole concept of alteratives is based on the premise that in a normally healthy person, disease symptoms are the external signs of activated internal defenses and, as such, should be stimulated and not suppressed.

Wild Ginger, as an example, acts as an alterative when it is used to stimulate sweating in a fevered state. Without a fever or physical exertion, Wild Ginger tea will increase intestinal, lung, and kidney secretions. With fever or exercise, the buildup of heat from combustion, and the dilation of peripheral blood supply, Wild Ginger takes the defense response to the next stage—breaking a sweat. You might have sweated eventually anyway, but you may be one of those people who doesn't perspire easily, and a diaphoretic such as Wild Ginger will act as an alterative for you by stimulating the next stage of defenses sooner than you would have on your own.

The term alterative is sometimes inaccurately used as a synonym for "blood purifier," particularly by nature-cure neo-Thomsonians such as Jethro Kloss, Arnold Ehret, and John Christopher. "Blood purifier" is a term better applied to the liver, spleen, and kidneys, not to some dried plant.

ALTERNATE Having plant parts, particularly leaves, arranged alternately along a stem, as opposed to in pairs or whorled.

ANABOLIC Promoting anabolism. Specifically, an agent or function that stimulates the organization of smaller substances into larger ones. Examples: making a starch out of sugars, a protein out of amino acids, or making triglycerides out of fatty acids are anabolic functions. Anabolic steroids are internal or external substances that will induce increased body size or mass. The opposite of catabolic.

ANALGESIC A substance that relieves pain. (Examples: aspirin, Balsam Poplar.)

ANESTHETIC A substance that decreases nerve sensitivity to pain. (Examples: nitrous oxide, Peppermint.)

ANTIBODY These are immunologic proteins, usually made from immunoglobulins, that are capable of binding to, and rendering inactive, foreign substances that have entered the skin envelope and have been deemed dangerous. They may be synthesized anew in the presence of a previously encountered substance (antigen); they may be present in small amounts at all times in the bloodstream; or they may be present in the tissues in a more primitive form designed to react to a broad spectrum of potential antigens. The latter may be responsible for some allergies.

ANTICHOLINERGIC An agent that impedes the impulses or actions of the nerves or fibers of the parasympathetic ganglia, competing with, and blocking, the release of acetylcholine at what are called the muscarinic sites. Cholinergic functions affected are those that induce spasms and cramps of the intestinal tracts and allied ducts. (Examples: atropine, Belladona, Silk Tassel.)

ANTICOAGULANT A medication or natural compound that slows or prevents the formation of blood clots. (Eamples: Heparin [endogenous], Dicumarol, and warfarin [drugs].)

ANTIDEPRESSANT Literally, substances meant to oppose depressions or sadness, and generally heterocyclic types such as Elavil, MAO inhibitors like phenelzine, or lithium carbonate. This category of substances formerly included stuff like amphetamines and other stimulants; but the only plants in this book that could fit the current definition for antidepressant activity would be Hypericum— and perhaps Devil's Club.

ANTIFUNGAL An agent that kills or inhibits fungi, and, in my usage here, an herb that inhibits either a dermatomycosis like ringworm or athlete's foot, or one that inhibits *Candida albicans* either externally as a douche or internally as a systemic antifungal. (Examples: Nystatin, griseofulvin, White Sage.)

ANTIGEN A substance, usually a protein, that induces the formation of defending antibodies. Example: bacterial toxins, Juniper pollen (in allergies). Autoimmune disorders occur when antibodies are formed against normal proteins created within the body.

ANTIHISTAMINE An exogenous agent that inhibits the release of histamine, the amino acid derivative that stimulates vasodilation and permeability under many circumstances, particularly tissue irritation. The most common type of antihistamine, the H1 receptor antagonist, produces many moderate side effects, and the H2 receptor antagonist cimetidine is even more problematic. That they are so commonly used can lull both physician and patient into trivializing their iatrogenic potential. Histamines, which are most abundant in the skin, respiratory, and GI tract mucous membranes, help heal; using antihistamines to inhibit the healing response for the whole body simply in order to lessen the acute but physiologically superficial symptoms of something like hay fever is to risk many subtle side effects.

ANTIMICROBIAL An agent that kills or inhibits microorganisms.

ANTIOXIDANT A substance that prevents oxidation or slows a redox reaction. More generally, an agent that slows the formation of lipid peroxides and other free-radical oxygen forms, preventing the rancidity of oils or blocking damage from peroxides to the mitochondria of cells or cell membranes. (Examples: vitamin E, *Larrea* (Chaparral), Balsam Poplar.)

ANTIPHLOGISTINE An agent that limits or decreases inflammation; an antiinflammatory or antihistamine.

ANTISPASMODIC A substance that will relieve or prevent spasms, usually of the smooth muscles of the intestinal tract, bronchi, or uterus. (Examples: barbiturates, Silk Tassel.)

ANTIVIRAL An agent that experimentally inhibits the proliferation and viability of infectious viruses. In our domain of herbal medicines, some plants will slow or inhibit the adsorption or random initial attachment of viruses, extend the life span of infected target cells, or speed up several aspects of immunity, including complement, antibody, and phagocytosis responses. Herbal antivirals work best on respiratory viruses such as influenza, adenoviruses, rhinoviruses, and the enteric echoviruses. Touted as useful in the alphabet group of slow viruses (HIV, EBV, CMV, etc.), they really help to limit secondary concurrent respiratory infections that often accompany immunosuppression.

APHTHOUS STOMATITIS Little ulcers or canker sores on the surface of the tongue, lips, and cheek mucosa. In adults, they are often related to gastric reflux and dyspepsia.

AROMATICS Chemically, molecules containing one or more benzene rings, but in our usage, plant compounds which, upon contact to the air, form gases which can be smelled: volatile oils. (Examples: menthol, Peppermint oil.)

ARRHYTHMIA An abnormal or irregular rhythm, usually in reference to the heart.

ARTERIAL Blood that leaves the heart. When it leaves the right ventricle, it is venous blood; and when it leaves the left ventricle, through the aorta, it is fresh, hot, oxygenated red stuff—my use of the term in this book. After it has passed out to the capillaries and started to return, it is venous blood.

ARTERIOSCLEROSIS The condition of blood vessels that have thickened, hardened, and lost their elasticity—"hardening of the arteries." Aging and the formation of blood-derived fatty plaques within or directly beneath the inner lining of the arteries are the common causes. Many of the large arteries aid blood transport from the heart by their rebound elasticity, "kicking" it out; smaller ones have muscle coats that need to contract and relax in response to nerves. All this is compromised when there is arteriosclerosis.

ARTHRITIS Literally, inflammation of one or more joints, usually with pain and sometimes with changes in the structure. Osteoarthritis is a chronic condition of loss in the organization of joint cartilage, with gradual calcification of the gristle, formation of spurs, and impaired function. Rheumatoid arthritis is an autoimmune disorder, with chronic inflammation and eventual distortion of the joints; the victim experiences a lessening of good health, worsening metabolic imbalance, allergies, and general stress (emotional, physical, and dietary).

ASTRINGENT An agent that causes the constriction of tissues, usually applied topically to stop bleeding, secretions, and surface inflammation and distension. Some, such as gallotannins, may actually bind with and "tan" the surface layer of skin or mucosa. (Examples: a styptic pencil, Yerba Reuma.)

ATOPIC A type of inherited allergic response involving elevated immunoglobulin E. Sometimes called a reagin response, it means that you have hay fever, bronchial asthma, or skin problems like urticaria or eczema. It can be acquired, sometimes after hepatitis or extended contact with solvents or alcohol, but if your mama sneezed and your daddy itched, you will probably have one form or another of the above stuff at different times of your life. Solution: since you can't change your stripes, keep in balance and avoid, if possible, the distortions of constant medications, both prescription and over-the-counter.

AWN A terminal or lateral bristle on a seed or plant organ.

AXIL The upper angle formed by a leaf or branch with a stem. Things that pop out in the axils are called AXILLARY.

BALSAMIC Soft or hard plant or tree resins composed of aromatic acids and oils. These are typically used as stimulating dressings and aromatic expectorants and diuretics. This term is also applied loosely to many plants that may not exude resins but which have a soothing, pitchy scent. (Examples: Balsam Poplar, Yerba Santa.)

BASAL At or near the base, and, if leaves, those that sprout directly from the root or crown.

BENIGN PROSTATIC HYPERTROPHY, OR HYPERPLASIA The benign buildup in the prostate of "warts" or epithelial neoplasias that can block or interrupt urination, and which are usually concurrent with moderate prostate enlargement, having a dull ache on urination, ejaculation, and/or defecation. The diagnosis is medical, since the same subjective conditions can result from cancer of the prostate. It is common in men over fifty and can be the result either of diminished production of complete testosterone or poor pelvic circulation. Alcohol, coffee, speed, and antihistamines can all aggravate the problem.

BILIOUSNESS A symptom-picture resulting from a short-term disordered liver, with constipation, frontal headache, spots in front of the eyes, poor appetite, and nausea or vomiting. The usual causes are heavy alcohol consumption, poor ventilation when working with solvents, heavy binging with fatty foods, or moderate consumption of rancid fats. The term is genially archaic in medicine; people who are bilious are seldom genial, however.

BIODIVERSE The state of life interdependency that is possible when large and small plants, soil organisms, insects, and fuzzy beasts exist in the ebb and flow created by the natural environment. Cut down the trees once and you lessen the biodiversity drastically. Wait fifty years and cut again and you have a small fraction of the life-form variety that you started with; the old diversity will never return—never.

BIOMASS The actual amount of existing material within a species or genus.

BIOSPHERE Literally, the part of the earth that supports life; more broadly, a large community of life-forms sharing a similar environment, such as a rain forest or prairie grassland.

BIPINNATE A pinnate compound leaf whose leaflets, in turn, are stems that have pinnate leaflets.

BITERNATE A compound leaf divided in threes, whose leaflets are in turn divided in pairs.

BITTER TONIC A bitter-tasting substance or formula used to increase a deficient appetite, improve the acidity of stomach secretions (and protein digestion), and slightly speed up the orderly emptying of the stomach. A good bitter tonic should possess little, if any, drug effect, only affecting oral and stomach functions and secretions. Dry mouth, bad gums, teeth problems with bad breath in the morning, and weak digestion, often with constipation, are the main symptoms. A bitter tonic has little effect in normal digestion.

BORBORYGMUS The bubbling, gurgling passage of gas across the transverse colon.

BPH Benign prostatic hypertrophy, or hyperplasia.

BRACTS Reduced or modified leaflets that are usually associated with flowers or an inflorescence, generally subtending or beneath the floral parts.

BRADYCARDIA A distinctly slow heartbeat, which may be a normal idiosyncracy or a functional or organic disease. Bradycardia is usually defined as a pulse below sixty beats a minute, or seventy in children.

BRONCHITIS Inflammation of the mucus membranes on the bronchi, usually caused by an infection but sometimes induced by allergies or chemical irritations.

BUFFERING SYSTEM The several blood factors that enable the acid waste products of metabolism to be carried in the alkaline blood without disrupting its chemistry. These include carbolic acid, carbonates, phosphates, blood proteins, and even hemoglobin. You can almost say that the blood is an acid sponge.

BURSITIS Inflammation of a bursa, the lubricating sac that reduces friction between tendons and ligaments or tendons and bones. The more common types of bursitis are of the shoulders, the elbows, the knees, and the big toe (a bunion).

CALYX The outer set of sterile, floral leaves; the green, clasping base of a flower.

CANDIDIASIS Generally, a disorder caused by *Candida (Monilia) albicans*. This is the most important member of the genus, a common yeastlike fungus found in the mouth, vagina, and rectum, as well as on the outside skin. It is a common cause of thrush in infants and vaginal yeast infections. In recent years much attention has been given to the increased numbers of people who have developed candidiasis in the upper and lower intestinal tract. Formerly only found in extremely debilitated patients, this condition is now known to occur as a result of extended antibiotic therapy and anti-inflammatory treatment. Most anti-inflammatory drugs are really immunosuppressants, and this rather benign and common skin and mucosal fungus can move deeply into the body when resistance is drug-depressed, or the normal, stable competition between fungus and bacteria is altered as the result of the treatment of the bacterial infection. The constant presence of the candida has been implicated in many chronic allergic states, occurs commonly in autoimmune and slow virus conditions, and is aggravated in people with problems with sugar metabolism.

CAPILLARY The smallest blood or lymph vessel, formed of single layers of interconnected endothelial cells, sometimes with loosely attached connective tissue basement cells for added support, and, in some tissues, a few smooth muscle cells for special contractions. Capillaries allow the transport across their membranes and between their crevices of diffusable nutrients and waste products.

Blood capillaries expand and contract, depending upon how much blood is needed in a given tissue and how much is piped into them by the small arteries that feed into them. They further maintain a strong repelling charge that keeps blood proteins and red blood cells pushed into the center of the flow.

Lymph capillaries have many open crypts that allow free absorption of interstitial fluid that has been forced out of the blood; these capillaries further tend to maintain a charge that attracts bits of cellular garbage too large to return through the membranes of exiting venous capillaries.

CARDIOGLYCOSIDES Sugar-containing plant substances that, in proper doses, act as heart stimulants. (Examples: digitoxin, stropanthin.)

CARDIOTONIC A substance that strengthens or regulates heart metabolism without overt stimulation or depression. It may increase coronary blood supply, normalize coronary enervation, soften rigid arteries (thereby decreasing back-pressure on the valves), or decrease adrenergic stimulation. (Examples: magnesium, Hawthorn.)

CARPEL A simple pistil or one of the modified leaflets forming a compound pistil.

CATABOLIC The part of metabolism that deals with destruction or simplification of more complex compounds. Catabolism mostly results in the release of energy. (Examples: the release of glucose by the liver, the combustion of glucose by cells.)

CAULINE Belonging to the stem, as in cauline leaves that emerge from the stem.

CENTRAL NERVOUS SYSTEM A collective term for the brain, spinal cord, their nerves, and the sensory end organs. More broadly, this can even include the neurotransmitting hormones instigated by the CNS that control the chemical nervous system, the endocrine glands.

CHRONIC A disease or imbalance of long, slow duration, showing little overall change and characterized by periods of remission interspersed with acute episodes. The opposite of acute.

CHRONIC FATIGUE SYNDROME (CFS) is a recently designated semidisease, often attributed to EBV (the Epstein-Barr virus) or CMV (Cytomegalovirus) infections, characterized by FUOs (fevers of unknown origin) and resulting in the patient feeling miserable. In most of us, the microorganisms involved in CFS usually provoke nothing more than a head cold; in some individuals, however, they induce a long, grinding, and debilitating disorder, characterized by exhaustion, depression, periodic fevers—a crazy-quilt of symptoms that frustrates both the sufferer and the sometimes skeptical physician.

CHYLOMICRONS These are organized blobs of fats, synthesized in the submucosa of the small intestine out of dietary lipids and cholesterol, carried out of the intestinal tract by the lymph, and slowly released into the bloodstream. In the capillaries, the triglycerides inside the chylomicrons are absorbed into the tissues for fuel or storage, and the outside cholesterol and phospholipid transport-cover continues through the blood to be absorbed by the liver for its use. This sideways approach takes (ideally) a large part of dietary fats into the lymph back alleys, spreading their release into the bloodstream out over many hours, thereby avoiding short-term blood fat and liver fat overload. To synthesize the maximum amount of dietary fats into chylomicrons, you need well-organized emulsification and digestion of lipids by the gallbladder and pancreas.

CIRCUMBOREAL Plants that are found worldwide, encircling the lands around the north pole.

CMV Cytomegalovirus.

CNS Central nervous system.

COLIFORM BACTERIA Intestinal bacilli that are gram-negative, sugar-digesting, and both aerobic and anaerobic. They are usually from the family Enterobacteriaceae; *Escherichia coli* is the best known of the group.

COLITIS Colon inflammation, usually involving the mucus membranes. Mucous colitis is a type with cramps, periods of constipation, and copious discharge of mucus with feces. Ulcerative colitis has pain, inflammation, ulceration, fever, and bleeding interspersed at various times—a long and serious illness.

COLLOID Gooey substances, usually proteins and starches, whose molecules can hold large amounts of a solvent (usually water) without dissolving. In lifeforms, virtually all fluids are held suspended in protein or starch colloids (hydrogels). (Examples: cell protoplasm, lime Jell-O.)

COMPOUND Leaves that are made up of leaflets, such as pinnate and palmate leaves.

CONGESTION The accumulation of an excess volume of fluid, including blood, in an organ or tissue. I use it in the subclinical definition, with fluid buildup as a consequence of unremitting inflammation, with edema of the parts, and resultant venous *and* lymphatic drainage, impairment, causing a distinctly less organic and more functional problem: thick and boggy tissues from excess inflammation.

CONJUNCTIVITIS Inflammation of the mucus membranes that line the eyeball and the eyelid.

CONTUSION A bruise, characterized by a trauma in which the skin is not broken but underlying blood vessels are busted, causing a deep or lateral hematoma, with disorganized blood and interstitial fluid buildup.

CORDILLERA The mountain ridge that spans North America, from Mexico through the Rocky Mountains into Alaska.

CORM The fleshy, bulblike, solid base of a stem, often rising out of a tuber or bulb.

COUNTERIRRITANT A substance applied to the skin to produce an irritating, heating, or vasodilating effect, in order to speed local healing by increasing circulation of blood, radiating the heat inward to inflamed tissues deep below the skin. It can also be used to induce reflex stimulation to seemingly unrelated internal organs. (Examples: mustard plaster, Poplar Bud oil.)

CRENULATED (OR CRENATE) Leaves having rounded, scalloped teeth along the edges.

CROHN'S DISEASE Also called regional enteritis or regional ileitis, this is a nonspecific inflammatory disease of the upper and lower intestine that forms granulated lesions. It is usually a chronic condition, with acute episodes of diarrhea, abdominal pain, loss of appetite, and loss of weight. It may affect the stomach or colon, but the most common sites are the duodenum and the lowest part of the small intestine, the lower ileum. The standard treatment is, initially, anti-inflammatory drugs, with surgical resectioning often necessary. The disease is autoimmune, and sufferers share the same tissue type (HLA-B27) as those who acquire ankylosing spondylitis.

CRUDE DRUG A dried, unprocessed plant, properly referring to one that was or is an official drug plant or the source of a refined drug substance. A **CRUDE BOTANICAL**, on the other hand, is one of our herbs that has no official standing. (Examples: Digitalis leaves [crude drug], White Sage [crude botanical].)

CYSTITIS An inflammation, often infectious, of the urinary bladder. It usually arises from a distal infection of the urethra or prostate.

CYTOKINE Also lymphokine, a broad term for a variety of proteins and neuropeptides that lymphocytes and macrophages use to communicate between themselves, often from long distances. They stimulate organization and antibody responses, seem to induce the bone marrow to proliferate the type of white blood cells needed for immediate resistance, and generate sophistication and fine-tuning for an overall strategy of resistance. A lymphocyte FAX.

CYTOMEGALOVIRUS (CMV) This subtle, worldwide microorganism is a member of the herpes virus group. It is large for a virus, contains DNA, and has a complex protein capsid. It forms latent, lifelong infections, and, except for occasional serious infections in infants and malnourished youngsters, seldom produces a disease state. With increased use of immunosuppression therapies for conditions ranging from arthritis to cancer to organ transplants, the incidence of adults with major infections of CMV increases yearly.

With herpes, EBV, and candida, CMV is one of a number of endogenous, normally benign bugs that is afflicting what has jokingly been referred to as *Homo medicus,* that is, overmedicated members of industrialized societies, particularly in the U.S. with its arcane, high-tech medical procedures.

CYTOPROTECTANT A substance or reaction that acts against chemical or biological damage to cell membranes. The most common cytoprotectant actions are on the skin and the liver (hepato-protectant), although there has been recent research involving lymphocyte T-cell cytoprotectants.

DECIDUOUS A plant that drops its leaves in the fall or, in some cases, during drought.

DIABETES Properly diabetes mellitus, it is a disease characterized by high blood sugar levels and sugar in the urine. Diabetes is really several disorders, generally broken down into juvenile onset and adult onset. The first, currently called insulin-dependent diabetes mellitus (IDDM or Type I), is somewhat hereditary, and results from inadequate synthesis of native insulin or sometimes from autoimmunity or a virus, and occurs most frequently in tissue-types HLA, DR3, and DR4. These folks tend to be lean.

The other main group is known as noninsulin-dependent diabetes mellitus (NIDDM or Type II). It is caused by a combination of heredity, constitution, and lifestyle, where high blood sugar and high blood fats often occur at the same time, and where hyperglycemic episodes have continued for so many years that fuel-engorged cells start to refuse glucose, and the person is termed insulin-resistant. These folks are usually overweight, tend to have fatty plaques in their arteries, and usually have chunky parents.

DIAPHORETIC A substance that increases perspiration, either by (1) dilating the peripheral blood vessels, (2) directly stimulating by drug action the nerves that affect the sweat glands, or by (3) introducing a volatile oil into the bloodstream that performs both tasks. (Examples of the three types: (1) California Bayberry, (2) Desert Milkweed, (3) Wild Ginger.)

DIARRHEA A watery evacuation of the bowels, without blood.

DIASTOLIC The lower number of a blood pressure reading signifying the myocardial and arterial relaxation between pump strokes. Too close to the higher number (systolic) usually signifies inadequate relaxation of the heart and arteries between heartbeats.

DIE-OFF The phenomenon of killing so many infectious organisms so quickly that the amount of dead biomass itself causes liver overload, allergic reactions, or a mild foreign-body response. It can occur with antibiotic therapy, treatment of candidiasis, and even with use of some herbal antivirals. Outside of prescription antifungals, it is seldom acknowledged as a medical problem. If you use a liver stimulant, diaphoretic, and diuretic, you will increase the efficiency of transport, catabolism, and excretion, and lessen the effects of die-off.

DIURETIC A substance that increases the flow of urine, either by increasing permeability of the kidneys' nephrons, increasing blood supply into the nephrons, or increasing the blood into each kidney by renal artery vasodilation.

DIVERTICULOSIS Having congenital pouches of the type found in many organs, particularly the colon, that are benign, but, being little cul-de-sacs, are likely to become inflamed from time to time. Diverticulitis is the term for inflamed diverticula.

DUODENUM This is the beginning of the small intestines, and it empties the stomach. It is 9 or 10 inches long, holds about the same amount of food as the digestive fundus or bottom of the stomach, and, through a papilla or sphincter, squirts a mixture of bile and pancreatic juices onto the previous stomach contents. These juices neutralize the acidic chyme; the pancreatic alkali and bile acids form soap to emulsify and aid fat digestion; and the duodenum walls secrete additional fluids and enzymes to admix with the pancreatic enzymes to initiate the final upper digestive investment. The duodenal wall secretes blood hormones to excite gallbladder and pancreas secretions, and, if overwhelmed, can inhibit the stomach from sending anything else down for a while, until they can catch their collective breath.

DYSCRASIA Presently a term referring to improper synthesis of blood proteins by the liver, especially clotting factors. Formerly it was used to describe an improper balance between blood and lymph in an organ or the whole person. Archaically, it referred to an imbalance between the four humors: blood, phlegm, yellow bile, and the postulated black bile.

DYSENTERY Severe diarrhea, usually from a colon infection, and containing blood and dead mucous membrane cells.

DYSPEPSIA Poor digestion, usually with heartburn and/or regurgitation of stomach acids.

EBV Epstein-Barr virus.

ECLECTICS The name commonly applied to the American School Physicians, a distinct group of physicians who trained in their own schools, were licensed as M.D.s, and specialized in low-tech, nonhospital rural health care—the country doc with a black bag. Besides standard medical procedures, they used a more wholistic approach to disease. They lost the licensing wars and are no more.

ECTOMORPH A thumbnail description of the somatotype who is dominated by the ectoderm, specifically the skin, nervous system, and endocrine glands. Less arcane, a tall and thin person, with long limbs, narrow chest, and a somewhat oversensitive nervous system.

ECZEMA A chronic dermatitis, more common in those with thin skin or allergies of an atopic or IgE-mediated type, and often clearly and distinctly aggravated by emotional stress.

EDEMA A localized or systemic condition in which the body tissues contain an excessive amount of fluid. Systemic edema can be as mild as premenstrual water retention (I mean mild by comparison) or involve loss of blood proteins or kidney and heart failures. Local edema is the result of extensive or extended inflammation, with blood protein leakage and the loss of interstitial colloid.

ELECTROLYTES In my context, acids, bases, and salts that contribute to the maintenance of electrical charges, membrane integrity, and acid-alkaline balance in the blood and lymph.

EMPHYSEMA A pulmonary condition with loss of elasticity in the alveoli and the interalveolar septa—the meat-foam and their interleaving sheaths that you fill up when you breathe. If a septum gets too stretched over time, several of the little sacs will coalesce together, decreasing the surface area for oxygen and carbon dioxide exchange. If enough of these sacs lose their separateness, breathing gets harder because each breath accomplishes less interchange of gases, resulting in emphysema. Caused by years of bad asthma, tobacco smoking, chemical damage, and other chronic lung disorders, it can be halted but not reversed.

ENDEMIC Confined to a limited geographic or ecologic niche.

ENDOMETRIOSIS The presence of endometrial tissue outside of the uterus. The endometrium is the mucous membrane inner lining of the uterus, with glandular cells and structural cells, both responding to estrogen by increasing in size (the proliferative phase); if there is endometrial tissue outside of the uterus, the tissue expands and shrinks in response to the estrus cycle, but shedding the menstrual phase can be difficult.

The most common type of endometriosis is found in the fallopian tubes; the endometrial tissue can shed and drain into the uterus, but *it hurts!* It's funny, but little tiny ducts, like the ureters, bile ducts, and fallopian tubes—they *really* cramp. The colon and uterus are big muscular tubes and, when cramped up, cause rather strong pain. When one of those little bitty things gets tenesmus, your face gets white (or light tan), you start to sweat, shiver, and revert to a fetal position.

Endometriosis that occurs around the ovaries or inside the belly is a purely physical and medical condition, but fallopian presence of endometrium usually reaches its peak in the early thirties; it can be helped by ensuring a strong estrogen *and* progesterone balance, thereby decreasing the tendency to form clots in the tubes, and to experience severe cramps every month.

ENTIRE A leaf with a straight, untoothed margin.

EPIPHYTE An air plant, growing on or with other plants but not in any way parasitic.

EPSTEIN-BARR VIRUS A large, ubiquitous, and normally benign, herpeslike virus with both DNA and capsid. It is sometimes implicated in mononucleosis and at least two types of lymphomas. It has been recently directly connected with the symptom picture called chronic fatigue syndrome (as has been CMV) and can produce many ill-defined (but subjectively distressful) symptoms, including fatigue, fevers of an unknown origin (FUO—love those acronyms!), and emotional lability. Immunosuppression, from whatever cause, allows the syndrome to occur.

ESOPHAGUS The dense, muscular tube, 9 to 10 inches long, that extends from the back of the throat (pharynx) to the stomach.

EXPECTORANT A substance that stimulates the outflow of mucus from the lungs and bronchial mucosa.

EXTRASYSTOLE A premature contraction of the heart. It can be caused by nervousness, indigestion, a tired and enlarged heart—anything up to an overt organic heart disease.

FEBRILE Feverish.

FIBROIDS An encapsulated tumor made up of disorganized and irregular connective tissue. Also called a leiomyoma or fibromyoma (or myofibroma, for that matter). A uterine fibroid is benign, there may be one or many, they grow slowly, have unknown causes, and may or may not cause painful menses or mid-cycle bleeding. Much depends on where they are in the uterus and whether or not they extend far enough into the cavity to impair and thin out the endometrium (if they do, they cause distress).

FLATUS Intestinal or stomach gas. If it rises upwards, it is an eructation (burp or belch); if it descends, causing borborygmus (love that word), you are flatulent (fartish).

FLAVONOID From *flavus*, Latin for yellow. A 2-benzene ring, 15-carbon molecule, it is formed by many plants (in many forms) for a variety of oxidative-redox enzyme reactions. Brightly pigmented compounds that make many fruits and berries yellow, red, and purple, and that are considered in European medicine to strengthen and aid capillary and blood vessel integrity, they are sometimes (redundantly) called bioflavonoids.

FOMENTATION A hot, wet poultice used on painful, inflamed areas. The usual form is a towel dipped in tea and applied hot or warm to the swollen tissue, being changed when it cools.

FUNCTIONAL An imbalance of response, without permanent tissue damage.

GANGLIA (singular: ganglion) Colonies of neurons outside the brain and spinal cord sometimes acting to control local functions. These latter are little affected by normal stress conditions. (Example: the solar plexus, made of two separate ganglions.)

GARBLE Rummaging through and cleaning out herbs; sorting.

GARDNERELLA Formerly *Haemophilus,* this is an anerobic bacteria that is a main contributor to bacterial vaginosis. It is sometimes sexually transmitted, but can stick around for years as a passive part of the vaginal flora, only to flare up. It seems to occur in up to a quarter of relatively monogamous women, but in half of women with multiple male partners. As bacterial vaginosis, Gardnerella is one of the three main causes of vaginal discharges, along with *Trichomonas* and *Candida albicans.* Antibiotic therapy for male partners seems of only marginal value, and the distinguishing characteristic of the infection is nearly no *Lactobacillus* vaginal presence, the main part of the flora that retains the lactic acid and peroxide balance so important in a healthy vagina. Live culture yogurt and douches help the problem.

GASTRITIS Inflammation of the stomach lining, with either congested and boggy membranes or inflamed membranes. It may be caused by bacteria and yeast, or chemical irritation like alcohol, but most frequently it is the result of emotional stress and inappropriate patterns of eating.

GASTROENTERITIS Inflammation of the stomach and small intestines. It is more frequently infectious than simple gastritis and is often accompanied by fever and general malaise.

GASTROESOPHAGEAL REFLUX The involuntary regurgitation of stomach contents or surface acids into the throat, with heartburn; it can be simple or serious.

GLUCOSIDE A plant compound containing a glucose and another substance, the bioactive part. A special-case glycoside.

GLYCOSIDE A plant compound containing one or more alcohols or sugars and a biologically active compound. The sugar part is called a glycone, the other stuff is called an aglycone. The important things to remember about some glycosides is that they may pass through much of the intestinal tract, with the hydrolysis of the molecule only occurring in the brush borders of the small intestine. The result is that the bioactive part, the aglycone, is absorbed directly into the bloodstream, and is often not floating around the intestinal tract contents at all.

Quinones are irritating and even toxic when ingested, but when taken as glycosides, they are absorbed directly into the bloodstream, where they are not dangerous (in moderation), and get excreted in the urine, where they inhibit infections. Plants like Madrone, Uva Ursi, and Manzanita work in this fashion. Some plant-derived heart medicines are only safe in proper doses because they, too, are glycosides, and they can be carried safely bound to proteins in the bloodstream, whereas if the aglycone were in the free form in the gut it might be either toxic or be digested directly into an inactive form.

GOUT A disease that causes episodes of acute arthritis and inflammatory swelling in one or more joints. Gout usually starts in a well-used, oft traumatized joint like the right big toe or knee, and usually starts in the night, during the time that Traditional Chinese Medicine calls "liver hour," 2:00 to 4:00 A.M. (allowing for daylight saving time). The inflammation is caused by uric acid crystals that have lodged in the joint's white blood cells and is started by hyperuricemia. Most folks with gout have a hereditary tendency to poorly excrete uric acid in urine as they get older, and it stays in the blood until . . . gout.

GRAM-POSITIVE/NEGATIVE Gram's Method is a staining procedure that separates bacteria into those that stain (positive) and those that don't (negative). Gram-positive bugs cause such lovely things as scarlet fever, tetanus, and anthrax, while some of the gram negs can give you cholera, plague, and the clap. This is significant to the microbiologist and the pathologist; otherwise I wouldn't worry. Still, knowing the specifics (toss in anaerobes and aerobes as well), you can impress real medical professionals with your knowledge of the secret, arcane language of medicine.

GRANULOCYTES These are a group of white blood cells that have many and well-pigmented granules, and derive from the bone marrow myeloblasts. The classic ones are neutrophils, eosinophils, and basophils, but should also include mast cells. Also, macrophages start out as agranulocytic monocytes but get *lots* of granules when they grow up. The granules are sources of digestive, immunologic, and inflammatory proteins.

HEMATURIA The presence of blood in the urine.

HEMOSTATIC A substance that stops or slows bleeding, used either internally or externally. (Examples: styptic pencil, Yerba Reuma.)

HEPATITIS An inflammation of the liver. It can be caused by an infection or by a simple liver toxicity, such as a three-day binge with ouzo, metaxa, and Ripple chasers.

HERPES A small group of capsid-forming DNA viruses, sometimes divided into Type I (forming vesicles and blisters on the mouth, lips—generally above the waist) and Type II (usually sexually transmitted, with symptoms mostly below the waist). Both types form acute initial outbreaks, go dormant, reactivate, and so forth. For most folks, frequent outbreaks are clear signs of stress or immuno-suppression. Both types are dangerous for infants.

HIATUS HERNIA An upwards protrusion of the stomach through the diaphragm wall. It is particularly common in women in their fourth and fifth decades.

HISTAMINE The defense substance responsible for most inflammation. It is synthesized from the amino acid histidine and is secreted by mast cells, basophils, and blood platelets. It stimulates vasodilation, capillary permeability, muscle contraction of the bronchioles, secretions of a number of glands, and attracts eosinophils, the white blood cells that are capable of controlling the inflammation. Mast cell histamine release is what can cause allergies.

HIV Human immunodeficiency virus, the retrovirus that is at least partially responsible for AIDS. At this writing (1993) it is not clear what other disorders besides AIDS may come from HIV infections. AIDS is a syndrome, partially (perhaps totally) produced by HIV. As with EBV, it is quite possible that the virus may cause only moderate immunosuppression in some people, while in others it will progress further to AIDS. The jury (all of them/us) is still out.

HOMEOPATHY Almost two centuries old, it is a system of medicine in which the treatment of disease (symptom pictures) depends on the administration of minute doses (attenuations) of substances that would, in larger doses, produce the same symptoms as the disease being treated. Homeopaths don't like that "disease" word, preferring to match symptoms, not diagnostic labels. Although by no means harmless, homeopathic doses are devoid of drug toxicity. Many practitioners these days prefer high, almost mythic potencies, sometimes resorting to "laying on of hands" to attain the alleged remedy. When M.D.s used homeopathy frequently (turn of the century), they preferred low potencies or even mother tinctures (herbs!), which I find quite reasonable (naturally).

HYBRID This is produced by a cross-fertilization between two species. This happens a lot more often than botanists would like, since a species is presumed to have distinct genetic characteristics and shouldn't do this hybridizing thing as often as it does. Most of the dozen or so species of Silk Tassel are really genetically the same, and the three hundred species of Aconite worldwide are all capable of hybridizing as well.

HYDROCELE An organized mass of serous or lymphatic fluid, usually encapsulated by connective tissue. An internal blister. The term is usually applied to a hydrocele of the testes, but a breast cyst is also a hydrocele.

HYPEREXTENSION The excessive extension of a limb or joint, usually followed by pain and some inflammation.

HYPERGLYCEMIA Elevations of blood glucose, either from the various types of diabetes, excessive sugar intake (short term) or from adrenalin or stimulant causes.

HYPERSECRETORY Oversecretion of fluids by a gland. It may occur from irritation, infection, or allergy, as in the nasal drooling in a head cold or hay fever, or, as in gastric hypersecretion, from a functional imbalance in the chemical and neurologic stimulus of the stomach lining.

HYPOTHALAMUS A part of the diencephalon of the brain, it is a major actor in the limbic system. This is a functional, not anatomic, system in the brain that influences and is influenced by emotions. Call the limbic system an ad hoc committee that decides how things are going today, based on past, present, potential, and myriad informational inputs from the meat. The hypothalamus gathers the data and sets the levels of the pituitary thermostat. The pituitary does what the hypothalamus tells it to do, and our whole chemical nervous system responds to the pituitary, which responds to the hypothalamus, which, along with the rest of the limbic system, decides the kind of day we need to get ready for. And to think that some doctors used to (and still) scoff at a "psychosomatic disorder."

IATROGENIC Illness, disease, or imbalances created by medical or nonmedical treatment that were not present before treatment. In medicine the therapy is blamed (not the therapist) and changed to something else. In alternative medicine it may be called a "healing crisis" and deemed good for you. *Beware:* if the therapy makes you feel worse in a new way, it is almost always the wrong therapy.

IBS Irritable bowel syndrome.

IgE Immunoglobulin E is a type of antibody produced by IgE plasma cells. These are specialized B-cell lymphocytes that make free-floating antibodies for what is termed humoral resistance. IgE is peculiar for several reasons. It is not made to be specific against only one antigen like other gamma globulins, but instead can bind with a number of dangerous proteins. Further, IgE travels to mast cells, sticks to their surfaces, and when antigens get stuck to the IgE, the mast cells secrete inflammatory compounds like histamine. Since IgE is a generalist, coded for a number of potential toxins, not just a single substance, it can decide that Juniper pollen and cat dander are antigens . . . and you have an allergy.

Elevated production of IgE is often inherited, which is why allergies run in a family—and why, once you have an allergy, the mast cells and IgE can decide that, for the duration, a whole bunch of other stuff causes hypersensitivity reactions, stuff that wouldn't normally bother you without an ongoing allergy.

ILEUM The lower two-thirds of the small intestine, ending in the ileocecal valve and emptying into the cecum of the colon. The last foot of the ileum is the only absorption site available for such important dietary substances as vitamin B_{12}, folic acid, some essential fatty acids, fat soluble vitamins, and recycled bile acids.

IMMUNITY The ability to resist infection and to heal. The process may involve acquired immunity, the ability to learn and remember a specific infectious agent, or innate immunity (the genetically programmed system of responses that attack, digest, remove, and initiate inflammation and tissue healing).

IMMUNOSTIMULANT An agent that stimulates either innate or acquired immunity. In the U.S., immunotherapy is relegated to experimental medicine, but a number of plant substances are used in Europe as immunostimulants. The presumption of immunostimulation is that you increase native resistance and let it run its course.

American Standard Practice, with all good intentions, tends to aggressive procedures, and feels empowered only when intervening *against* not *with* physiologic responses. Medicine is undoubtedly the only approach to many problems, but in the U.S. we all tend to forget that our brand of standard practice is uniquely aggressive and invasive amongst the industrialized nations.

IMMUNOSUPPRESSANT An agent that acts to suppress the body's natural immune response. This is totally understandable in tissue and organ transplants, and in some dangerous inflammatory conditions, but nearly all anti-inflammatory medications are immunosuppressant, including cortisone, antihistamines, and even aspirin. Some medical radicals are convinced that the chronic viral and fungal disorders of our age are partially facilitated by such medications.

INTERSTITIAL FLUID The hydrogel that surrounds cells in soft tissues. It is a mucopolysaccaride starch gel, and the serum that leaves the blood capillaries flows through this gel, some to return to the exiting venous blood, some to enter the lymph system. There is an old medical axiom: the blood feeds the lymph, and the lymph feeds the cells. Interstitial fluid that flows through the starch colloid is this lymph.

IRRITABLE BOWEL SYNDROME This is a common and benign condition of the colon, taking different forms but usually characterized by alternating constipation and diarrhea. There is often some pain accompanying the diarrhea phase. The bowel equivalent of asthma, its main cause is stress, often accompanied by a history of GI infections. Adrenalin stress slows the colon and causes constipation, followed by the cholinergic rebound overstimulation of the colon. It is also called spastic colon, colon syndrome, or even chronic colitis.

ISOTONIC Having the same salinity as body fluids. You can make a quart of water isotonic by adding a slightly rounded measuring teaspoon of table salt.

KLEBSIELLA A genus of bacteria in the Enterobacteriaceae. *K. pneumoniae* is implicated in much pneumonia, particularly when it is a secondary infection following a simple chest cold.

LACTOBACILLUS A genus of gram-positive, acid-resistant bacteria in the Lactobacillaceae family. We know of lactobacillus because of its use in making yogurt and the conventional wisdom of taking it in one form or another after antibiotic therapy, but it is an integral part of the colon and mouth flora, and is the critical acidifying agent in vaginal flora. There is a growing body of rather ignored data showing the value of regular consumption of a lactobacillus-containing food in immunosuppression, slow virus, and candidiasis conditions.

LANCEOLATE A leaf that is lance-shaped.

LATERAL At or on the side, usually from a stem.

LEAFLET A small leaf that is part of a compound leaf.

LINIMENT A liquid containing therapeutic agents for topical application. It may be an alcohol, oil, or water preparation.

LUTEINIZING HORMONE (LH) This is a sugar-bearing protein manufactured by the anterior pituitary. Like a lot of the pituitary hormones, it surges on and off, since constant secretion would overload and deaden receptors. In women, it builds up after menses, stimulating the release of estrogen from the ovaries. Estrogen in turn stimulates the hypothalamus to increase its stimulation of LH from the pituitary, until, a day or two before ovulation, they produce a guitar-amp feedback, and the cells that produce LH start to surge follicle-stimulating hormone (FSH). The egg pops, being replaced by the corpus luteum, which produces progesterone for the next ten to twelve days.

Progesterone inhibits and lowers LH levels, as well as inhibiting levels of estrogen already being produced by the young follicle that will produce next month's egg. In men, LH is responsible for stimulation of testosterone, although FSH and the testes hormone inhibin are responsible for both the production of sperm and controlling testosterone.

LYMPHATIC Pertaining to the lymph system or lymph tissue, the "back alley" of blood circulation. Lymph is the alkaline, clear intercellular fluid that drains from the blood capillaries, where the arterial blood separates into thick, gooey venous blood and lymph. It bathes the cells, drains up into the lymph capillaries, through the lymph nodes for cleaning and checking for bad stuff, up through the body, and back to recombine with the venous blood in the upper chest. Blood in the veins is thick, mainly because part of its fluid is missing, traveling through the tissues as lymph.

Lymph nodes in the small intestine absorb most of the dietary fats as well-organized chylomicrons. Lymph nodes and tissue in the spleen, thymus, and tonsils also organize lymphocytes and maintain the software memory of previously encountered antigens and their antibody defense response. Blood feeds the lymph, lymph feeds the cells, lymph cleanses the cells and returns to the blood.

MACROPHAGE This is a mature form of what is released from the marrow as a monocyte. A macrophage lives long, can digest much detritus, and is able to wear particles of odd food on its outer membrane. This allows T-cell and B-cell lymphocytes to taste the particle (an epitope) and form an antibody response. Further, these macrophages, traveling as monocytes, will take up permanent residence in many tissues, providing them with immunity. They line the spleen, form the cleansing Kupffer cells in the liver, make up the "dust cells" that protect the lungs, protect the synovial fluids of the joints, and form the microglial cells that provide protection to the brain and nerve tissue—on and on, the macrophages cleaning up messes and acting as the intermediates between innate and acquired immunity.

MAST CELLS These are a group of cells that line the capillaries of tissues that come in contact with the outside, like skin, sinus, and lung mucosa. They, like their first cousin basophils, are produced in the red bone marrow and migrate to the appropriate tissues, where they stay. They bind IgE, supply the histamine and heparin response that gives you a healing inflammation, and cause allergies.

MENSTRUUM The solvent used in extraction. For a dry tincture, the menstruum might be 50% alcohol and 50% water.

MESENCHYMAL CELLS Literally, those derived from embryonic mesoderm; practically, those in a tissue that give it structure and form. Opposite of parenchymal.

MESOMORPH In somatotyping, a mesoderm-muscle-structural-dominant person. The Incredible Hulk syndrome.

METABOLISM The sum total of changes in an organism in order to achieve a balance (homeostasis). Catabolic burns up, anabolic stores and builds up; the sum of their work is metabolism.

METABOLITES A by-product, waste product, or endotoxin produced as the result of metabolism.

MITTELSCHMERZ Abdominal pains that occur midway between menstrual periods and which are caused by ovulation.

MONONUCLEOSIS Properly, infectious mononucleosis, a viral infection of the lymph pulp most frequently caused by the Epstein-Barr virus. The spleen, lymph nodes, and (sometimes) the liver are involved. The general symptoms are fever, sore throat, exhaustion, and abnormal white blood cells.

MUCUS MEMBRANES The mucosa, forming a continuous layer that protects the internal membranes from the outside, where the external environment goes into or through the body, as in both the cavities (respiratory system and genital-urinary system) and the intestinal tract. The external skin and the internal mucosa meet at the orifices, forming mucoepithelial membranes.

MYALGIA Tenderness or pain of the muscles themselves; muscular rheumatism.

MYENTERIC PLEXUS Broadly, the several neuron masses, ganglia, and nerve fiber plexus that lie in the walls of the intestinal tract, particularly the small intestine. They monitor and stimulate local muscle and glandular functions as well as blood supply, with little interface or control by the central nervous system or the autonomics. Each synapse away from the CNS gives greater autonomy, and these nerves only listen to God . . . and food. This means the small intestine is relatively free of stress syndromes.

NARCOTIC A substance that depresses central nervous system function, bringing sleep and lessening pain. By definition, narcotics can be toxic in excess.

NEURALGIA Pain, sometimes severe, that manifests along the length of a nerve and arises in the nerve itself, not in the tissue from which the sensation is felt.

NEUROPATHY A disease of the central or peripheral nervous systems. In more common reference, a neuropathy is primarily a disorder of peripheral nerves. CNS diseases are often life threatening; neuropathies are generally disorders of the control and sensory nerves out in the body.

NEUTROPHILS Another name for polymorphonuclear leukocytes, the most common type of blood-carried white blood cell, and the first mobile resistance cell to come to the rescue in injury.

NITROGENOUS A compound or molecule that contains nitrogen; in my context, a substance that is or was a part of protein metabolism.

NUCLEOPROTEIN A molecule that is formed from a structural protein that is combined with nucleic acid, and generally found in cell nuclei and other proliferative points in cells. Upon cell death, nucleoproteins, unlike others, cannot be catabolized and recycled efficiently; instead, part of the protein is degraded to purines, and thence to uric acid. Uric acid, unlike urea, is an excretory dead end.

NURSE LOGS In old-growth forests, these are ancient downed trees that rot so slowly that they themselves become the fundus and growth media for new and growing trees and other life-forms.

OIL, FIXED These are lipids, esters of long-chain fatty acids and alcohols, or generally related oily stuff. If you drop some fixed oil on a blotter, it just stays there—forever. (Example: olive oil.)

OIL, VOLATILE The aromatic, oxygenated derivitives of terpenes that can be obtained from plants (in our case), usually by distillation. Unlike a fixed oil that has no scent (unless rancid), volatile oils are *all* scent. (Example: oil of Peppermint.)

OPPOSITE Plant parts, usually leaves, that form pairs at nodes.

ORCHITIS Inflammation of the testes, manifested by swelling and tenderness, usually infectious, sometimes from trauma.

ORGANIC DISEASE A disease that started as, or became, impairment of structure or tissue. The smoker may have coughing and shortness of breath for years, and suffer from functional disorders; when the smoker gets emphysema, it is an organic disease.

PALMATE Having a leaf shaped like a hand.

PANCREAS This is a gland situated above the navel in the abdominal cavity that extends from the left side to the center, with its head tucked into the curve of the duodenum. It is about 6 inches long, weighs 3 or 4 ounces, secretes pancreatic enzymes and alkali into the duodenum in concert with the gallbladder and liver, and secretes the hormones insulin and glucagon into the blood.

Insulin acts to facilitate the absorption of blood glucose into fuel-needing cells, and glucagon stimulates a slow release of glucose from the liver, primarily to supply fuel to the brain. That most cherished organ uses one-quarter of the sugar in the blood and has no fuel storage.

PANICLE A compound flower head that forms a raceme.

PARASYMPATHETIC A division of the autonomic (involuntary) nervous system that controls normal digestive, reproductive, cardiopulmonary, and vascular functions and stimulates most secretions. This subsystem works as a direct antagonist to the sympathetic division, and organ functions balance between them.

PARENCHYMAL These are cells in a tissue or tissues in an organ that are concerned with function. These are the characteristic cells or tissues that do the actual stuff. The importance to us is that parenchymal tissues expend much vital energy in their functions and are less tolerant of a degraded environment than the structural mesenchyme. A congested and impaired organ like the liver of a heavy drinker has so much regular disfunction that eventually the more tolerant and metabolically less particular mesenchymal cells become more common, and the distressed, overworked, and metabolically compromised parenchymal cells become a minority. The structural cells can multiply with ease in a poor environment, the more delicate functional cells cannot—and you end up with the type of cirrhosis sometimes termed mesenchymal invasion disease. The point of this is that the sooner you return an organ or tissue back to the healed state, the more likely you are to have a healthy balance between the structural and functional.

PEDICEL The stem of a flower within a floral cluster.

PEDUNCLE The stem or stalk of a single flower or a whole floral cluster.

PELVIC INFLAMMATORY DISEASE (PID) Also called salpingitis, the term is applied to infections of the fallopian tubes that follow or are concurrent with uterine and cervical infections. Gonorrhea and chlamydia are the most common organisms, and the infection is usually begun through sexual contact; an IUD can induce inflammation sufficient to allow an endogenous organism to start the infection. PID after birth, on the other hand, is usually the result of staph or strep infections that can infect injured membranes.

PETIOLE A leafstalk or stem, or an unexpanded section.

PHAGOCYTOSIS The act of absorbing and digesting fragments, detritis, or whole organisms, as an amoeba does. Granulocytes do this in the body.

PINNAE The leaflets or primary division of a pinnate leaf.

PINNATE A compound leaf, having the leaflets arranged on each side of the stem.

PINNATIFID A leaf that is pinnately cleft, but into lobes that do not reach the midrib, and not into separate leaflets.

PINNULE A division of a pinna.

PISTILLATE A female flower that has pistils but no stamens.

PITUITARY An endocrine gland somewhat behind the eyes and suspended from the front of the brain. The front section, the anterior pituitary, makes and secretes a number of controlling hormones that affect the rate of oxidation; the preference for fats, sugars, or proteins for fuel; the rate of growth and repair in the bones, connective tissue, muscles, and skin; the ebb and flow of steroid hormones from both the gonads and adrenal cortices. It does this through both negative and positive feedback. The hypothalamus controls these functions, secreting its own hormones into a little portal system that feeds into the pituitary, telling the latter what and how much to do. The hypothalamus itself synthesizes the nerve hormones that are stored in the posterior pituitary, which is responsible for squirting them into the blood when the brain directs it to. These neurohormones act quickly, like adrenalin, to constrict blood vessels, limit diuresis in the kidneys, and trigger the complex responses of sexual excitation, milk let-down in nursing, and muscle stimulus in the uterus (birthing, orgasm, and menstrual contractions), prostate, and nipples.

PLATELET AGGREGATION Platelets are the small, rather uniform fragments of large bone marrow cells that aid the blood in coagulation, hemostasis, inflammation, and thrombus formation. Mild subclotting and sticking is a common early condition that can lead to thrombosis, atherosclerosis, and strokes, and can be helped by an aspirin a day, better fat digestion, and Red Root.

PORTAL CIRCULATION This is a type of circulatory bypass used when substances in blood or fluid need to be kept out of the general flow. A portal system begins in capillaries and ends in capillaries, and nothing leaves it intact. The hypothalamus sends hormones into the portal system between it and the pituitary, and the pituitary responds to it by secreting its own hormones, but dissolving the hypothalamus ones. Blood that leaves the intestinal tract, spleen, and pancreas (partially) goes into the liver's portal system and does not leave that organ until it has been thoroughly screened and altered.

POSTPARTUM After birthing.

PROGESTERONE This is the hormone secreted after ovulation by the corpus luteum. It is a steroid (a cholesterol with a funny hat), enters receptive cells to stimulate their growth, and acts as an anabolic agent. Estrogen should be viewed as the primary coat underneath the cycles during a woman's reproductive years, with progesterone, its antagonist, surging for ten or twelve days in ovulatory months.

Most of the actions of progesterone cannot occur without estrogen having previously induced the growth of progesterone-receptive cells. In the estrus cycle, estrogen stimulates the thickening of membranes (the proliferative phase), and progesterone stimulates their sophistication into organized and secreting mucosa (the secretory phase). The new secretions contain anticoagulants, antimicrobials, and rich mucus fluids. If there is pregnancy, the uterine membranes are fully structured for the long haul; if menses occurs, the thickened tissues can erode away without clotting, becoming infected, or flow poorly. If there is not enough estrogen, the corpus luteum will not mature. If the corpus luteum is weak, menses becomes disorganized, clotty, and painful.

PROSTATE This is a walnut-sized gland that surrounds the beginning of the urethra in men. It secretes the alkaline transport fluid that mixes with sperm from the testes to form semen. The prostate needs adequate anabolic steroid stimulation for its health and growth, especially testosterone. Because of diminished healthy hormone levels, pelvic congestion, and decreased blood (and hormone) circulation, or because of sexually transmitted or urinary tract infections, a male may get prostatitis. (See BENIGN PROSTATIC HYPERTROPHY.)

PROTEOLITIC An enzyme or agent that speeds up the breaking down or digestive hydrolysis of proteins into smaller proteins, peptides, polypeptides, oligopeptides, amino acids, and all that delicious nitrogenous slurry-stuff.

PURINES These are waste products or metabolites of nucleoproteins. They are not recyclable and are broken down further to an excretable form, uric acid. High purine presence in a tissue signifies a recent high turnover in nucleoproteins from injury or cell death, which is why some purines, such as allantoin, will stimulate cell regeneration. Many plants contain allantoin, most noticeably Comfrey. Some foods are heavy purine producers and can elevate uric acid levels. These include organ meats, seafood, legumes, and such politically correct foods as spirulina, chlorella, and bee pollen. Caffeine and theobromine are purine-based alkaloids and can mildly increase uric acid, but they pale beside algae, pollen, and glandular extracts from the chiropractor.

PYRROLIZIDINE ALKALOID A type of alkaloid found in many plants of the Composite and Borage families, once termed a *Senecio* alkaloid. Some of the pyrrolizidine group have been shown to cause several types of liver degeneration and blood vessel disorders. Several deaths have been attributed to improperly identified plant usage of a *Senecio,* and some of the desert Boraginaceae annuals and *Senecio* annuals are overtly toxic. Young leaves and spring roots of Comfrey hybrids should be avoided as well.

RACEME A flowering spike or cluster where the flowers are borne along the peduncle on pedicels of similar length.

RAY FLOWERS The margin flowers on a composite head, usually sterile, that resemble single petals. (Example: the white "petals" of a Daisy.)

REFLEXED Turned down or curved backwards.

REGRANULATION Granulation is the forming of connective tissue fibroblasts, epithelium and inflammatory cells around the nucleus of new capillaries in tissues that have been burned or scraped. This delicate tissue is often reinjured, and regranulation is a slower process with more formation of scar tissue. Some plant resins will quickly stimulate the process, increase the complexity of healing, and lessen fibroblast scar formation.

RESINS These are wax-containing plant oils, often secreted to fill in injured tissues, much like a blood clot, sometimes used to protect leaves from loss of water through evaporation or to render them unpalatable. (See BALSAMICS.)

RHEUMATOID Broadly, having dull aching in joints, muscles, eyes, and so forth. In a more literal sense, it is having an autoimmune response, usually between certain IgM and IgE antibodies, that may have started as a bacterial infection or as some autoimmune reaction. The severity is increased under emotional, physical, dietary, and allergic stress—or any stress.

Hans Selye showed a few years ago that once a chronic disease response occurs, *any* stress above metabolic tolerance will aggravate the chronic disease, which is why some people, stressed by cold, wet weather, must avoid it; but someone else is stressed by legumes, still another person gets upset (and stressed) by watching too much CNN. You know best what stresses you; it's not fair to ask a doc to find it out for you. Rheumatoid arthritis is so named because it somewhat resembles the joint inflammations that can occur in rheumatic fever, a different disease started by a strep infection.

RHINITIS Simply, inflammation of the sinus membranes, sometimes extending to the eyes and ears. It may be caused by a head cold, hay fever, or a chemical irritant.

ROULEAU A group of red blood cells arranged together like a roll of coins, usually only noticed on a slide. Since red blood cells in a reasonably healthy person should have a mutually repelling membrane charge, this means that something like an inflammatory response or an elevation of liver-synthesized lipids is occurring. Inflammation makes the blood "sticky," and the lipids from the liver lower the charges. Remember, of course, that I am talking about subclinical imbalances—such things as rouleau can accompany some pretty gnarly diseases. *Our* kind of rouleau can give you a headache or make your hands and feet cold because it's hard to push rolls of coins through little bitty capillaries.

SACRAL NERVES These are five pairs of CNS nerves that exit through the sacral foramen and sacral hiatus, and bring information in and out of the spinal cord. Much of their function relates to the sciatic nerve, and they bring information in from the skin dermatomes of the heel, back of the legs, buttocks, and the pelvic floor.

SALICYLATES Esters or salts of salicylic acid, such as aspirin, and including glycoside forms such as salicin.

SALPINGITIS Inflammation of the fallopian tubes. (See PELVIC INFLAMMATORY DISEASE.)

SAPONIN Any plant glycoside with soapy action that can be digested to yield a sugar and a sapogenin aglycone. Many (but not all) saponins can be toxic and speed up hemoglobin degradation. Many of the plants in this book contain saponins, although only Amole Lily could cause this type of response—and that's used as a soap. (Examples: Sarsaparilla, California Spikenard.)

SCAPE A long flower-bearing stem or peduncle that arises from the ground. It is leafless, or the leaves are reduced to bracts.

SCIATICA This is neuralgia of the sciatic nerve. These are the two largest nerves in the body, composed of the tibial and common peroneal nerves, bound together and containing elements of the lowest two lumbar and upper three sacral spinal cord nerves. Sciatica is felt as severe pain from the buttocks, down the back of the thighs, often radiating to the inside of the leg, even to the point of parasthesia or prickly numbness. Although tumors can cause the problem, far and away the most common causes are a lower back subluxation (responding to adjustment) or pelvic congestion and edema (responding to laxatives, exercise, and decreasing portal vein and lymphatic congestion).

SEBORRHEA A disorder of the sebaceous glands, with changes in the amount and quality of the oils secreted. Although it can occur in any part of the body, seborrhea of the scalp (dandruff) is most common.

SEMINAL VESICLES These are a couple of spongy glands, 1½ to 2 inches long, that secrete high-sugar, acidic, and thick, ropy colloid into the ductus deferens (containing sperm from the testes) during ejaculation. The two fluids empty into the prostate, where they are mixed with alkaline prostatic fluids to form semen.

SEPAL A leaf or segment of the calyx.

SHIGELLOSIS An acute, self-limiting intestinal infection, with diarrhea, fever, and abdominal pain, caused by one of the *Shigella* genus of gram-negative bacteria. The infection is contracted through food prepared by infected individuals or by direct contact with them. Raw sewage contamination can also be a source.

SPADIX A short, flowering spike on a thick, fleshy axis.

SPATHE A specialized bract, usually large, that encloses a flower cluster or spadix—especially in the Araceae family.

SPLEEN The large organ lying to the left of, below, and behind the stomach. This organ is partially responsible for white blood cell formation (red blood cells in childhood), and it is lined with resident macrophages that help it filter the blood, remove and recycle old and dead red blood cells, and send this all up to the liver in the portal blood. The liver, in fact, does most of the recycling of splenic hemoglobin derivatives. The spleen initiates much resistance and immunologic response, being made mostly of lymph pulp, and it stores and concentrates a large number of red blood cells. These can be injected into the bloodstream for immediate use under flight or fight stress, since the spleen is covered with capsule and vascular muscles that constrict in the presence of adrenalin or sympathetic adrenergic nerve stimulus.

STAMENS The male, pollen-producing organs in flowering plants. A staminate flower is only male, with pistillate (female) flowers on the same or different plants. Most flowering plants have both parts on the same flower, although they may mature at different times to avoid self-pollination.

STAPH This is short for *Staphylococcus aureus* and *S. epidermidis,* the two types that are likely to cause disease. They are gram-positive, nonmotile bacteria that are aerobic—unless they need to be anaerobic. Staph of various types are responsible for boils and carbuncles; they may be involved in impetigo, toxic shock syndrome, endocarditis, osteomyelitis, and urinary tract infections; they stay around hospitals and veterinary clinics waiting to get you. They are also a normal part of the mouth, throat, and skin flora in a third to a half of all of us, causing no problems, but just waiting. Staph has always been with us—some even eat our antibiotics.

STEROID HORMONE These are fats similar to, and usually synthesized from, cholesterol, starting with Acetyl-CoA, moving through squalene, past lanosterol, into cholesterol, and, in the gonads and adrenal cortex, back to a number of steroid hormones. Nearly all of the classic hormones are proteins or smaller peptides; they don't get inside a cell (the membrane keeps them out); instead, they bind to, and initiate, cell changes from the outside. The exceptions are thyroxine (from the thyroid) and the steroid hormones. They move *into* the cell, bind with receptors, and initiate changes in the way a cell regenerates itself or synthesizes new compounds.

Because the steroid hormones stimulate cell growth, either by changing the internal structure or increasing the rate of proliferation, they are often called anabolic steroids. Estrogen, an ovarian steroid, when secreted into the bloodstream, will be bound within a short time by internal receptors inside those cells that need estrogen for their growth; the unused portion is broken down, mostly in the liver. Since luteinizing hormone from the pituitary is surged in pulses an hour apart, the estrogen is also surged from the reacting ovaries, and by the time more estrogen is available, the binding cells *need* more; their program of synthesis has run out and needs to be started again. Of course, most steroid hormone reactions are less measured than this, but you get the idea.

STEROIDS, PLANT The previous subject is obviously an endless one, but as this is the glossary of an herb book, let me assure you, virtually no plants have a direct steroid hormone-mimicking effect. There are a few notable exceptions with limited application, like Black Cohosh and Licorice.

Plant steroids are usually called phytosterols, and, when they have any hormonal effects at all, it is usually to interfere with human hormone functions.

B-sitosterol, found in lots of food, interferes with the ability to absorb cholesterol from the diet. Corn oil and legumes are two well-endowed sources that can help lower cholesterol absorption. This is of only limited value, however, since cholesterol is readily manufactured in the body, and elevated cholesterol in the blood is often the result of internal hormone and neurologic stimulus, not the diet. Cannabis can act to interfere with androgenic hormones, and Dandelion phytosterols can both block the synthesis of some new cholesterol by the liver and increase the excretion of cholesterol as bile acids; but other than that, plants offer little direct hormonal implication.

The classic method of synthesizing pharmaceutical hormones involved using a saponin, diosgenin, and a five-step chemical degradation, to get to progesterone, and another, using stigmasterol and bacterial culturing, to get to cortisol. These are chemical procedures that have nothing to do with human synthesis of such hormones, and the plants used for the starting materials—Mexican Wild Yam, Agave, and Soybeans—are nothing more than commercially feasible sources of compounds widely distributed in the plant kingdom. A clever biochemist could obtain testosterone from potato sterols, but no one would be likely to make the leap of faith that eating potatoes makes you manly (or less womanly), and there is no reason to presume that Wild Yam (*Dioscorea*) has any progesterone effects in humans. First, the method of synthesis from diosgenin to progesterone has nothing to do with human synthesis of the corpus luteum hormone; second, oral progesterone has virtually no effect since it is rapidly digested; and third, orally active synthetic progesterones such as norethindrone are test-tube born, and never *saw* a Wild Yam.

STIPULES A little leafy appendage formed at the juncture of a leaf and the main stem.

STOLONIFEROUS A plant that tends to form lateral roots, sometimes green and potentially stemming, sometimes blanched and tending to root from the nodes—or both.

SUBACUTE Having characteristics of both acute and chronic. This is the state in a disease when most of the aches and pains have subsided and you are likely to overdo things and not completely recover. The chest cold that lingers for weeks as a stubborn cough is a subacute condition, as is the tendonitis that lingers because you won't stop playing tennis long enough to completely heal.

SUBCLINICAL This is *our* turf, the period of time when a potential disease is still potential, and a functional imbalance or tendency has not caused any organic disruption. Those years of poor digestion, heartburn, and the systematic suppression of upper intestinal function by adrenalin stress have not become overt gastritis, ulcers, or IBS. You have symptoms of distress (subclinical) but no real, ripened clinical disease.

SYMPATHETIC A division of the autonomic or involuntary nervous system that works in general opposition to the parasympathetic division (q.v.). Many of the sympathetic functions are local, specific, and involve secretion of acetylcholine, like any other of your normal nerves—stimulating or suppressing a specific muscle, gland, or whatever. A certain number of these nerves, however, unlike any others in the body, secrete epinephrine (adrenalin) and are called adrenergic.

Since the adrenal medulla also secretes the same substances into the bloodstream as a hormone, all the muscles or glands that are affected by the adrenergic sympathetic nerves also react *in toto* to the epinephrine secreted into the blood. This forms the basis for a potentially lifesaving emergency fight or flight response and is meant for short, drastic activities.

A chronic excess of the adrenergic response, however, is a major cause of stress—and a major contributor to many types of chronic disease. The more you use a particular nerve pathway or affect a particular group of functions, the more blood, fuel storage, and mitochondria are produced to strengthen that group of actions. Using adrenergic energy excessively gives literal dominance to those things that are stimulated or suppressed, and the effects of adrenalin stress linger in the body after the adrenalin is long gone. Since one of the first subjective symptoms of subclinical malnutrition, metabolic imbalances, and environmental pollution is irritability of the central nervous system, hypersympathetic function acts as an intermediate between poor diet, pollution, and disease.

SYSTOLIC The measurement of arterial blood pressure at the point of heart contraction (greatest pressure); the higher of the two BP numbers, with diastolic (q.v.) being the lower.

TACHYCARDIA Abnormally fast heartbeat.

TANNINS A group of simple and complex phenol, polyphenol, and flavonoid compounds, bound with starches, and often so amorphous that they are classified as tannins simply because at some point in degradation they are astringent and contain variations on gallic acid. Produced by plants, tannins are generally protective substances found in the outer and inner tissues of plants, often breaking down in time to phlebotannins and, finally, humin. All of the tannins are relatively resistant to digestion or fermentation, and either decrease the ability of animals to easily consume the living plant, or, as in deciduous trees, cause the parts of the plant to decay so slowly that there is little likelihood of infection to the still-living parts of the plant resulting from rotting dead material around its base. All tannins act as astringents, shrinking tissues and contracting structural proteins in the skin and mucosa. Tannin-containing plants can vary a great deal in their physiological effects and should be approached individually.

TERNATE Divided into threes.

TERPENES Any of a group of hydrocarbons that are made up of building blocks of isoprene (C_5H_8) or similar five-carbon units, with a monoterpene made up of two units (example: limonene and pinene), a sesquiterpene made up of three units (example: humulene, a Hops aromatic), and a diterpene made up of four units. The terpenes, in our context, are the primary constituents in the aromatic fractions of our scented plants.

THOMSONIAN That school of medical philosophy and therapy founded by the American messianic nature therapist Samuel Thomson (b. 1769). Thomson's great axiom was, "Heat is life, and cold is death." He lived in New England, which explains some of this. He and the later Thomsonians made great use of vomiting, sweating, and purging to achieve these ends—crude by present standards, but saner than the standard practice medicine of the times. The Thomsonians split vehemently from the early Eclectics before the Civil War; the latter, larger group preferred to train true professional physicians as M.D.s. The first group disavowed any overt medical training ("physicking").

Many of the practices of Jethro Kloss (*Back to Eden*) and John Christopher are neo-Thomsonian, and much of what still goes on in the old guard of alternative therapy is what Susun Weed calls the "Heroic Tradition" (no compliment intended). Rule of thumb: If you see Lobelia and Capsicum together in a formula, along with recommendations for colonics, it's probably something Sam Thomson did first.

TINEA Dermatomycosis; any number of skin fungus infections, such as ringworm, athlete's foot, and so forth. It is generally slow to acquire and hard to get rid of.

TMJ Abbreviation for temporomandibular joint. These are the two joints that connect the jawbone to the skull under the zygomatic arch. TMJ syndrome involves pain in the joint, clicking in the joint from degradation of the sinovial fluids, and sharp, shooting pain when chewing. The two main causes are malocclusion (improper tooth alignment) and tension. Some people grind their teeth, others clench their jaws, perhaps from the inability to say what is felt. Chiropractors and osteopaths love helping these folks, some even specializing in TMJ work.

TOMENTOSE Having woolly hairs.

TONIC A substance taken to strengthen and prevent disease, especially chronic disease. Formerly, tonics were widely available both as over-the-counter and prescription formulas. Unfortunately, the increased sophistication of medicine has led to the abandonment of preventative or strengthening approaches that utilize the innate abilities of an organism (like ourselves) to right itself with a little prodding in the correct direction. The last several decades have seen increased focus on disease-at-a-time medicine, with more and more patients receiving treatment at acute care facilities like hospitals and clinics, circumstances that delegate against preventative or tonic approaches.

TRIFOLIATE Having three leaflets in a compound leaf, like a clover.

TRIGONE This is the triangular basement muscle of the urinary bladder. It differs in structure and nerves from the top of the bladder, the detrusor muscle, which expands as the bladder fills, and contracts during urination under parasympathetic nerve stimulus. The trigone does not expand, is under sympathetic nerve stimulus, and supplies the rigidity and sphincter support for the urethra in front and the ureters in back.

TRIMESTER The three three-month sections of a pregnancy.

TRIPINNATE Thrice pinnately compound leaf.

TUBER A short, fleshy, underground part of a stem or root. (Example: potato, Western Peony.)

UMBEL A flowering head where the pedicels (individual flower stems) all spring from one point, usually the end of the peduncle. Compound umbels, found in some Umbelliferae, have umbels branching from peduncle umbels that themselves are branching from the main stem.

URATES The salts of uric acid, found in the urine, some kidney stones, and (unfortunately) in gouty joints.

URETHRITIS Any inflammation of the urethra, whether from external irritation, overly acidic or scalding urine, passage of stones, or an active infection of the canal. (See CYSTITIS.)

URIC ACID The final end product of certain proteins in the body or from the diet, especially the nucleoproteins found in the nucleus of cells. Unlike the much smaller protein waste product urea, which is mostly recycled to form many amino acids, uric acid is an unrecyclable metabolite. It is a bent nail that won't re-straighten, and it must be excreted—nucleoprotein to purine to uric acid to the outside in the urine or the sweat. (See GOUT, PURINES.)

URINARY TRACT (UT) The kidneys and the lower urinary tract, which includes the ureters, bladder, and urethra.

U.S.P.–N.F. *United States Pharmacopeia* and *National Formulary.* The *U.S.P.* was first published in 1820 and ever ten years thereafter until the Second World War, after which it has been revised every five years. It has always been meant to define the physical, chemical, and pharmaceutical characteristics of the most accepted and widely used drugs of the time, and to set the standards for purity. The *N.F.* was first published in 1888, and, up until 1980, in the same year as the *United States Pharmacopeia.* Since 1980, both have been issued in the same volume.

The *National Formulary* was originally intended as a list of the official recipes for pharmaceutical formulas; characteristics of those drugs or plants used in the formulas or that were still recognized as secondary drugs; and the substances needed for the manufacturing of drugs but that were not active, like gelatin or pill binders. With the decreased use of tonics and less invasive medications after the Second World War, the *National Formulary* became primarily a text defining the inactive substances used in drug manufacturing; the *United States Pharmacopeia* now lists the active substances; and all the rich heritage of tonics, elixirs, bitters, syrups, and alternate preparations has disappeared from the short memory span of Standard Practice Medicine. If an herbalist wanted to practice as a pharmaceutical antiquarian, the *U.S.P.*s and *N.F.*s of the years between 1890 and 1950 would supply virtually every needed formula and herbal preparation that a Western herbalist would ever need—it's all there (and all forgotten). To a great degree, the contemporary herbal renaissance is reinventing the wheel.

VAGINITIS An inflammation of the vagina, either from simple tissue irritation or from an infection.

VAGINOSIS A vaginal infection characterized by a smelly discharge and the presence of Gardnerella, Mycoplasma, and other anaerobic bacteria, with the lack of *Lactobacillus* species.

VAGUS NERVE Also called the pneumogastric nerve, this is the tenth cranial nerve, with many fibers leading to parasympathetic ganglia in internal organs, and can be considered the presynapse starter for the upper parts of the parasympathetic functions.

VASODILATION, PERIPHERAL The increase of blood into the skin, resulting from the relaxation of the small arterioles that lead into the capillary beds of the edges of the body. This is a gentle way to lessen early high blood pressure, decreasing the difficulty of pushing columns of arterial blood through miles of capillaries. (Examples: Wild Ginger, California Bayberry.)

VENEREAL WARTS Caused by human papillomavirus (HPV) and also known as condylomata acuminata, anal warts, and genital warts. It is nearly always transmitted from person to person by sexual contact, can increase the risk for women of cervical cancer, and occurs in near epidemic proportions in sexually active teenage women.

WHEAL An inflammatory response to mild skin irritation, with a well-defined, raised redness, lasting for perhaps an hour and then disappearing. The cause is usually atopic allergies in an IgE-excess person, although mild, subclinical adrenocortical deficiency can be another factor.

XEROPHYTE A plant that is adapted to, and needs, dry desert climate or is particularly hardy in periodic droughts.

SELECTED REFERENCES AND FURTHER READING

BOTANY

Andersen, B., and A. Holmgren. *Mountain Plants of Northeastern Utah*. Logan, Utah: Utah State University,1985.

Belzer, Thomas J. *Roadside Plants of Southern California*. Missoula, Mont.: Mountain Press Publishing, 1984.

Benson, Lyman, and Robert A. Darrow. *Trees and Shrubs of the Southwestern Deserts*. 3d ed. Tucson, Ariz.: University of Arizona Press, 1981.

Boren, Marjorie D., and Robert R. Boren. *Mountain Wildflowers of Idaho*. Boise, Id.: Sawtooth Publishing, 1989.

Elias, Thomas S. *The Complete Trees of North America*. New York: Van Nostrand Rheinhold, 1980.

Heller, Christine. *Wild Flowers of Alaska*. Portland, Ore.: Graphic Arts Center, 1966.

Hitchcock, C. Leo, and Arthur Cronquist. *Flora of the Pacific Northwest*. Seattle, Wash.: University of Washington Press, 1973.

Horn, Elizabeth L. *Wildflowers 1: The Cascades*. Beaverton, Ore.: Touchstone Press, 1972.

Hulten, Eric. *Flora of Alaska and Neighboring Territories*. Stanford, Calif.: Stanford University Press, 1968.

Jaeger, Edmund. *Desert Wild Flowers*. Stanford, Calif.: Stanford University Press, 1956.

Jepson, Willis. *Manual of the Flowering Plants of California*. Berkeley, Calif.: University of California Press, 1960.

Kearney, Thomas, and Robert Peebles. *Arizona Flora*. Berkeley, Calif.: University of California Press, 1964.

Lackschewitz, Klaus. *Vascular Plants of West-Central Montana*. Ogden, Utah: U.S. Forest Service Intermountain Research Station, 1991.

Mason, Charles, and Patricia Mason. *A Handbook of Mexican Roadside Flora*. Tucson, Ariz.: University of Arizona Press, 1987.

Moss, E. H. *Flora of Alberta*. Toronto, Ontario: University of Toronto Press, 1959.

Munz, Philip A. *A California Flora*. Berkeley, Calif.: University of California Press, 1968.

———. *A Flora of Southern California*. Berkeley, Calif.: University of California Press, 1974.

Patterson, Patricia A., Kenneth E. Neiman, and Jonalea R. Tonn. *Field Guide* to *Forest Plants of Northern Idaho.* Ogden, Utah: U.S. Forest Service Intermountain Research Station, 1985.

Peck, Morton E. *A Manual of the Higher Plants of Oregon.* Portland, Ore.: Binford and Mort, 1941.

Ricket, Harold W. *Wild Flowers of the United States.* Vols. 4 and 6. New York: McGraw-Hill Book Company, 1973.

Shreve, Forrest, and Ira Wiggins. *Vegetation and Flora of the Sonoran Deserts.* 2 vols. Stanford, Calif.: Stanford University Press, 1964.

Spellenberg, Richard. *The Audubon Society Field Guide to North American Wildflowers, Western Region.* New York: Alfred A. Knopf, 1979.

Stocking, Stephen K., and Jack A. Rockwell. *Wildflowers of Sequoia and Kings Canyon National Parks.* Three Rivers, Calif.: Sequoia Natural History Association, 1989.

Sudworth, George B. *Forest Trees of the Pacific Slope.* Reprint. New York: Dover Publications, 1967.

Taylor, Ronald J. *Northwest Weeds.* Missoula, Mont.: Mountain Press Publishing Company, 1990.

Taylor, Roy L. *Vascular Plants of British Columbia.* Vancouver, British Columbia: University of British Columbia, 1977.

Underhill, J. E. (Ted). *Roadside Wildflowers of the Northwest.* Blaine, Wash.: Hancock House, 1981.

Vines, Robert A. *Trees, Shrubs and Woody Vines of the Southwest.* Austin, Tex.: University of Texas Press, 1960.

Whitson, Tom D., et al. *Weeds of the West.* Laramie, Wyo.: University of Wyoming, 1991.

Wiggins, Ira. *Flora of Baja California.* Stanford, Calif.: Stanford University Press, 1980.

Willis, J. C. *A Dictionary of the Flowering Plants and Ferns.* Cambridge, England: Cambridge University Press, 1988.

Young, Dorothy King. *Redwood Empire Wildflower Jewels.* Healdsburg, Calif.: Naturegraph Publishers, 1970.

BOTANICAL MEDICINE AND ETHNOBOTANY

Alstat, Edward K., comp. *Eclectic Dispensatory of Botanical Therapeutics.* Portland, Ore.: Eclectic Medical Publications, 1989.

Balls, Edward K. *Early Uses of California Plants.* Berkeley, Calif.: University of California Press, 1962.

British Herbal Pharmacopeia. London: British Herbal Medicine Association, 1977.

Chesnut, V. K. *Plants Used by the Indians of Mendocino County California.* 1902. Reprint. Fort Bragg, Calif.: Mendocino County Historical Society, 1974.

Culbreth, David. *A Manual of Materia Medica and Pharmacology.* 1927. Reprint. Portland, Ore.: Eclectic Medical Publications, 1983.

Duke, James. *Handbook of Medicinal Herbs.* Boca Raton, Fla.: CRC Press, 1986.

Ellingwood, Finley. *American Materia Medica.* 1917. Reprint. Portland, Ore.: Eclectic Medical Publications, 1983.

Erichsen-Brown, Charlotte. *Use of Plants for the Past 500 Years.* Aurora, Ontario: Breezy Creeks Press, 1979.

Ethnobotany of the Thompson Indians of British Columbia. Washington, D.C.: Bureau of American Ethnology, Smithsonian Institution, 1927–28.

Felger, R. S., and M. B. Moser. *People of the Desert and the Sea.* Tucson, Ariz.: University of Arizona Press, 1985.

Felter, H. Wicks. *Eclectic Materia Medica.* 1919. Reprint. Portland, Ore.: Eclectic Medical Publications, 1983.

————, and John U. Lloyd. *Kings American Dispensatory.* 2 vols. Portland, Ore.: Eclectic Medical Publications, 1983.

Ford, Karen. *Las Yerbas de la Gente.* Ann Arbor, Mich.: Museum of Anthropology, University of Michigan, 1975.

Foster, Steven, and James A. Duke. *A Field Guide to Medicinal Plants.* Boston: Houghton Mifflin, 1990.

————, and Yue Chongxi. *Herbal Emissaries.* Rochester, Verm.: Healing Arts Press, 1992.

Gagnon, Daniel, and Amadea Morningstar. *Breathe Free.* Wilmot, Wis.: Lotus Press, 1991.

Grieve, Maud. *A Modern Herbal.* 2 vols. 1931. Reprint. New York: Dover Publications, 1971.

Gunther, Erna. *Ethnobotany of Western Washington.* Rev. ed. Seattle, Wash.: University of Washington Press, 1973.

Harper-Shrove, F. *Prescriber and Clinical Repertory of Medicinal Herbs.* Devon, England: Health Science Press, 1952.

Hellson, J. C., and M. Gadd. *Ethnobotany of the Blackfoot Indians.* Ottawa, Ontario: National Museums of Canada, 1974.

Herbal Pharmacology of the People's Republic of China. Washington, D.C.: National Academy of Sciences, 1975.

La Herbolaria Medica Tzeltal-Tzotzil en los Altos de Chiapas. Ciapas, Mexico: Gobierno del Estado de Chiapas, 1990.

Hocking, George M. *A Dictionary of Terms in Pharmacognosy.* Springfield, Ill.: Thomas, 1955.

Kuts-Cheraux, A. W. *Naturae Medicina and Naturopathic Dispensatory.* Des Moines, Ia.: American Naturopathic Physicians and Surgeons Association, 1953.

Lewis, Walter H., and Memory P. F. Elvin-Lewis. *Medical Botany*. New York: John Wiley, 1977.

Lloyd, John Uri. *Elixirs and Flavoring Extracts*. New York: William Wood, 1892.

Mabey, Richard. *The New Age Herbalist*. New York: Macmillan, 1988.

Martindale's Extra Pharmacopia. 25th ed. London: Pharmaceutical Press, 1967.

Martinez, Maximo. *Las Plantas Medicinales de Mexico*. 4th ed. Mexico City: Botas, 1959.

Millspaugh, Charles. *American Medicinal Plants*. 1892. Reprint. New York: Dover Publications, 1974.

Moerman, Daniel E. *Medicinal Plants of Native America*. 2 vols. Ann Arbor, Mich.: Museum of Anthropology, University of Michigan, 1986.

Moore, Michael. *Medicinal Plants of the Mountain West*. Santa Fe, N.M.: Museum of New Mexico Press, 1979.

―――. *Medicinal Plants of the Desert and Canyon West*. Santa Fe, N.M.: Museum of New Mexico Press, 1989.

―――. *Los Remedios: Traditional Herbal Remedies of the Southwest*. Santa Fe, N.M.: Red Crane Books, 1990.

―――. *A Brief Herbal Materia Medica*. Albuquerque, N.M.: Southwest School of Botanical Medicine, 1991.

―――. *Herbal Repertory in Clinical Practice*. 3d ed. Albuquerque, N.M.: Southwest School of Botanical Medicine, 1991.

―――. *Herbal Tinctures in Clinical Practice*. 2d ed. Albuquerque, N.M.: Southwest School of Botanical Medicine, 1991.

―――. *Herbal Energetics in Clinical Practice*. Albuquerque, N.M.: Southwest School of Botanical Medicine, 1992.

Murphey, Edith Van Allen. *Indian Uses of Native Plants*. Fort Bragg, Calif.: Mendocino County Historical Society, 1959.

Powell, Eric F. *The Modern Botanical Prescriber*. London: L. N. Fowler, 1965.

Priest and Priest. *Herbal Medication*. London: L. N. Fowler, 1982.

Schofield, Janice J. *Discovering Wild Plants*. Bothell, Wash.: Alaska Northwest Books, 1989.

Stubbs, R. D. "Investigation of the Edible and Medicinal Plants Used by the Flathead Indians." Master's thesis, University of Montana, 1966.

Stuhr, Ernst. *Manual of Pacific Coast Drug Plants*. Corvallis, Ore.: Ernst Stuhr, 1933.

Train, Percy. *Medicinal Uses of Plants by Indian Tribes of Nevada*. 1941. Reprint. Lawrence, Mass.: Quaterman Publications, 1982.

Turner, Nancy J. *Ethnobotany of the Okanagan-Coville Indians of British Columbia and Washington*. Victoria: British Columbia Provincial Museum, 1980.

————. *Ethnobotany of the Nitinant Indians of Vancouver Island.* Victoria: British Columbia Provincial Museum, 1983.

Uphof, J. C. *Dictionary of Economic Plants.* 2d ed. Lehre, Germany: J. Cramer, 1968.

Ward, Harold. *Herbal Manual.* London: L. N. Fowler, 1969.

Weiss, Rudolf Fritz. *Herbal Medicine.* Beaconsfield, England: Beaconsfield Publishers, 1988.

Willard, Terry. *The Wild Rose Scientific Herbal.* Calgary, Alberta: Wild Rose College of Natural Healing, 1991.

————. *Textbook of Advanced Herbology.* Calgary, Alberta: Wild Rose College of Natural Healing, 1992.

————. *Edible and Medicinal Plants of the Rocky Mountains and Neighboring Territories.* Calgary, Alberta: Wild Rose College of Natural Healing, 1993.

Wilson, Cloyce. *Useful Prescriptions.* Cincinnati, Ohio: Lloyd Brothers Pharmacy, 1935.

Wren, R. C. *Potter's New Cyclopedia of Botanical Drugs and Preparations.* Devon, England: Health Science Press, 1975.

MEDICAL AND TECHNICAL

Churchill's Medical Dictionary. New York: Churchill Livingstone, 1989.

Foye, William O. *Principles of Medical Chemistry.* Philadelphia: Lea and Febiger, 1974.

Harrison's Principles of Internal Medicine. 12th ed. New York: McGraw-Hill, 1991.

The Merck Index. 11th ed. Rahway, N.J.: Merck and Co., 1989.

The Merck Manual, 15th ed. Rahway, N.J.: Merck and Co., 1987.

Seeley, Rod. R., Trent D. Stephens, and Philip Tate. *Anatomy and Physiology.* St. Louis, Mo.: Times Mirror/Mosby College Publishing, 1989.

Taber's Cyclopedic Medical Dictionary. 13th ed. Philadelphia: F. A. Davis, 1977.

Trease, G. E., and W. C. Evans. *A Textbook of Pharmacognosy.* 10th ed. London: Tindall and Cassell, 1972.

Tyler, Varro E., Lynn R. Brady, and James E. Robbers. *Pharmacognosy.* 7th ed. Philadelphia: Lea and Febiger, 1976.

White, Abraham, Philip Handler, and Emil L. Smith. *Principles of Biochemistry.* 4th ed. New York: McGraw-Hill Book Company, 1968.

INDEX OF PLANT NAMES

Primary plants are capitalized, Latin and Spanish names are in italics.
Drawings are in bold.

THE AUTHOR

Respected herbalist Michael Moore has been a teacher of herbology for more than two decades. He is the director and an instructor for the Southwest School of Botanical Medicine, a trade school for professional herbalists in Albuquerque, New Mexico. Previously he directed the School of Clinical Herbology and co-founded the Institute of Traditional Medicine in Santa Fe, New Mexico. Moore leads seminars throughout the West and has given classes for Continuing Education credits for New Mexico and Colorado Pharmaceutical Associations, the medicine schools at the University of New Mexico and the University of Arizona, the New Mexico Acupuncture Board, and the National College of Naturopathic Medicine. Moore is the author of three previous books on herbs, *Medicinal Plants of the Mountain West, Medicinal Plants of the Desert and Canyon West,* and *Los Remedios: Traditional Herbal Remedies of the Southwest.*

THE ILLUSTRATOR

Mimi Kamp started working with plants as a child growing up in western Pennsylvania. Not long after graduating from Grinnell College in Iowa in 1965 (B.A. Art, B.A. English), she began studying in the Pacific Northwest with older women herbalists, spending long hours in the woods, long hours with books. She worked in a Seattle clinic, where she collected herbal data with Joy Gardner and later illustrated some of Joy's books. In Seattle she also studied acupuncture and polarity therapy. She began working with southwestern plants when she moved to Arizona in 1976, studied with Michael Moore, did botanical illustrations for some of his books, and began traveling to many areas of the U.S. and Mexico to collect and study herbs. She then started a small but well-supplied tincture business as well as an herbal consultation practice and has been working with flower essences. She is a co-founder of Desert Alchemy flower essence company and is presently forming her own flower essence research project. She lives with her three girls in a homemade adobe house near Bisbee, Arizona.

MICHAEL TIERRA is a California State Licensed Acupuncturist with an Oriental Medical Doctor's degree, author of *Way of Herbs, Planetary Herboloby,* and the *East West Herbal Correspondence Course.*

CASCADE ANDERSON GELLER, Herbalist, is a Northwest native plant specialist. She was an assistant professor of botanical medicine at the National College of Naturopathic Medicine in Portland, Oregon, from 1978–1992.